P9-DUX-288

Cambridge History of Medicine
EDITORS: CHARLES WEBSTER AND CHARLES ROSENBERG

Mystical Bedlam

Mystical Bedlam

MADNESS, ANXIETY, AND HEALING
IN SEVENTEENTH-CENTURY ENGLAND

Michael MacDonald

Department of History
University of Wisconsin at Madison

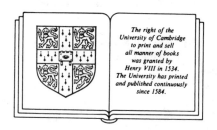

The right of the
University of Cambridge
to print and sell
all manner of books
was granted by
Henry VIII in 1534.
The University has printed
and published continuously
since 1584.

CAMBRIDGE UNIVERSITY PRESS

CAMBRIDGE

NEW YORK   NEW ROCHELLE

MELBOURNE   SYDNEY

Published by the Press Syndicate of the University of Cambridge
The Pitt Building, Trumpington Street, Cambridge CB2 1RP
32 East 57th Street, New York, NY 10022, USA
10 Stamford Road, Oakleigh, Melbourne 3166, Australia

© Cambridge University Press 1981

First published 1981
First paperback edition 1983
Reprinted 1985, 1988

Printed in the United States of America

Library of Congress Cataloging in Publication Data
MacDonald, Michael, 1945–
Mystical Bedlam.
(Cambridge history of medicine)
Bibliography: p.
Includes index.
1. Psychiatry—History—17th century. 2. Mental illness—Great
Britain—Public opinion—History—17th century. 3. Mental
illness—Great Britain—History—17th century. 4. Family—Great
Britain—History—17th century.—I Title II. Series.
[DNLM: 1 Mental disorders—History—England.
2. Psychiatry—History—England. WM II FE5 M13m]
RC438.M27   362.2'0942   80-25787
ISBN 0 521 23170 I hardcovers
ISBN 0 521 27382 X paperback

To the memory of my father
and to
the mentally disturbed patients
of Richard Napier

Contents

APPENDIXES

Tables, figures, and maps

Preface

Anyone who writes about the history of insanity in early modern Europe must travel in the spreading wake of Michel Foucault's famous book *Madness and Civilization*. Foucault believes that medieval and Renaissance madmen were voyagers both in reality and in imagination, fools whose hermetic wisdom signified to the sane the animality of the human and the humanity of vice.[1] The dawn of the age of reason, was, he argues, a catastrophe for the living metaphors of unreason.[2] The insane were secluded in asylums, where they were chained and brutalized, their animality no longer a lesson but a badge of their inhumanity. The imprisonment and degradation of the insane was the consequence of a shift in the mentality of European society. In the new world of profit and wage labor, madmen became merely another variety of pauper, antagonistic to bourgeois values and terrifying to the authorities. Foucault insists upon the ideological origins of the great confinement, as he calls the rise of institutionalization, and he believes that its causes were the same all over Europe.[3]

The great value of Foucault's work lies in his insight that madness was a speculum in which normal people saw their own image reversed and distorted. Its major weaknesses are that abstractions confront abstractions in his book and his description of how real men and women thought and acted is often vague or fanciful. It is easier to grasp the shape of Foucault's personal vision of history than it is to see how actual people interpreted madness and how they treated the insane persons whom they encountered. Much of what Foucault has to say seems to me to be correct, in spite of his rejection of the prevailing standards of historical discourse, and some of it is brilliant. Although the arguments in this book sometimes parallel Foucault's, they are nevertheless philosophically and methodologically at odds with his approach to history.[4] I have not attempted to rewrite *Madness and Civilization* in a plain and tangible form accessible to English and American readers.[5] I have instead set myself the different task of discovering how popular beliefs about insanity and healing illuminate the mental world of ordinary people. Both the scope of this study and the evidence it examines contrast sharply with Foucault's perspective and sources. He focuses his attention on the ways in which madmen were perceived and treated by intellectuals and officials all over Europe; I have concentrated on the views and actions of two thousand obscure rustics who were treated for mental disorders by an astrological physician in early seventeenth-century England. Their stories lack the sound and fury of the sources Foucault favors, but they do provide a unique opportunity to find out what insanity meant in the lives of people who actually experienced or observed it. I have endeavored to place the experiences and beliefs of these ordinary people in their immediate historical context by analyzing them in light of other contemporary accounts of madness and healing in medical and legal documents, diaries and autobiographies, scientific and religious writings, and imaginative literature. The advantage of this approach is that it reveals the social conditions and beliefs that actually shaped people's understanding of mental disorder and their responses to the insane; its disadvantage is that it obscures the effects of broad social and intellectual changes that influenced the history of madness all over Europe. Although I am aware of the perils of parochialism and have tried to avoid them where possible, I confess that I prefer methodologically to establish first what happened in England, then to compare afterward those findings with conditions and events in other countries, rather than to limit the investigation to themes that transcend national, or rather cultural, boundaries. Furthermore, the thoughts and actions of humble men and women are interesting and important in themselves; it was they, after all, who experienced mental disorders, both as patients and as relatives and neighbors who sought medical care for the insane and took legal action to confine lunatics and protect their property.

Because this is a book about popular beliefs and traditional practices, I have used common words to describe the maladies discussed in it. The language of popular psychology in the seventeenth century was rich and complex, but it was not very precise. The correspondence between the words that denoted the varieties of insanity and the conditions they described was seldom exact, and it would be wrong to impose a terminology on contemporary ideas that lent them spurious consistency. The perils of anachronism seem to me to outweigh the virtues of verbal precision, especially as the best way to attain precision would be to resort to modern psychiatric jargon. Throughout this book I have therefore preferred terms that are commonly used by laymen today or that were used by ordinary people in the seventeenth century to technical language that has never been part of popular speech. This may trouble readers anxious to fit the ideas discussed here into modern categories, and I have considered the advantages and disadvantages of avoiding twentieth-century psychiatric concepts at greater length in Chapter 4, which analyzes popular stereotypes of mental disorder. My aim has been to devise a rhetoric that would convey seventeenth-century beliefs readily by calling to mind our own parallel experiences, the everyday words and notions that shape laymen's understanding of insanity.

In early modern England, ordinary villagers viewed mental disorders as part of the galaxy of misfortunes that threatened their health and happiness. Traditional cosmological and religious beliefs enabled them to locate insanity in the universe of natural and supernatural events. They believed that individual experiences and social actions resonated on several planes of existence simultaneously. These resonances could be classified using popular religious and scientific lore, and the associations created by invoking these concepts made their experiences meaningful and comprehensible. Thoughts, feelings, and actions were, for example, often divided into contrasting categories of good and evil, normal and abnormal, and linked with the appropriate supernatural agencies and theological concepts as divine or diabolical, acts of grace or sins. The traditional symbolism of the psychomachy, the struggle between angels and demons for Everyman's soul, provided the iconography for representing these contrasting states in art and, as we shall see, in life. Mental states and behavior could also be explained in purely natural terms by appealing to astrological and medical ideas. Astrologers helped their clients to relate emotional disturbances and mad behavior to astronomical events, and physicians provided their patients with diagnoses that classified mental disorders as types of sickness. Although personal convictions and professional allegiances often made individuals favor one form of categorization over another, all of the various ways of understanding a particular misfortune or problem could be comprehended into a single cosmological model, familiar to us as the "Elizabethan world picture." It is doubtful that humble people grasped all of the complexities of contemporary cosmology, but it is certain that they habitually employed its categories, paralleled the natural and supernatural, mingled medical ideas and popular religion. Moralists frequently exploited and reinforced these venerable modes of thought by arguing that all sins, violations of God's rules for human behavior, were forms of madness, transgressions of society's standards of proper conduct. This was more than a mere rhetorical stratagem: It was an appeal to the widespread belief that madness was, if not sinful, more diabolical than divine. I shall argue in this book that contemporary social conditions and popular religion exerted a powerful influence on beliefs about insanity and methods of caring for the insane. The fusion of the social and the moral, of the natural and the supernatural, was characteristic of interpretations of mental disorder in the early seventeenth century. To emphasize the importance of the eclectic mixture of religious, magical, and scientific thought typical of the age, I have borrowed for this book the title of the most famous of the sermons paralleling spiritual maladies with varieties of madness.

Writing a history of mental disorder from this perspective has presented unusually difficult theoretical and methodological problems, and I have been fortunate to have received the advice of many scholars more learned and experienced than I. Two masterly historians supervised me during the preparation of the doctoral thesis on which this book is based. Paul Seaver taught me my craft and gave me the confidence to pursue the most complex and interesting problems I was capable of solving. I shall always remain his apprentice; through his advice and example he has set standards of workmanship and artistry, as a writer and a teacher, that I can hope to emulate but never to excel. Keith Thomas guided my research in England and showed me how to combine rigorous historical discipline with broad intellectual concerns. He made it possible for me to write the kind of book I could only imagine by myself. He told me about the manuscripts of Richard Napier; he alerted me to hundreds of complementary sources; he read earlier versions of the manuscript and saved me from many foolish and careless errors. My debt to his published work is evident on every page of this book; my debt to his thoughtful suggestions and great learning is even more pervasive, but it cannot be displayed in footnotes nor adequately acknowledged here.

Lawrence Stone examined the material about family life and shared his immense knowledge of the relevant literature with me. I have benefited greatly from his astringent criticism and generous encouragement; he has caused me to sharpen both my arguments and my enthusiasm. Alan Macfarlane exchanged ideas and citations with me when I was beginning my research. He will recognize many passages and references, the fruits of our early conversations, too numerous to acknowledge individually in the notes. Steven Feierman, Paul Slack, and Charles Webster read my thesis and gave me many acute ideas about how to turn it into a book. Laura Engelstein and Kirk Willis helped me to make the text more readable and accurate. Thomas Barnes, Walter King, Richard Neugebauer, Michael Shepherd, and Carol Weiner took extraordinary pains to answer my questions and suggest problems to investigate. Another historian, Carol Dickerman, read all the worst passages in the drafts of this book, endured countless conversations about Richard Napier and his clients, helped me to count cases in Napier's notebooks, and checked the accuracy of most of the quotations and notes. Academics' wives are doomed to perform such vexatious tasks, but I have been doubly fortunate, not only because I had expert assistance, affectionately volunteered, but because I can repay my debt to her in kind. She has made our peripatetic workshop a very happy place in which to live and labor.

The staffs of several institutions have been no less generous than my teachers and colleagues. Although I was unable to obtain permission to examine the early records of Bethlem Hospital, no other collection was closed to me, and many archivists and librarians were extremely helpful. The Bodleian Library, the Public Record Office, the British Library, the Buckinghamshire County Record Office, and the Bedfordshire County Record Office provided me with books and manuscripts. I am grateful for their permission to use and cite documents in their care. Without the many kindnesses of the staff of Duke Humfrey's Library, especially Colin G. Harris, this book could not have been written at all. St. John's College and Corpus Christi College made my residence at Oxford pleasurable and convenient. The Foreign Area Fellowship

Program of the (American) Social Science Research Council and the American Council of Learned Societies supported my research financially; and the Mabelle McLeod Lewis Fund, the National Institute of Mental Health, Stanford University, and Reed College provided grants-in-aid to defray some of the costs of calculation and composition. While I was working on the revisions of the manuscript, I had the privilege of being a research associate at the Wellcome Unit for the History of Medicine at Oxford. Charles Webster, Margaret Pelling, and the other members of the unit provided my wife and me with an ideal blend of friendship and intellectual stimulus. Finally, the staff of the history department of the University of Wisconsin at Madison typed three versions of this book and gave me their candid opinions about passages they found snappy, boring, or illiterate. Their help was indispensable, and I am beholden to everyone who worked on the project, especially to Jane Mesler and Karen Isenberg, who had to endure my demands firsthand.

However badly I may have behaved sometimes under fire, I am grateful to these men and women for exposing my mistakes and misapprehensions, and for showing me how to correct them. If they have been unable to eliminate all my errors, it is because I sent them forth as battalions, not as solitary spies.

M. MacD.

Note on quotations, citations, and dates

The spelling, capitalization, and punctuation of quotations from works written before 1800 have been modernized. Although modernization removes nuances of meaning from the writing of some authors, it greatly clarifies the sense of others. The most frequently cited writer in this book, Richard Napier, was a wayward speller and a worse penman. Preservation of his orthography would have resulted in hundreds of conjectural readings of words whose meaning is plain even if their spelling is not. For the sake of readability and consistency, therefore, I have altered texts that had not been previously edited to conform with modern English usage.

The number of sources consulted in writing this book was so large that it proved impractical to list them all, and a bibliography of works cited would be redundant. A listing of manuscript sources and their locations has been provided at the end of the book. An index of printed sources has been included to permit the reader to locate readily the first citations of printed sources.

Dates are given Old Style, except that the year is taken to begin on 1 January. This method of dating was employed by Napier, and approximate dates for many of the citations to cases in his practice notes may be obtained by consulting the list of manuscript sources.

1

Insanity in early modern England

Madness is the most solitary of afflictions to the people who experience it; but it is the most social of maladies to those who observe its effects. Every mental disorder alienates its victims from the conventions of action, thought, and emotion that bind us together with the other members of our society. But because mental disorders manifest themselves in their victims' relationships with other men and women, they are more profoundly influenced by social and cultural conditions than any other kind of illness.[1] For this reason the types of insanity people recognize and the significance they attach to them reflect the prevailing values of their society; the criteria for identifying mental afflictions vary between cultures and historical periods. The response to the insane, like the reaction to the sufferers of physical diseases, is also determined by the material conditions, social organization, and systems of thought that characterize a particular culture and age. The methods of caring for mentally disturbed people, the concepts that are used to explain the causes of their maladies, and the techniques that are employed to relieve their anguish are all determined more by social forces than by scientific discoveries, even today. Two central problems, therefore, confront historians of insanity. First, they must show how ideas about mental disorder and methods of responding to it were adapted to the social and intellectual environment of particular historical periods. Second, they must identify changes in the perception and management of insanity and explain how they were related to broader transformations in the society.

The history of mental disorder in early modern England is an intellectual Africa. Historians and literary scholars have mapped its most prominent features and identified some of its leading figures, but we still have very little information about the ideas and experiences of ordinary people. Both the unfortunates who actually suffered from mental afflictions and the men and women who tried to help them still inhabit *terra incognita*.[2] Their story, the social history of insanity between the Reformation and the Industrial Revolution, falls into two distinct eras divided by the cataclysm of the English Revolution. During the late sixteenth and early seventeenth centuries, the English people became more concerned about the prevalence of madness, gloom, and self-murder than they had ever been before, and the reading public developed a strong fascination with classical medical psychology. Nevertheless, conventional beliefs about the nature and causes of mental disorders and the methods of psychological healing continued to reflect the traditional fusion of magic, science, and religion that typified the thinking of laymen of every social rank and educational background. The enormous social and psychological significance of the family shaped contemporary interpretations of insane behavior and determined the arrangements that were made to care for rich and poor lunatics alike. This book explores these traditional beliefs about insanity and healing practices and charts the social and intellectual forces which formed them. But it also describes some of the features of the subsequent age and notes the shifting conditions that eventually destroyed the older system of therapeutic eclecticism and family care. During the century and a half following the great upheaval of the English Revolution, the governing classes embraced secular interpretations of the signs of insanity and championed medical methods of curing mental disorders. They shunned magical and religious techniques of psychological healing. Private entrepreneurs founded specialized institutions to manage mad people, and municipal officials established public madhouses. The asylum movement eventually transferred the responsibility for maintaining lunatics out of the family and into the asylum. Madmen were removed from their normal social surroundings and incarcerated with others of their kind; lunatics lost their places as members of a household and acquired new identities as the victims of mental diseases.[3]

Interest in insanity quickened about 1580, and madmen, melancholics, and suicides became familiar literary types. Scientific writers popularized medical lore about melancholy, and clergymen wrote treatises about consoling the troubled in mind. Gentlemen and ladies proclaimed themselves melancholy; physicians worried about ways to cure the mentally ill; preachers and politi-

cians denounced sinners and dissenters as melancholics or madmen. Anxious intellectuals claimed that self-murder was epidemical, and they argued about its medical and religious significance.
Introducing the first comprehensive treatise about suicide in 1630,
the famous Puritan divine, William Gouge, wrote:

I suppose that scarce an age since the beginning of the world hath afforded more examples of this desperate inhumanity, than this our present
age; and that of all sorts of people, clergy, laity, learned, unlearned, noble, mean, rich, poor, free, bond, male, female, young and old. It is
therefore high time that the danger of this desperate, devilish and damnable practice be plainly and fully set out.[4]

Heightened concern about the nature and prevalence of mental
disorders was fostered by the increasing size and complexity of
English society. Population growth and economic change increased the numbers of insane and suicidal people and overburdened the capacity of families and local communities to care for
the sick and indigent.[5] Renaissance humanism set new standards
of conduct for the nobility, and the turbulent and incomplete triumph of Protestantism fragmented English society into religious
groups with sharply differing views about how people ought to
behave. The adequacy of traditional codes of conduct was subjected to intense criticism by learned reformers and religious
zealots, and both humanist intellectuals and Puritan clergymen
were naturally concerned about the causes and significance of abnormal behavior. Although they often looked to the same sources
for ideas about insanity, one can say in general that religious conservatives elaborated classical medical psychology, whereas Puritan evangelists revitalized popular religious psychology and set it
in a Calvinist theological framework.

   In spite of the increased interest in insanity and the growing
controversy about its religious implications, the perception and
management of mental disorders did not change fundamentally
before 1660. Contemporary ideas about the varieties of mental
maladies and their characteristic signs were rooted in ancient science and medieval Christianity, and the typology of insanity was
similar all over Western Europe. Within the broad framework of
medical and religious thought, however, popular stereotypes of
mental disorder were adapted to fit English conditions. For example, widely held beliefs about the behavior of mad and troubled

people and the immediate causes of their misery reflected the psychological significance of the family in the lives of ordinary villagers. Descriptions of the symptoms of violent madness placed great emphasis on irrational threats toward members of one's immediate family. Traditional legal prohibitions against suicide aimed to prevent it by emphasizing the responsibility of potential self-murders for their family's welfare. Common complaints about the causes of overwhelming anxiety and despair included unrequited love, marital strife, and bereavement. This preoccupation with the family was the consequence of its elemental importance in English society. The household was the basic social unit, and at every level of society it performed a myriad of functions. Within the walls of great houses and cottages children were reared and educated, the sick and infirm were nursed and maintained, estates were managed and goods were manufactured. Most households were very small. Except among the wealthy, whose entourages often included dozens of servants, clients and kin, households normally consisted only of a married couple, their young children, and, in many cases, a servant or apprentice. The small size of domestic groups and the high rate of geographical mobility in early seventeenth-century England greatly enhanced the part that the nuclear family played in the emotional lives of people of low and middling status.

The social importance of the family was also recognized in the arrangements for maintaining mad and troubled people. Only a handful of the insane in a nation of five million souls were cast into an asylum before the English Revolution. Bedlamites swarmed through the imaginations of Jacobean playwrights and pamphleteers, but the famous asylum was in truth a tiny hovel housing fewer than thirty patients. Bethlem Hospital was the only institution of its kind, and its inmates languished there for years, living in squalid conditions without adequate medical treatment.[6] Private institutions to house the insane did not begin to proliferate until the last half of the seventeenth century, municipal asylums to rival Bedlam were not founded in major cities for another century, and county lunatic hospitals were not established until after 1808.[7] Tudor and Stuart governments responded to increasing concern about insanity by refurbishing traditional institutions to help families bear the burden of harboring a madman. The welfare of rich lunatics was guarded by the Court of Wards and Liveries, which exercised the crown's feudal right to manage the affairs of minors who inherited land as tenants-in-chief.[8] Children, idiots, and lunatics were siblings in the eyes of the law, because they all lacked the capacity to reason and so could not be economically and legally responsible.

The Court of Wards was notorious for selling its favors to the highest bidder, allowing guardians who purchased wardships to ruin their charges' estates and bully them into profitable marriages. But toward lunatics the court behaved with uncharacteristic delicacy, repudiating rapacity in favor of family and legitimacy. King James instructed the court to ensure that lunatics "be freely committed to their best and nearest friends, that can receive no benefit by their death, and the committees, bound to answer for . . . the very just value of their estates upon account, for the benefit of such lunatic (if he recover) or of the next heir."[9] The order was obeyed. The court usually appointed relatives or friends of mad landowners to see that they were cared for and their property preserved.[10] Naturally, there were some sordid struggles for the guardianship of rich lunatics, and sometimes men hurled false accusations of insanity at wealthy eccentrics in hopes of winning a rich wardship. But the court was unusually scrupulous about investigating chicanery when it concerned lunatics, and abuses appear to have been rare.[11] Before a landowner was turned over to a committee of guardians, a jury of local notables was assembled to certify that he had been too mad to manage his estates for a year and more. Such juries relied on common sense and common knowledge to establish that a person was insane, but their chief preoccupation was to discover whether he could perform the necessary economic chores to preserve the family property.[12]

The court and the men who acted as inquisitors and guardians on its behalf behaved more virtuously toward the estates of lunatics than those of minor heirs because there was little profit in the wardship of the insane. Lunacy was regarded as a temporary state and the law decreed that when the madman recovered he should have restored to him all of his property, save the amount the guardians expended for his care.[13] And because lunatics were unreasoning creatures, they could not contract marriages, perhaps the most valuable aspect of the wardship of minors. Legal rules and low incentive to break them effectively protected the rights of insane landowners, and when the Court of Wards was abolished during the Revolution cries were heard that lunatics were now vulnerable to the greed of unscrupulous guardians as never before—surely the unique expression of regret about the disappearance of the court.[14] Soon after the Restoration, the crown transferred the jurisdiction over the estates of lunatics to Chancery.[15]

The chief concern of the crown's policy toward insane landowners was to preserve the integrity of their estates so that their lineages would not be obliterated by the economic consequences of their madness. Paupers had no property or social standing to protect, but the Tudor and Stuart state tried also to assist poor lunatics by providing financial relief for their families. After 1601 the government obliged parishes to treat impoverished madmen as "deserving poor," people who, like orphans and cripples, were unable to work through no fault of their own.[16] Michael Dalton's standard handbook for Justices of the Peace explains: "The person naturally disabled, either in wit or member, as an idiot, lunatic, blind, lame, etc., not being able to work . . . all these . . . are to be provided for by the overseers [of the poor] of necessary relief, and are to have allowances proportionable and according to the continuation and measure of their maladies and needs."[17] These allowances were paid out of the funds from local taxation for poor relief, and they were intended to prevent humble families from starvation and fragmentation because the lunatic's labor was lost. A 1658 order by Lancashire justices to provide for Isabell Breatherton illustrates the way the system worked in practice:

> It is ordered by this court that the . . . churchwardens and overseers of the poor within the parish of Wimwick shall . . . take into consideration the distracted condition of Isabell, wife of James Breatherton of Newton and provide for her or allow unto her said husband weekly or monthly allowances as her necessity requires, so as she may be kept from wandering abroad or doing any hurt or prejudice either to herself or otherwise [18]

As the population grew and the economy became more specialized in the sixteenth and seventeenth centuries, poverty became a major social problem. Municipal governments experimented with new kinds of institutions, such as hospitals and workhouses, in an attempt to find some solution to the increasingly alarming situation, and the crown began slowly to imitate some features of these experiments. In 1609, for example, counties were ordered to establish houses of correction to confine the able-bodied poor and train them for gainful employment; compliance was slow, but by the 1630s every shire had such an institution.[19] Lunatics were sometimes housed in these local Bridewells, but it appears that incarceration was regarded as an exceptional and undesirable expedient. Lancashire officials were reluctant to confine madmen to the county's house of correction if they could avoid it, preferring to leave them in the care of their families whenever possible.[20] For the poor as for the rich, therefore, the Tudor and early Stuart state left the care and management of the insane largely in the hands of their families and attempted to lessen the social and economic impact of lunacy by helping families either directly through the Court of Wards or indirectly through the parishes.

Early seventeenth-century methods of explaining the natural and supernatural causes of insanity and relieving the suffering of its victims were marked by a traditional mingling of magical, religious, and scientific concepts. Individual cases of mental disorder might be attributed to divine retribution, diabolical possession, witchcraft, astrological influences, humoral imbalances, or to any combination of these forces. Cures were achieved (in theory) by removing the causes of the sufferer's disturbance, and the means to combat every kind of malign effect were dispensed by a bewildering array of healers. Insane men and women were treated by specialists, such as humanistic physicians, who practiced a single method of psychological healing, or they were consoled by eclectics, such as medical astrologers or clerical doctors, who combined remedies from several systems of therapy. The profusion of causal explanations for insanity and of healing methods was not simply the result of the inchoate state of the medical profession. It was also a practical manifestation of the popular confidence that magic, religion, and science could be reconciled. Medieval and Renaissance cosmology provided a systematic model for making such a reconciliation, and on a less sophisticated plane popular religious thought fused religious and magical beliefs.

Classical medical psychology became very popular among the educated classes during the sixteenth and seventeenth centuries. It was disseminated by the physicians, who were increasingly articulate and well-organized, and by humanist intellectuals, who were often clerics and medical amateurs. The reading public ingested psychological theory as avidly as it did the exotic new drugs flooding into England from abroad.[21] Although the remedies

sanctioned by natural scientific theories were no more effective
than religious or magical treatments for mental disorder, the medical approach eventually prevailed over supernatural explanations
for the causes of madness. In the early seventeenth century the
natural and supernatural approaches coexisted uneasily, championed by rival groups of professionals, to be sure, but not yet incompatible to many minds. Humanistic physicians battled to secure a monopoly over the care of sick and insane people and to
make their trade proof against the interloping of clerical doctors,
apothecaries, surgeons, astrologers, and village wizards.[22] Writing in 1612, a famous physician of Northampton, John Cotta, denounced the "ignorant practisers" his profession hated. The worst
offenders were "ecclesiastical persons, vicars, and parsons, who
now overflow this kingdom with this alienation of their own
proper office and duties and usurpation of others', making their
holy calling a linsey wolsey, too narrow for their minds, and
therefore making themselves room on others' affairs, under pre-
tense of love and mercy."[23] Although he admits that astrology is a
useful tool for understanding the diseases of mind and body, Cotta
complains that many astrologers exceed the uses of their art, "sufficient and profitable unto physic," and "fish for a name and fame
among the common and eas[il]y deceived vulgars with the glorious bates of prodigious precepts."[24]

Cotta's complaints were justified. Medical practice was a natural extension of ministers' duty to relieve the afflictions of their
flocks, and a great many rural rectors and vicars provided various
kinds of medical services for their parishioners. Medicine was an
essential aspect of the astrologers' art, and occultists of every degree of rank and learning, from highly educated university graduates to illiterate village wise folk, used astrology as a tool for medical diagnosis and prognostication. The doctors could do little to
prevent clergymen from practicing their craft, because the church
and the universities had the power to license medical practitioners,
and neither was likely to concur that learned clerks who practiced
medicine were as culpable as ignorant quacks. Humanistic physicians could not possibly supply all the medical needs of the English people, and so long as clerical doctors, and indeed astrologers and cunning men and women, did not slaughter their patients
and garnered reputations for effective treatments, the authorities
were inclined to grant them licenses to practice medicine legally.

In London and its suburbs, however, the College of Physicians were empowered to fine unlicensed practitioners, and the privilege was used to harass popular astrologers and empirics.[25] Among their most notable victims was the famous astrologer, Simon Forman, who quarreled with the college for decades until his death in 1611.[26] The doctors' efforts to persuade the public that scientific medicine was the only legitimate basis for healing made little headway before the English Revolution: Professional eclecticism and therapeutic pluralism continued to characterize the treatment of physically ill and mentally disturbed people.

During the course of the seventeenth century, religious controversy and the shock of revolution accelerated the triumph of medical explanations for insanity among the governing classes. The Anglican hierarchy repudiated popular demonology for theological reasons, only to discover that Jesuits and Puritans eagerly took up the struggle against the Fiend and his minions.[27] Radical Protestants developed new means for casting out devils and uplifting downcast hearts and used them to proselytize as well as to console. They insisted that misery, anxiety, and sadness were the emblems of sin, the normal afflictions of the unregenerate, and they taught that the surest means to overcome them was spiritual self-discipline and godly fellowship. Insanity was the epitome of conduct unguided by a pious and responsible personality. "My neighbours were amazed at this my great conversion," wrote John Bunyan, "from prodigious profaneness to something like a moral life; and truly so well they might for this my conversion was as great as for a Tom of Bethlem to become a sober man."[28] The Puritans produced a literature of anxious gloom in which despair normally preceded conversion, and they naturally bruited about their ability to relieve such suffering. During the Revolution the sects – especially the Quakers – employed their powers of exorcism and spiritual healing to prove by miracles their divine inspiration and refute the charges of the "hireling priests."[29] The orthodox elite seized the healer's gown in which the radicals clothed themselves and turned it inside out, calling religious enthusiasm madness and branding the vexations of tender consciences religious melancholy.[30]

These events coincided with remarkable achievements in physical science and anatomy, and they helped to accomplish the end that physicians had been unable to attain by propaganda and persecution. They prompted the ruling elite to embrace secular explanations for mental disorders and to repudiate magical and religious methods of healing them. The secularization of the elite's beliefs about insanity affected their notions about the nature of mental diseases as well as the causes of such afflictions. Their skepticism about the divine revelations of radical prophets and the healing miracles of Nonconformist thaumaturgists was reflected in Restoration and Augustan reformulations of the popular stereotypes of insanity. John Locke's influential remarks about madness enhanced the anti-enthusiasts' claims by making delusions of thought and perception the signs of the most acute forms of insanity, rather than of the milder disorder, melancholy. The orthodox elite accepted this new interpretation of the significance of delusions, and it became a shibboleth of eighteenth-century views of insanity.[31] The educated classes' gradual rejection of traditional religious ideas about suicide in favor of the medical theory that it was the outcome of mental disease was also fostered by orthodox hatred of religious enthusiasm. Throughout the eighteenth century dissenting sects continued to exorcise people who believed that they were possessed by the Devil. Anglican spokesmen argued that the age of miracles was long past, and the Devil rarely if ever swayed the minds and inhabited the bodies of people in modern times. This argument corroded the traditional stereotype of suicide, which depicted self-murder as a religious crime, committed at the instigation of the Devil, who often appeared personally to urge his victims on to self-destruction.[32]

The rejection of the supernatural beliefs and thaumaturgy of the sectaries fostered scorn for religious and magical therapies. Although the methods of psychological healing practiced by the Dissenters were often effective, the governing classes abandoned them in favor of medical remedies for mental disorders, techniques that were widely recognized to be unpleasant, ineffective, and theoretically insupportable. Magical remedies against supernatural harm, such as astrological amulets, charms, and exorcisms, were discarded by reputable practitioners. By the end of the seventeenth century a loose hierarchy of prestige had been established among the various types of healers who treated insanity, and at its apex were the humanistic physicians, who viewed madness and gloom as natural disorders. The dominance of secular interpretations of insanity among the eighteenth-century governing classes was embodied in the asylum movement. Beginning about 1660, scores of entrepreneurs founded private madhouses to care for the insane, and beginning about a century later, some municipal governments established receptacles for pauper lunatics. The therapeutic practices of the new asylums were based mainly on medical theories and remedies. The supportive and nonviolent healing techniques employed by the Nonconformist sects were not reintroduced into the curative repertories of respectable mad doctors until the end of the eighteenth century, when the so-called moral therapy movement was inaugurated at the Quaker asylum, the York Retreat.

The governing classes' repudiation of supernatural explanations of the signs and causes of insanity and their rejection of magical and religious therapies were not readily accepted by the mass of the English people. Throughout the eighteenth century ordinary villagers continued to believe that witches and demons could drive men mad and that the Devil could possess the minds and bodies of his victims. They sought the help of a ragtag regiment of increasingly disreputable astrologers and folk magicians to protect them against these evils. The exorcisms and religious cures of the Nonconformist sects, and particularly of the Methodists, appealed to the strong popular attachment to traditional supernaturalism. The deepening abyss between elite attitudes toward insanity and popular beliefs was not simply the consequence of the enlightened scientism of the educated classes. Medical theories about mental disorders were contradictory and controversial; medical therapies were notoriously difficult to justify either theoretically or empirically. They appealed to an elite sick of sectarian enthusiasm because they lacked the subversive political implications that religious psychology and therapy had acquired during the seventeenth century. As the eighteenth century progressed, more and more people were subjected to incarceration in madhouses and to medical brutality. The abolition of family care for lunatics and the abandonment of therapeutic pluralism were the consequences of religious conflict, political strife, and social change. The lunacy reformers of the early nineteenth century drew an exaggerated, but nevertheless genuinely horrified, picture of the terrible suffering that the asylum movement and rise of medical psychology inflicted on the insane.[33] This book seeks to add another dimension to their well-known description of conditions after the English Revolution by showing how beliefs about insanity and healing practices before 1640 had been integrated into the mental world and social lives of ordinary people.

2

A healer and his patients

Like the buried remains of ancient nomads, the sources for the study of insanity before the age of asylums are scattered and hidden in unlikely places. Accounts of mad and melancholy Englishmen, real and imagined, can be found in a profusion of records, papers, and books, but no great concentrations await a fortunate archeologist. Even in the most prolific records that have been located, the surviving documents of the Court of Wards, coroners' inquests, and medical practice books, traces of the mentally disturbed are buried in the much vaster debris left by the sane. Because one cannot survey the remains of the whole culture, it is necessary to select one area for close scrutiny and then to assess its relationship to the rest by collecting as many diffuse scraps of evidence from the same period as can be readily found. The basic source for this book is the voluminous medical practice notes of a seventeenth-century astrological physician named Richard Napier. I have analyzed the more than two thousand descriptions of insane and troubled people in his manuscripts from several perspectives.[1] The results of this investigation have been supplemented by accounts of mental disorder and its treatment in coroners' inquests, court records, diaries, medical and religious treatises, plays, and popular literature. Because the foundation of this work is the labor of a single man, it is essential to know something of his life and methods.

Richard Napier's portrait hangs in a hall facing a cabinet of oddities in the Ashmolean Museum at Oxford. Dressed in rich clerical black and wearing a cap embroidered with gold thread and pearls, he stares obliquely at Powhatan's mantle, displayed a few yards away. He appears to be reflecting on the manic and indiscriminate

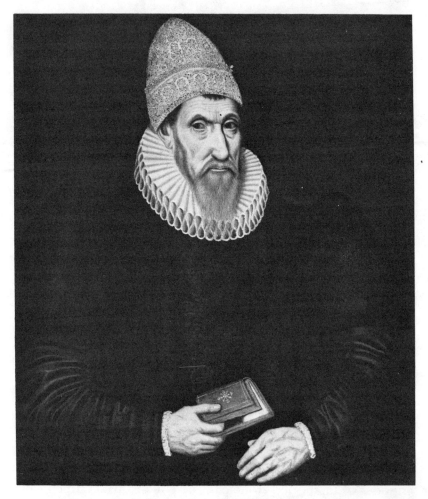

Plate 1.   The Reverend Richard Napier, alias Sandy. By courtesy of
the Ashmolean Museum, Oxford.

energies of the man who bequeathed all the curious objects that
surround him to the University of Oxford, Elias Ashmole. For
had not Ashmole hoarded ancient coins and tricked the Trades-
cants out of their collection of New World artifacts, Napier's own
papers, the records of his life's work as an astrologer, alchemist,
physician, and divine, would not have survived. Ashmole was a
generation younger than Napier and, together with his gayer,
drunker friends William Lilly and John Aubrey, revered the ob-

scure physician as a magus, a practitioner of prophetic and healing magic who was the embodiment of the hermetic tradition in England after John Dee's death. He purchased Napier's manuscripts, a congeries of medieval alchemical works, the books and papers of Simon Forman, magical manuscripts collected by Forman and Napier, and Napier's own notes about medicine, alchemy, magic, and religion and had them expensively bound and numbered. Napier's medical notes alone filled sixty volumes. Near the end of his life Ashmole decided to leave his vast collections of objects and papers to the university, founding a new museum to house them. Faced with the task of cataloguing this miscellany, an Oxford librarian complained that the antiquarian should have sent more books about Roman coins and buried Napier's astrological papers. But the terms of the bequest were honored, and the astrological and medical notes were carefully preserved, as was Napier's portrait, destined to share a hallway with the bric-a-brac of the collection, deemed unsuitable for display in the statelier galleries of the Ashmolean.[2]

The picture is bad art but good caricature. The sitter's stern visage mirrors his sober enthusiasm for learning and medicine and his sullen intelligence and piety. His hollow cheeks and facial furrows were not earned on coital escapades like Simon Forman's, nor on binges of political pamphleteering and practical joking like William Lilly's, nor on colossal drinking sprees like John Aubrey's.[3] Once, about 1610, Napier "in a merriment" stole his friend Forman's horse and the purloined beast kicked him in the leg. The memory of his blackened limb was still fresh ten years later when he recorded the "accidents" or notable events of his life in a calculation of his astrological nativity, and he apparently learned the perils of frivolity from it. No other trace of raucous play or verbal wit enlivens his thousands of pages of notes, professional and personal. His jottings for the nativity confirm the painter's somber vision: "Extreme fearful by nature to declaim or preach"; "very fearful of spirits and orating and timorous by nature and much afflicted with mopish melancholy . . . and mightily no mind to marry but a great mind to all manner of studies and arts; a weak brain"; "very earnest in dispute."[4] Napier was a shy and scholarly man whose excellences were intellectual, not a weak brain at all but not, perhaps, a brilliant mind. The painter calls attention to Napier's arcane studies. His subject wears a richly worked cap and clutches a small book, possibly the attributes of a hermetic adept. This was the facet of Napier's life that preoccupied Ashmole and Aubrey when they plundered his papers for cabalistic secrets, astrological and medical instruction. In his brief life of Napier, Aubrey gives an indolent summary of what they learned. His piety and occult wisdom were so great that he could conjure angels: He communicated with the Miltonic angel, Raphael, and received trivial and profound knowledge from him. The gossipy Aubrey can recall that the Archangel predicted John Prideaux's elevation to the bench of bishops. Greater truths prove harder to remember: "There are also several other queries to the Angel as to religion, transubstantiation, etc., which I have forgot. I remember one is whether the good spirits or the bad be most in number? R[esponsum] R[aphael] is: 'the Good.'" If that revealed theology is ever to be found again, a good spirit will have to be conjured once more, for the passages Aubrey recalls so dimly have disappeared.[5]

Represented by a poor portrait and this odd fragment of biography, Napier's reputation was soon but a lesser curiosity among the collections of Ashmole and Aubrey. The picture has been ignored; the sketch has been ridiculed and scissored apart by modern scholars scoffing at a credulous, cranky quack.[6] Among his contemporaries Napier's standing was far higher. The tens of thousands of patients who trekked to Napier's home between 1597 and 1634 were attracted by his fame as an astrological physician. The theologians who visited him and wrote long queries about disputed points for his comments knew him as a pious and learned churchman. The alchemists and "mathematicians" who learned their arts from him respected his mastery of chemical and magical secrets. He was a fabulous polymath who combined all the skills to minister to men's troubled minds and bodies with a zeal for the kind of learning Frances Yates calls Rosicrucian, occult studies employing alchemical, hermetic, cabalistic, Neoplatonic, and Christian lore.[7]

Richard Napier was one of the last Renaissance magi. He lived on the cusp between two eras dominated by the antagonistic forces of magic and science. In the sphere of the educated elite, old ideas were exploded or deprived of their brilliance by new intellectual novas and fresh discoveries. The influence of Neoplatonism waned as scientific materialism waxed. The natural magic of the cabala and the hermetic texts was exploded by Casaubon's discovery that the antiquity of their authorities was bogus.[8] Astrology faded as the new astronomy grew more brilliant and visible. Alchemy gradually lost its philosophical and magical aura and only its scientific core survived. The forces of religious opposition warred with one another. Calvinism dominated the religious cosmos of the late sixteenth century and flared anew during the Civil War, but as its luminosity declined the constellation of conforming Anglicans and the new Arminian nova overpowered its influence and then in turn were eclipsed by the cool and rational religion of the Restoration. All of these changes were accompanied by sublunary tempests: the great storm of witchcraft prosecutions, the battle betweeen the Galenist physicians and their astrological and Paracelsian competitors, the Anglican attack on exorcists, the religious struggles of the seventeenth century, and the eruption of antagonistic political and cosmological ideas during the Interregnum. These new ideas did not determine the allegiances of ordinary people or even of intellectuals. The stars did but incline: The actual course of change was shaped by political strife, social change, and religious passion.[9] For Richard Napier, living during the decades of intensifying controversy, these events meant that the synthesis of magic, religion, and science he practiced was in imminent peril. Separated from his age by a vast expanse of time, we can see that his quest for the superior wisdom offered by angelic magic, astrology, alchemy, and Christian Neoplatonism was often shadowed by intimations of change and hostility that were already ominously visible.

To the rather anachronistic minds of his younger admirers, Lilly, Aubrey, and Ashmole, his mastery of the practical cabala, the magic that elevated the priestly philosopher to the realms of the archangels, was his greatest intellectual and spiritual achievement. And these occult pursuits were certainly his greatest passion because they united all of his strongest interests, astrology, alchemy, ancient learning, and theology. The pious magic that he practiced was very similar to the hermetic arts of John Dee. Like Dee, he sought magically to attain knowledge about religion and science he could not get from solely human sources. Like Dee, he found the means to conjuring in the works of Lull, Agrippa, the *Key of Solomon*, *Picatrix*, and a library of other medieval texts of baffling authorship and provenance believed by Napier and his colleagues to have been composed in Biblical times. Like Dee, he suffused all of his necromancy with a personally purifying faith, and the climax of his long rituals of prayer, fasting, and magical ritual was actual conference with an archangel.[10] Some evidence that his friends were right, that his magic was successful, survives. The most dramatic document is a smeared and blotted sheet containing a prophesy, hastily scribbled, delivered to the pious scribe by the Archangel Raphael himself. A great plague and lethal dearth would strike the world in 1609 and 1612, slaughtering Londoners but permitting some to survive in the villages near Napier's home.[11]

The world was spared and London waited until 1625 for the next great visitation of the pestilence. We cannot know whether this and other failures corroded the magician's faith that the angelic presence was good and genuine. Nor do we know when his conferences with spirits began, how often they occurred, and whether he ceased to practice angelic magic. Simon Forman probably kindled his interest in conjuring, but it was surely Napier's acquaintance with John Dee that induced him to practice it. He met Dee's son Arthur in 1602 and records a dinner with the doctor himself two years later at which Dee "entreated for Raymond Lull" and showed Napier an alchemical text.[12] Lilly maintains that Napier knew Dee well, and it is from him and Aubrey that testimony about the frequency of Napier's seances comes.[13] They claim easy familiarity between the magus and Raphael and assert that Napier asked the Angel's opinion about each of the medical cases he treated. Traces of prophesy do occur in Napier's practice notes, but it is often difficult to know whether the many queries about his clients' health, about theology, and about people's personal futures were made as questions for the spirit, as astrological problems, or simply as matters for close study.[14] Like Dee, Napier was attracted by a kind of magic that put "the conjurer in direct contact with the angelic or intellectual world," rites that "come out very clearly as priestly magic, and [in which] the highest dignity of the Magus is seen to be the Magus as priest, performing religious rites and doing religious miracles."[15] Aware of Dee's misfortunes, Napier was careful to leave few traces of his secret arts in his main body of papers and did not imitate him by broadcasting his success.[16]

In an age when demons and fairies, witches and their familiars, were the visible companions of sober husbandmen, ministers, and gentlefolk, it was not mad delusion to see the unseen world. But Protestants of every stripe agreed that to invoke it was profoundly wrong. Satan, the master of protean illusions, was the author of angelic forms; the men who raised such apparitions, even for pious purposes, were the worst kind of witches. The magician sought to protect himself from evil, asking even in the act of conjuring that God

give leave and license, strength, faith, authority and divine power to call to our sight and hearing to our help and instruction thy holy angel Raphael or any other that shall better please Thee . . . That so we may be truly and perfectly certified and instructed touching those things wherein we stand in doubt good and necessary to be known, and because the subtle serpent, Satan, . . . with his wicked ministers oftentimes intrude themselves, as though they were angels of light . . . We beseech thee to reprove him and to cut short that he may have no power to delude us.[17]

Sensitive to the sin of idolatry and sensible to the extreme power of the Devil and the extreme weakness of man, no Puritan would have hesitated to condemn this magic, no matter how well intentioned. Jealous of the established church's monopoly over legitimate spiritual power, no member of the Anglican orthodoxy would openly permit such activities. Keith Thomas has remarked that although a few English churchmen with Neoplatonic enthusiasms endorsed hermetic magic, even the Anglican proponents of ritual and ceremony were wary of it: "For the most part the tone of the Anglican Church was profoundly hostile to any kind of conjuration or spirit-raising."[18] No wonder Napier was alarmed when a crazy and malevolent neighbor once called him a conjurer. The penalty for necromancy was death.[19]

And here is an enigma, for this obscure and rustic Faustus was simultaneously a learned and orthodox Anglican minister. Whatever the official position of his church on his secret dealings, his public and sincerely won reputation was that of an extremely pious and conservative theologian. The child of a younger son of the Scottish Napiers, lairds of Merchiston, Richard had a long and thorough education in theology at Oxford. He seems to have entered the university in 1577, when he was eighteen; he received his B.A. in 1584 and his M.A. in 1586; he was elected a fellow of Exeter College in 1580, a post he held until 1590. He left Oxford in that year and became a minister and the rector of Great Linford in northern Buckinghamshire, a tiny hamlet in which he worked until his death in 1634.[20] Even if he himself had not told us that preaching terrified him, we would have Lilly's testimony that one Sunday, his anxiety overmastering him, he broke down in the pulpit and was forced to abandon his public duties, employing ever afterward a curate to perform the necessary tasks of serving his congregation's souls.[21] A shy and scholarly exile from the university he loved, he busied himself with theology, alchemy, and above all astrological medicine, finding in the service of men and women's bodily and mental afflictions a vocation that suited him brilliantly and that he practiced for almost forty years, from 1597 until 1634. He treated tens of thousands of patients for every kind of malady and became a famous healer at a time when it was not unusual for clergymen to be physicians as well. By the last decade of his life he counted earls among his clients and knights and baronets among his friends. He made his prodigal nephew and namesake, heir to his practice and property, a rich man. The beautiful rectory he remodeled testifies that his practice and the living were lucrative.[22] Still, piety mattered more to him than riches, and he preferred the company of clergymen to that of noblemen.

He gave most of what he got from his enormous medical practice to the poor, according to Aubrey.[23] But the biographer's compulsive hyperbole cannot be reduced to historical reality, because Napier recorded his gifts to paupers only at New Year's and at times when he felt unusually pious or repentant. His fees were rather small, and he forgave them for the poor – that much is clear from his early notes. He had no head for the profits and the losses, and even when he had the help of a business agent to keep track of them he was insufficiently greedy to be precise: "My man William and I did reckon up our books, and I came short in my reckoning and we had great babblement," he once wrote ruefully.[24] Avarice was not among his sins. Nor was the kind of pride enjoyed by the creatures of the great. He met his noble patients through his brother, a Levant trader who grew prodigiously rich, became a baronet, and insinuated himself into the Duke of Buckingham's circle. When the nobility first noticed him, after 1615, he was flattered by their overtures of friendship: "I went to Grafton to see the Duke [?of Lennox]. He did take me by the hand after that I was going hence twice, but still prevented."[25] His deference was doubled a few years later when his brother and his aristocratic cronies twice arranged for him to kiss the king's hand and Prince Charles's – he proudly scribbled descriptions of the meetings in his diary.[26] But Napier was not overawed by the nobility nor eager for their favor. When Buckingham and his mother entreated him to cure the duke's lunatic and adulterous brother, Viscount Purbeck, Napier evaded the scandalous imbroglio as long as prudence allowed.[27] His contact with the Villiers and their clients in the years that followed made him acid about the clan; he wrote that Buckingham was "full of bribery" and blamed Purbeck's madness on his mother, whom the physician hated.[28] He scolded another great lady, perhaps Purbeck's estranged wife, accusing her of raging at her father and husband and denouncing them behind backs, in language that bears no trace of respect for aristocratic dignity.[29]

As an astrologer, an alchemist, a conjurer, he had as much to fear from the attentions of the great as he could gain from them. Anxiety and pride are mingled in his description of a conversation a friend of his overheard at Oxford in 1620: "My Lord Chancellor extolled me and the Earl of Exeter's son called me conjurer, and . . . my Lord Wentworth commended me and pleaded for my memory. The Lord that knoweth the secret of all hearts reward him and all his family for it and deliver me from my enemies, visible and invisible, and all slanderous tongues and make me patiently to undergo all crosses."[30] Napier was delivered from his visible enemies – he was never prosecuted for his magical arts – but his escape probably owed as much to his reputation as a conforming theologian and his friendships with important clergymen as it did to his connections with powerful courtiers.

Napier was a champion of his generation's orthodoxy. Educated at a time when tepid Calvinism was the tenor of the church's crucial doctrines, his views about salvation and free will echo Archbishop Whitgift's. While men are free to do good works "of nature," he wrote to one of his nephews, they cannot "do such acts as tend to the salvation of their souls."[31] For salvation, he explains elsewhere, depends on "God's promise, who hath out of his infinite free love promised to reward every man according to his deeds . . . for God maketh the good deeds and works of his saints to be inferred of merit."[32] He wrote vigorous refutations of Catholic doctrines, apparently unpublished treatises and notes on the errors of the "Pontificans."[33] Surrounded by recusant noblemen attended by a Jesuit priest early in the 1620s, he was plainly upset by their beliefs and tried to wean their protectors, Purbeck and his mother, the Countess of Buckingham, from their hated creed.[34]

But his sharpest conflicts were with Puritans.[35] He thought that God was generous with the saving grace that allowed men to perform good works and he repudiated the precise Calvinist's anxiety about the surety of salvation. In letters to Henry Jackson (the editor of Hooker), to his nephew Richard Napier, and to an anonymous clergyman, he developed an argument for the validity of the Ancient Fathers, the councils of the church, and the "public spirit of the church" against the personal interpretations of the scriptures on which Cartwright and the "Puritan writers" grounded their rejection of the episcopacy and the wearing of the surplice. The chief modern authorities he cites are the great Anglican apologists Jewel and Hooker.[36] Alarmed by Jackson's intimation that he was sympathetic to millenarianism, as many moderate Anglicans were, he wrote: "I condemn them as much as you or any man breathing" – noting, however, that not all the authorities condemned them utterly.[37] The moderate and conforming cast of his religious thought is mirrored in the views of the clerical friends who visited him at Great Linford. Many younger churchmen came to talk and use his vast library of theological tracts. Some of these men were young Oxford dons, and he helped one of them, Michael Jermin, to a spectacular pair of appointments as the chaplain of the Queen of Bohemia and King Charles. Like another more famous visitor, John Towers, the Laudian Dean of Peterborough, he suffered under the Puritan regime.[38] The bishop of Lincoln, John Williams, a political rival of Laud's but a staunch Anglican, was probably the learned rector's most powerful clerical friend.[39]

The region around Great Linford was thick with Puritan clergy, and in spite of his reluctance to declaim his views in public, Napier clashed with them on several occasions. His most illustrious antagonist was William Twisse, a Puritan divine famous for his lucid sermons and effective polemics. He attacked Napier publicly during a routine visitation at Olney in 1617, and the wounded victim later complained in his diary that Twisse had carried a friend and neighbor with him: "On visitation . . . Dr. Twist [*sic*] and Mr. Tyrringham assaulted me in disputation and Dr. T. scoffed at me."[40] The kind of issues they quarreled about were doubtless similar to the ideas Napier expressed in a pair of pamphlets aimed at Puritans, which proclaim his hatred of disunity in the church and dislike for the kind of scrupulousness that repudiated the wisdom of the past. His answer to "the apology of the schismatic ministers that refuse subscription and conformity which is required by the act of parliament" (1621) has unfortunately vanished, but we do possess his long defense of the edifying power of classical learning. He wrote the tract after the minister of Newport Pagnell criticized him for quoting Horace in a visitation sermon. He commends the "learning of the gentiles" for "their stories, apothegems, philosophy, poets, testimonies, their mythological and mystical fictions, though never so aptly and fitly applied."[41]

Scrabbling through the extant rubble of Napier's theological writings, it is difficult to reconstruct his ideas with enough exactitude to see how he joined his moderate and orthodox Anglicanism to the temple of magical tradition. But his profound respect for ancient authority is everywhere visible, and it was probably the apparent antiquity of the chief texts of the hermetic and Neoplatonic traditions that persuaded him that they could be used like the other kinds of "learning of the gentiles."[42] A defense of the religious legitimacy of astrology that Napier wrote but failed to publish argues conventionally that the stars incline but do not decide, and that the Lord is not constrained by astral determinism any more than the watchlike regularity of the natural movements of the universe prevents His providence from affecting this world. He characteristically supports his views with citations from what might be styled the "Hooker Library of Ancients and Romans," classical and medieval authors whom the mainstream of Anglican writers admired: Josephus, St. Basil and St. Augustine, Plato, Aristotle and Ptolemy, St. Thomas, Duns Scotus and Peter Lombard, all are plundered for quotations approving astrology.[43]

The touchstone of Puritan theology was the second commandment, which forbids men to make any "graven images," an injunction radical Protestants interpreted to embrace all religious paraphernalia that was not mentioned in the Bible. "Any forms of words, vestments, or implements used in worship services were considered idolatrous if they were not of scriptural provenance," explains Sears McGee.[44] The determinist cast of astrological thought was suspect, and any kind of magic that employed ritual objects and symbols was abhorrent to the Puritan mind.[45] Napier's notes for an apology for the use of images to achieve godly ends therefore provide some insights about his personal reconciliation of theology and magic. He collected a profusion of scriptural citations and remarks by the Ancient Fathers to demonstrate "the antiquity and original [*sic*] of images" and to prove that "it is not lawful to make an idolatrical image, yet it is lawful to make others, images not idolatrical" – a distinction no Puritan precisionist would ever have granted possible. Moreover, he continues, "if God give an art, then the use of that art must needs be lawful . . . Solomon sent for Hiram to work all manner of work of brass who was a man full of wisdom and knowledge to work, and he is not condemned for it."[46] Latter-day Hirams, such as Napier, who made brass amulets to protect their wearers against evil spirits could hope for the same indulgence.

If making amulets was lawful because the patriarchs were permitted to do so, then angelic magic based on texts that were believed to contain the secret wisdom of Solomon and even the unwritten revelations Moses received on Sinai should also be lawful. No fragments survive either among the secret manuscripts Ashmole separated from the main collection or in Napier's diaries to prove that he took this final step in a spiritually perilous path of reasoning. But his thinking about the safer topics of astrology and amulets points in this direction, and we know that his conception of the permissible sphere of natural reason was far broader than the Puritans'. Sounding much like Richard Hooker and John Jewel, he once wrote that theological "errors which are not fundamental and do not concern man's salvation," had to be defended "pertinaciously" to be heretical.[47] Magic was perhaps one of those matters that, even if proved unlawful, would be "not damnable because it doth not race and overthrow the foundation as being no way repugnant or contradictory to the scripture or any principle of faith grounded thereon."[48] The Anglican notion of "things indifferent" might therefore be construed to permit even conjuring, but only in the minds of men who accepted both the Biblical provenance and Neoplatonic principles of the hermetic texts. Few contemporaries would have accepted the legality of Napier's angelic magic during his lifetime.

The ancient science of astrological medicine, on the other hand, was still widely defended against its clerical critics in the early seventeenth century. Minds to which omnipotence seemed synonymous with unpredictability and regularity implied determinism were suspicious of figure casters. This attitude was naturally most common among Puritans, who possessed an awful sense of the power and inscrutability of the deity. But many clergymen and physicians were persuaded that the scientific foundations of astrology were valid and believed it to be a particularly useful tool for diagnosing mysterious diseases.[49] Notable churchmen such as Archbishop Laud and Bishops Sanderson and Thornborough were interested in astrology, and other important Anglicans or members of their immediate families consulted astrological physicians. Napier treated Bishop Williams, Archbishop Abbot's niece, and the Dean of Peterborough, for example.[50] Nor were individual Puritans always hostile to the astral science; during the Civil War a host of pious Independents and Presbyterians resorted to astrologers.[51] Although the London College of Physicians harassed astrologers whose popularity as doctors threatened their domination of medical practice in the city, an almanac-maker was twice president of the college during James's reign. The prestige of medical astrology did not decline significantly until after the Revolution, and even then popular clamor for the services of its practitioners kept it alive for another century.[52]

Most physicians regarded astrology as a tool of their art and not its basis. Napier was no exception. He became interested in practicing astrology in 1597, when on a visit to London he consulted the notorious Simon Forman about some property that had been stolen from Great Linford.[53] Forman possessed a mesmerizing personality and the sexual appetite of a goat, and he made himself the most popular astrologer of his time. His chaotic moods and exuberant immorality were precisely opposed to Napier's somber chastity, but soon Forman was instructing his new friend in every branch of the astrologer's art: finding lost and stolen goods, predicting marriages and diagnosing pregnancy, treating all the maladies of mind and body.[54] The master heaped fond abuse on his pupil, complaining that he had repeatedly instructed him to know "on which side" a disease was lodged, calling him a dunce, and declaring that a meat pie Napier sent him as a present tasted like "paste closed in boards."[55] In spite of such hectoring, the pious rector pursued his studies avidly and, as William Lilly remarked, soon "outwent Forman in physic and holiness of life" – the latter, of course, took no special gifts.[56] Many clergymen combined medical practice with pastoral care, and medicine was the branch of astrology that appealed most to Napier. He began to diagnose and treat sick neighbors in 1597, and as the year passed he confined himself more and more strictly to that activity, performing few of the kinds of divination that made some other astrologers popular. His reputation as a healer grew rapidly, and within a decade he was treating as many as two thousand patients a year; perhaps sixty thousand people journeyed to Great Linford to consult him during the thirty-seven years he practiced medicine.

Napier treated between five and fifteen patients a day, repeating with each of them a ritual of interrogation and annotation that invoked the axioms of astrological medicine. Seated before his practice book, Napier began every consultation with a fixed litany of questions. Who is the patient? Where does he live? How old is he? Is he present or has someone come to represent him, with or without his consent? When the precise coordinates of the patient's identity had been recorded, the astrologer noted the time and date and drew a cross-hatched box on the page. Deciphering the ephemeris at his elbow, he mapped the heavens at that moment, positioning the symbols of the planets and the signs of the zodiac along the celestial frame. The purpose of this astral cartography was to situate the patient in the cosmos, placing him at the vortex of the natural forces that impelled the universe, discovering the correspondences that linked microcosm and macrocosm. Astrological medicine presumed that the perturbations of the mind and body were mirrored in the motions of the stars, and the horoscope was an aid to discovering their nature and origins. If the correspondence was to be exact, the patient's symptoms had to be observed as precisely as the heavens, and below this horoscope of each client Napier carefully listed the sufferer's description of his malady or the signs reported by his representative. Now the astrological circumstances and the disease's manifestations could be compared, and remedies possessing the appropriate celestial and medical virtues selected.

Here is an account of the patients he treated in an easy day's work. On 12 April 1620 Napier met his first client at 9:30 A.M. She was Elizabeth Goodfellow, a fifty-one-year-old woman from the nearby village of Stanwick. After mapping the heavens for that moment, Napier recorded her symptoms. Since Christmas she

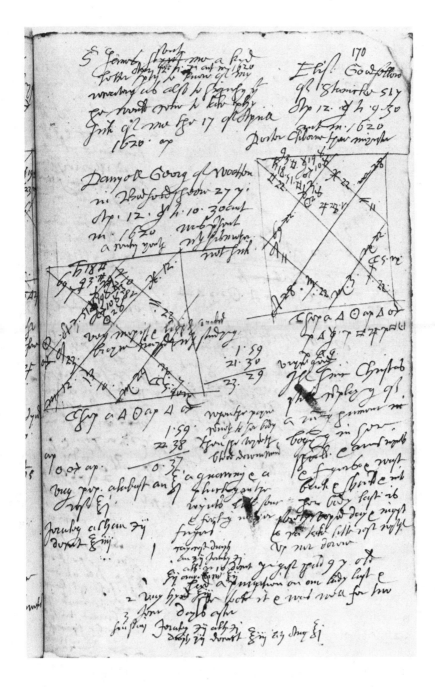

Plate 2. Case notes of Richard Napier for 12 April 1620. By courtesy of the Bodleian Library, Oxford.

had suffered a "running humor," a pain that began in her back and shoulders and then descended down her limbs and into her body. When that happened, he noted she "voideth blood downward." Her joints felt gnawed and plucked, her fingers were numb. Earlier in the year another healer had given her a purge, and for two days afterward she had gained some relief. As usual, Napier followed standard medical practice, prescribing substances that would repeat the purge, ordering her to be bled, and giving her an ointment to procure sleep, because she could "take little rest neither up nor down." Goodfellow was in many ways a characteristic patient and she received typical treatment.

Most of the men and women who sought Napier's care were suffering from physical maladies, often vague and lingering, and he seldom used remedies that could not be found in the pharmacopoeias of classical physicians. Rarely, he resorted to magical amulets, exorcism, and prayer to cure his troubled clients or used folk treatments that had been effective for others. The records for the rest of April 12 are typical cases of mental disorder. At 10:30, 12:30, and 1:00 he treated clients who were emotionally disturbed. Daniel Georg was "very mopish and lightheaded" because his brain was "crazed with studying"; Mistress Mathew and her husband were both "troubled in mind" – she because he was unkind, he for no apparent reason. All of them received purges, vomits, and bleeding, and Mistress Mathew was ordered to take a concoction of egg whites and milk, which she had told the physician she liked. At 2:30 he was confronted with William Whyting, a love-struck twenty-two-year-old who was "lunatic by fits but better at this time." The motions of Saturn were analyzed, perhaps to account for the ebb and flow of madness. Noting another healer's earlier failure to cure the young man, Napier wrote that one Mr. Gylsan had purged him a year before. Among these case notes are other jottings, one recording that a woman suffering from a "dead palsy" had been cured by someone who applied bags of fried oats to her affected limbs and another detailing a prescription for a rich man with an ulcerated tongue.[57]

Astrological physicians of Napier's caliber were not quacks. They presumed that the maladies of mind and body could be studied as systematically as the movements of the planets, and the techniques of recording and analysis made the best of them better empiricists than many physicians who spurned astrology. A letter to Napier from Arthur Dee, the son of the great John Dee and himself an astrological doctor, captures the critical attitude characteristic of the breed:

Concerning him whom I asked your opinion of in your brother Sandie's garden, whom I had in cure upon an empyema with a general consumption of his whole body, whom you judged almost past cure with these words to my question – "They are seldom or never helped" – yet it pleased God I [sic] recovered so perfect well and strong as that he . . . at this present is in better state of body than myself – Concerning the other question I propounded in Moorfields, *an fuisset gravida* [if she had been pregnant], we were both deceived, for it proved not so. I have sent you the figures to consider of it, and I have since found it by experience that it is not sufficient to find the lord of the fifth house with another planet, unless it be in the ascendant . . . I pray you to send me some receipts of worth found by your own practice.[58]

Dee's anxiety to perfect his art by comparing the predictions he drew from his horoscope with his medical experience is obvious in this letter. The same concern for accuracy prompted Napier to keep meticulous records and to pay close attention to the signs and usual courses of diseases. When he heard of the recovery or relapse of one of his patients he referred to his notes on the case and annotated his astrological charts and lists of symptoms. The figures Dee sent show that he had the same habit of reviewing the past histories of his clients and comparing the cases of people suffering from the same disease; Forman, Booker, and (more haphazardly) Lilly all kept extensive records of their practices.[59]

The practice books of doctors uninterested in astrology are typically brief and do not list their patients' ages or symptoms.[60] Because astrologers were visited by their clients in contrast to classically trained physicians who usually attended their patients, the famous astrologers treated many more people than physicians normally did, and the stress astrology laid on time, identity, and age prompted them to make systematic records. The enormous reputations gained by Napier and his peers may reflect the fact that their art encouraged them indirectly to become better prognosticators than most physicians. Seventeenth-century men and women were well aware of the feeble curative powers of contemporary medicine. What they expected above all from their doctors was that they distinguish fatal illnesses from harmless or transient maladies. Napier was persuaded that astrology assisted him to do this better than the diagnostic technique favored by classical physicians, uroscopy. When two clergymen asked him about the relative merits of the two techniques "his answer was that where his figure deceived him once, the urine did it ten times; and that sometime they would speak quite contrary things, but he always found in his figure most truth."[61] This is the outlook of a pragmatist and not a blind enthusiast, and it is probable that Napier was simply stating the fruits of his experience.[62] By encouraging habits of careful observation and record keeping by the physician, astrology probably did help him to be especially adept at recognizing the types and "critical days" of his clients' sufferings. Certainly the thousands of people who walked to Great Linford to seek Napier's help thought that he was an unusually skilled prognosticator; his reputation was sown and nurtured by satisfied customers.

A physician's reputation for medical sagacity is only one of the factors that attract clients to his practice, and some people may be equally repelled by his personality, prices, or beliefs. The characteristics of the group of patients a particular doctor treats are also affected by the location of his practice and the kind of people who live in the neighborhood. A recent study of psychiatric illnesses in medical practices located in London warns that investigations based on a single practice are not as useful as those based on a broader sample.[63] No doubt. But historians cannot simply enroll more doctors in their projects and must make do with the sources preserved by chance. Because there appear to be no other surviving medical records that are precisely comparable to Napier's practice notes, the eccentricities of his patients can only be identified by keeping his biases in mind and analyzing statistical profiles of his clients in light of what is known about contemporary society in the Midlands. A discussion of the demographic, social, and ecological circumstances of his clients, sane and insane, fills the last half of this chapter. Here it is sufficient to stress that his attitudes toward magic and religion probably discouraged Puritans from consulting him as freely as Anglican and religiously apathetic villagers.

Although most of Napier's patients were people of humble social standing and unlikely to be well informed about current controversies over the legitimacy of astrology, Puritan clergymen were certainly repelled by his use of magical amulets and by his strenuously anti-Puritan views. William Lilly reports that Napier once cured a girl of epilepsy by giving her a ring engraved with astral symbols. "Her parents acquainted some scrupulous divines with the cure of their daughter," Lilly continues, " 'The cure is done by enchantment,' they say, 'cast away the ring, it is diabolical, God cannot bless you if you do not cast the ring away.'" The frightened parents complied, but their daughter's fits returned. After a long time they retrieved the ring, and she wore it in good health for a year or two, "which the Puritan ministers there adjoining hearing, never left off till they procured her parents to cast the ring quite away." The cycle was repeated until Napier finally refused to make another amulet, snapping that "those who despised God's mercies were not capable or worthy of enjoying them."[64]

Puritans such as Twisse and Worcester, who preached nearby, knew Napier well, and they probably discouraged their followers from consulting him just as these "scrupulous divines" did.[65] Nor did Napier hide his impatience with Puritan scruples. He was very unsympathetic to people whose religious dilemmas were occasioned by "Puritanical" consciences. Men and women suffering from the kind of anxieties one writer calls "salvation panic" may have avoided Napier if they knew anything of his religious views.[66] Catholics, on the other hand, would not have been as disturbed by some aspects of his methods, exorcism for example, and in spite of his staunch antipapalism, many distinguished recusants did consult him.[67] Since the religious views of the majority of his clients cannot be known, the actual proportions of Puritans and Catholics among his clients cannot be calculated, but it would be prudent to assume that there were fewer of the former and more of the latter than one would have found in a random group collected from the region.

Napier's autobiographical jottings that he was "much afflicted with mopish melancholy" and "very fearful of spirits" suggest other ways in which his attitudes may have affected the complexion of his practice. A melancholy man might easily gain a reputation for special sympathy in treating the troubled in mind. But if that is so, they certainly did not avail themselves of his counsel very freely. The mentally disturbed form a tiny fraction of the clients he treated, less than 5%, and although comparisons are risky, they seem to be somewhat underrepresented in his prac-

tice.[68] No doubt his austerity and rigid morality, evident throughout his case notes and diaries, had something to do with that. He
was certainly perplexed by the problems of distinguishing mental
afflictions from the operations of witches and spirits. He collected
accounts of methods that indicated when a person had been bewitched, and he prepared amulets and exorcisms that would relieve both the mentally ill and the supernaturally afflicted. The
local villagers were terrified of spirits and witches, and his interest
in countermagic no doubt attracted many to consult him. Yet, as
we shall see in a later chapter, he was quite skeptical about individual claims of bewitchment and did not pander to the fears of the
multitude. His clients were no more credulous than the people of
Northamptonshire, Essex, and Lancashire whose fears fueled
witchcraft prosecutions.[69]

Napier lived during the last era in which a prestigious medical
practitioner could reconcile his beliefs in astrology, magic, religion, and science. Few ordinary people during the first half of the
seventeenth century thought that it was illegitimate to marry
physic and astrology, medicine and divinity, in spite of the efforts
of professional physicians to distinguish these arts. The doctors
eventually succeeded in branding astrologers as quacks, and the
clergy finally discredited magic among the elite – assisted, of
course, by the proponents of the new science. Much later, the
triumphant champions of scientific medicine made spectacular improvements in diagnosing and healing physical diseases. But it
would be anachronistic to project these triumphs backward into
the seventeenth century. In his own time Napier was not a bigoted
quack hawking magic to stupid rustics. The principal objection his
professional rivals, such as the physician John Cotta, had was that
men like Napier were eclectics, interloping on a monopoly they
hoped to establish over health care. Napier was popular because he
offered orthodox medical treatment, astrological diagnosis, and
spiritual counseling for low fees at a time when only the rich could
afford treatment by the humanistic physicians who were the fore-
fathers of modern medicine.[70] The tens of thousands of men and
women who journeyed in hope and fear to Great Linford during
the four decades he practiced medicine would have concurred in
the modest epitaph his curate entered in the parish register: "Mr.
Richard Napier, Rector, the most renowned physician both of
body and soul."[71]

AN EPIDEMIOLOGY OF MENTAL DISORDER

On one point common wisdom and medical science agreed in the seventeenth century. The likelihood that a man or woman would succumb to madness or melancholy depended upon both physiological predisposition and environmental stress. Some people were more apt to "take grief" or fear than others, and some circumstances were so oppressive that not even the most stolid soul could remain untroubled. Contemporaries also recognized that the physical differences between the sexes and the bodily changes effected by aging caused men and women to be vulnerable to different afflictions at various stages in their lives. Simon Forman, for example, had this to say about the importance of age and sex in diagnosing physical diseases:

Is there anything in the age; or is there any difference of diseases in respect of the age? . . . Yes, for there is as much difference in the ages as there is between a child and an elder body. For children are subject to the red gum, to worms, to the smallpox, to measles, to scabs, etc., which old folk are not. Again, young maids are subject to the green sickness, which old women nor children are not. Old men are subject to the gout, which children or young folks are not (or very seldom). And we see by experience that many diseases come in children that come not in middle-aged nor old folk, and many come in middle age that come not in children [sic] nor old age, and many come in old age that come not in children nor middle age, because in time in respect of age the humours do alter.[72]

Popular writers such as Lewis Bayly declared that at each stage in men's lives they were subject to different miseries because of their bodily ills and changing circumstances.[73] Medical authorities, emphasizing physiological differences more than social circumstances, remarked that mental disturbances were most common among young males and people who were middle-aged or old. For example, the celebrated anatomist of melancholy, Robert Burton, summarizing lore culled from authorities as venerable as Galen and Aretaeus, concluded that melancholy's victims were: "Of sexes both, but men more often, yet women misaffected are far more violent and grievously troubled . . . Of particular times: old age, from which natural melancholy is almost an inseparable accident, but this artificial malady is more frequent in such as are of a middle age."[74] Some social groups, such as indolent aristocrats, bored wives, and scholars, were also believed peculiarly vulnerable to emotional disturbances.[75]

But the early epidemiologists of mental disorder did not demonstrate any consistent link between the natural attributes and social conditions that contributed to psychological suffering and specific kinds of insanity. They succumbed instead to the enthusiastic urge to hoard together the manifold varieties of mental disease they identified into a single heap that included every type of human misery and folly. "Kingdoms and provinces are melancholy," Burton exclaimed, "cities and families, all creatures, vegetal, sensible and rational, . . . all sorts, sects, ages, conditions are out of tune . . . For indeed who is not a fool, melancholy, mad? . . . Who is not brain-sick? Folly, melancholy, madness are but one disease; delirium is a common name to all."[76] No wonder there were few statements about the prevalence of mental afflictions that commanded unanimous assent.

Modern studies are not much more consistent. Psychiatric epidemiologists and anthropologists all think that social and cultural factors affect the distribution of mental disorders among different groups and peoples, but both the statistics they exhibit and the explanations they give are frequently contradictory. The most careful works show that demographic attributes and social environment do affect the rates of disorder, and that sex, age, marital status, social status, and community solidarity all seem to play an important role in disposing people to some kinds of mental illnesses. The reasons for these variations are complex and disputed, but many investigators think that physiological differences and social factors determine the patterns of psychiatric consultation of different kinds of people and place special burdens of stress on some groups.[77] Both the contemporary and modern literature about mental disorder therefore suggest that a careful look at the social and environmental backgrounds of Napier's clients is in order.

The rest of this chapter examines the demographic characteristics of Richard Napier's mentally disturbed clients and the kinds of communities in which they lived. Although the social backgrounds of people suffering from particular symptoms were analyzed and compared, the results of that study will not be presented here. The only notable correlation between a type of mental affliction and a social variable shows that those who had the fashionable malady melancholy were in better company than the rest of Napier's patients, for it was a frequent complaint of aristocrats and gentlefolk. Otherwise, no difference of disease, neither madness nor mopishness nor trouble of mind, can be tied to a particular group of clients.[78] The focus in the pages that follow will therefore be on the entire pool of mentally disturbed people, and the aim of the discussion will be to identify characteristics special to them by comparing them with Napier's other patients and with the people in the region of his practice. The unit of analysis will be a case of mental disorder, defined for statistical purposes as one or more consultations with Napier for an episode of illness that included symptoms he regarded as mentally abnormal. Patients sometimes returned years later, with different complaints, so consultations more than one year apart have been treated as separate episodes of illness. There were 2,039 cases of mental disorder in Napier's practice by this definition, about 95% of which were experienced by people whom he never again treated for a psychological disorder.

Sex

All over the world today more women suffer from reported psychiatric maladies than men. Social scientists have offered a hectic profusion of explanations for the apparent psychological frailty of females, but nobody has advanced very much beyond the plausible assumption that women's numerical superiority among the ranks of the troubled and insane owes something to their subordination to men in the vast majority of human societies. Defective diagnoses, meaningless statistical comparisons, and crackpot moralizing characterize the most comprehensive surveys of the problem, and the best scholarship has concentrated on showing how the tyrannical pressure to conform to the sex roles of specific countries and groups influences the detection and management of female insanity.[79] For example, in the early 1960s Professor Michael Shepherd and his colleagues made a careful study of psychiatric disorders in London general medical practices and found that there as elsewhere women complained of more mental illness than men. They noticed that the female "prevalence rate" was almost twice as high as the male rate, and that an inordinate proportion of disturbed women were middle-aged. Commenting on this finding, they quote a nineteenth-century physician's speculation that men hate going to doctors and are less boggled by nervous and sexual excitement than women, and that "the blighted hopes, the ambitious cravings, the sensual as well as mental excesses" of middle age make that the most perilous stage of people's lives. They then conclude cautiously that differences between the readiness of the sexes to identify their suffering as illness and the variations in the social pressures to label men or women mentally sick, unable to perform their daily tasks, probably accounted for the prevalence of women in the practices they studied. Their quotation from an obsolete medical study is doubtless a subtle hint that they believe that whatever the true causes of the greater vulnerability of women to psychiatric disorders, they have not changed much since the nineteenth century.[80]

The role of women in English society today differs more in degree than in kind from the ideal of the Victorian middle class. Breeding and nesting are still regarded as the natural occupations of young and middle-aged women. The evidence that more than three centuries ago, the women among Napier's clients also suffered from more insanity, sadness, and anxiety than men is perhaps more surprising. He recorded 1,286 cases of mental disorder involving females and 748 cases concerning males. Five disturbed clients had sexually ambiguous names and their sex could not be guessed from the language of Napier's case notes. Expressed conventionally as the number of males per 100 females, the sex ratio of Napier's mentally disturbed clients was 58.2, a figure very similar to the ratios reported for modern medical practices in Britain. As Shepherd and his team of collaborators remark, a low sex ratio of mentally disturbed medical patients in a general practice may be caused by several factors, working singly or together. The doctor's medical personality, his character, his specialty, and his biases in diagnosing his patients, or the location of his practice in a demographically odd place may make the sex ratio in the practice peculiar. Socially conditioned habits of medical consultation or physical and social stresses particular to women may also affect the number of female mental patients the physician treats.[81] Did Napier's personal attitudes and habits attract women to his practice? Was his practice in a sexually odd area? Did women consult him medically more readily than men? Did they suffer more physical disease and emotional pressure than men?

Richard Napier was sexually indifferent toward women, openly contemptuous of their intellectual capacities, and strongly disinclined to specialize in female complaints.[82] Nothing in his manner or attitudes can have enticed women to reveal their emotional problems to him. Some astrologers were sexually rapacious and used their art as an aid in seduction. The energetic love life of the Casanova of the astrological consulting rooms, Simon Forman, shows that pure sex appeal could affect the composition of a practice like Napier's. But there is no evidence that Napier ever attempted to seduce any of his clients, and his hatred of illicit fornication and adultery makes it significant that he did not record a single assault on his chastity by a female patient in the fifteen thousand or so folios of diaries and practice notes he kept. His patients evidently thought he was unappetizing. Other astrologers, even when they did not exploit their clients sexually, found that it was profitable to cater to young women's obsession with their marital prospects and to specialize in the difficult business of determining whether women were pregnant and of predicting the unborn child's sex.[83] Napier did his share of such work, but it formed only a very small proportion of his medical practice. He sometimes predicted the romantic futures of his clients, but he confined himself largely to medical conundrums, such as deciding if women suffering irregular or vanished periods were sick, infertile, or pregnant. An unusual personal preoccupation with the mysteries of the feminine heart and body was not part of his professional strategy.

Although it is very plain that Napier's personality and astrological specialties did not lure women into his web, it is possible that his practice may still have been in a region overpopulated with females. There is not very much information available about the sex ratios of English towns and villages in the early seventeenth century, and none at all for counties, regions, and the country as a whole. Historical demographers have found that women, especially young unmarried women, seem to have collected in unusual numbers in cities and towns and probably to a lesser degree in country villages. There are two simple reasons for the low sex ratios of urban areas: Work for women as domestic servants was to be found mainly in cities, while jobs for men as agricultural laborers were scattered in the countryside; and the endemic pestilence that regularly exploded into epidemics in the cities and towns apparently killed men more readily than members of the biologically more durable sex. But even the concatenation of economic opportunity and bubonic plague did not produce a sex ratio as low as 58.2 in any English town. In early sixteenth-century Coventry disastrous circumstances lowered the sex ratio to 72; three other English cities less affected by depression and disease, Bristol, Lichfield, and London, had sex ratios of 80, 83, and 87 in 1695.[84] Very few of Napier's clients came from large urban settlements; most of them walked to Great Linford from the small villages and hamlets within a fifteen- or twenty-mile radius of that tiny village. The sex ratios in those places cannot normally have been even as low as 90. The large forest villages in nearby Northamptonshire were infamous as the haunts of paupers, vagrants, thieves, and witches, but not as Amazonias.[85] The peculiarities of the "population at risk," as the epidemiologists call potential medical patients, certainly did not by themselves account for the low sex ratio among Napier's mentally disturbed clients.

Feminine habits of consulting physicians and the greater vulnerability of women to physical and mental stress did affect the sexual balance of the group of tormented people Napier treated. Like the general practitioners Shepherd and his team studied in modern London, Napier spent a large amount of his time ministering to the physical ailments of women. The sex ratio of the clients who consulted him for all kinds of maladies in four sample years was 78.8.[86] Women sought medical treatment more often than men because they were more often ill. In addition to the afflictions men bore, women also suffered from diseases that tormented only their sex. Nutritional deficiencies afflicted young women with anemia. Gynecological ailments, which neither women's cunning nor scientific medicine could cure, caused many to suffer the "reds" or "whites," enduring pain, festering infections, and menstrual disorders until nature and time brought remission – if they did. Childbirth without anesthesia or asepsis was excruciating and dangerous: Difficult and botched deliveries often left women mangled, sterile, or lame – if they survived the infections that appear commonly to have followed dangerous labors. These afflictions were quite familiar in Napier's practice, and they can easily be seen to have contributed to the surplus of mentally disturbed women, for one out of five of them complained to the doctor of a gynecological or obstetrical problem in addition to her psychological distress.[87]

Because women like these were driven to seek medical help more often than men, perhaps they were readier to turn to a physician when they suffered emotionally. It is tempting to speculate that the habit of frequenting doctors was encouraged by a common prejudice that made it acceptable for women (but not men) to express their frustrations as sicknesses and for men (but not women) to express their frustrations as aggression and violence.[88] Unfortunately, although there is plenty of evidence that contemporary notions about the proper behavior of the sexes affected criminal styles, none of the contemporary literature I have read can be construed to say that illness, real or imagined, and the demand for medical care were somehow feminine or, conversely, unmasculine.

The extra burden of disease that women suffered not only led them to consult physicians more often than men did; it also contributed to their superabundance among the mentally tormented in a less direct manner. The protracted agony of many gynecological maladies and the debilitating lassitude of anemia must also have increased the mental stress women were forced to endure. Some doctors did recognize that there was a connection between female diseases and psychological disturbances, and they tried to persuade their fellow practitioners and the literate public that an ailment they called "suffocation of the mother" was widespread. They attributed bizarre symptoms, weird perceptions, and grand delusions to this illness and blamed them on the alleged propensity of the uterus to become a vagabond, leaving its proper place in the womb and wandering into the upper parts, near the passionate heart.[89] Speculative physiology thus invented a wild explanation for an observation verified by common experience, that women were more vulnerable than men to psychological stress because of illness.

Not all the stress that women suffered was caused by physical illness. As we shall see in a later chapter, 767 of Napier's mentally disturbed clients complained about intolerable dilemmas that corroded their happiness, and many of the people who were tormented by frustrating relationships and upsetting experiences were women. The fact that the sex ratio among these patients (just 52.3) was even lower than the ratios of the mentally disordered and the physically ill suggests that women were also more vulnerable than men to psychologically disturbing social situations. Their individual propensities to anxiety and sadness were en-

Table 2.1. *Age structure of Napier's sane and mentally disturbed patients (in percent)*

Age	Napier disturbed	Napier 1610 1620	Ealing 1599	Lichfield 1695	England 1695
0–9	0.7	6.6	20.6	27.3	27.7
10–19	8.0	11.7	28.8	20.6	20.2
20–29	33.2	24.1	13.4	15.3	15.5
30–39	24.7	20.4	12.7	15.7	11.7
40–49	16.9	16.9	7.0	8.8	8.4
50–59	9.4	10.7	10.5	6.0	5.8
60+	7.1	9.6	7.0	6.3	10.7
Totals	100.0	100.0	100.0	100.0	100.0

Sources: The figures for Napier's sane clients are calculated from the ages of 2,386 people who consulted him during 1610 and 1620. The figures for Ealing are from Peter Laslett, *The World We Have Lost,* 2nd ed. (London, 1971), p. 108; those for Lichfield and England are from King's estimates, tabulated by D. V. Glass, "Two Papers on Gregory King," in D. V. Glass and D. E. C. Eversley, eds., *Population in History* (London, 1965), pp. 181, 212.

hanced by patriarchal customs and values that limited their ability to remedy disturbing situations, even the catastrophes of family life, the only domain in which the female had any hope at all of influencing events. Gerrard Winstanley said: "If it be rightly searched into, the inward bondages of the mind, as covetousness, pride, hypocrisy, envy, sorrow, fears, desperation and madness, are all occasioned by the outward bondage that one sort of people lay upon another."[90] Napier and his troubled patients also believed that oppression made people miserable and even mad, but the bondage they found most troubling subordinated daughters to parents, wives to husbands, rather than peasants to lords.

Age

Conventional wisdom in Shakespeare's England declared that each stage of life produced its own peculiar affliction of body and soul, and that the vulnerability of men and women to disease and emotional suffering changed as their mental powers waxed and

Table 2.2. *Age structure of adults (in percent)*

Age	Napier disturbed	Napier 1610 and 1620	England 1695
20–29	36.3	29.5	29.8
30–39	27.0	24.9	22.4
40–49	18.6	20.7	16.1
50–59	10.3	13.1	11.3
60+	7.8	11.8	20.4
Totals	100.0	100.0	100.0

Sources: As in Table 2.1. Persons under 20 have been omitted and the percentages recalculated accordingly.

waned with age. Children and ancients sickened and died more often than young people and the middle-aged, and the turbulence of adult life and the bodily decay of old age caused the middle-aged and elderly to suffer more mental disease than other people, according to contemporary writers. Napier's clients, however, found youth much more dangerous emotionally than middle or old age. Almost exactly one-third of his troubled patients were in their twenties, as Table 2.1 shows, although the few comparative figures available suggest that only about 15% of the general population were in that age group. This is not a statistical mirage. Even when one corrects for the lack of children among Napier's mentally disturbed patients by disregarding people under twenty, young adults can still be seen to have been unusually numerous, as comparisons with a sample of Napier's physically ill clients and with Gregory King's estimates of English ages in 1695 show (Table 2.2). Many of these young people complained to their physician about the anxieties of courtship and marriage and the uncertainties of getting a living and bearing children, problems that accompanied the transition from youthful dependence on parents and masters to full independence as married adults. Contemporaries were well aware of the psychological stress young people endured. Although learned writers emphasized the frailty of aged minds, they also warned their readers about the dangers of lovers' melancholy and described the lacerating effects of marital strife, infant deaths, and economic misfortune.[91] These common stresses troubled hundreds of Napier's clients, and they will be discussed in detail in the next chapter.

The most striking feature of the distribution of ages among Napier's patients, both the physically ill and the mentally distressed, is the rarity of children among them. Paradoxically, seventeenth-century England swarmed with children even though they suffered mortal sicknesses appallingly often. In spite of mortality rates showing that disease slew as many as one-half of the boys and girls under five years old who were born in some cities, about 25% of the population was under ten and from 45% to 50% was under twenty.[92] Nations without modern technology and medicine need many children to assure an adequate supply of adults, and the youthfulness of the English population can be paralleled with the age structures of developing countries today. Because there were many children and because they were more often sick than middle-aged adults, it is surprising that less than 7% of Napier's patients were under ten and less than 20% were not yet twenty. Among psychologically disturbed clients, children were still scarcer: 0.7% were under ten, 7.5% under twenty. Why did parents bring their sick and troubled children for medical treatment so seldom?

Accustomed as they were to see infants and toddlers sicken and die, many parents must have regarded their children's illnesses with gloomy resignation. No expert was needed to diagnose the too familiar diseases that carried away most children, and a physician (or a witch-finder) must have seemed necessary only when the child's illness was unusually sudden or lingering, convulsive or mysterious. That is how many of the illnesses of Napier's youngest patients were described. Nor was there much point in purchasing costly medical treatments for children, because the remedies physicians used were either useless or harmful and often both. Thomas Phaer, the author of the earliest English book about pediatrics, advised his readers to avoid treating common children's diseases with physic: "The best and most sure help in this case is not to meddle with any kind of medicines but to let nature work her operations."[93] The Puritan diarist Adam Martindale loved his children, but when his daughter fell ill he decided not to take her to Bath for treatment because a physician friend told him that the costly therapy was probably ineffective and Martindale knew personally someone who tried the cure but died anyway. Such rea-

soning probably explains why affectionate parents like Ralph Josselin did not take their sick children to doctors and perhaps
accounts for the scarcity of children among Napier's clients.[94].

Even today after more than half a century of analysis and speculation about the emotional development of children, there are no
reliable figures about how many of them are insane or emotionally
disturbed. Shepherd and his collaborators, confronting the complex issues of defining mental disorder among the very young,
refused the jump and omitted persons under fifteen from their
study of the epidemiology of psychiatric disorder in London general practices.[95] No other work provides any persuasive information about childhood abnormality that would tell us how many
mad or troubled children one might expect to find in a modern
medical practice comparable to Napier's. Nevertheless, disturbed
children were strikingly rare among his clients, and contemporary
attitudes toward children's mental capacities suggest that seventeenth-century parents were less ready than we are to think that
their children were psychologically disturbed.

Napier treated only 13 cases of mental disorder involving children under ten, and not all these boys and girls were unmistakably
afflicted with maladies of the mind. The three youngest suffered
from physical illnesses as well as psychological problems, and
even if one adds the six ten-year-olds to the cases of childhood
disturbance, over half of these youngsters (10 out of 19) still cannot be classified as unambiguously insane, because Napier's practice notes list both mental and physical symptoms.[96] Opinion of
every variety and the practices of legal and religious institutions
assumed that children were incapable of reason, and their scarcity
among the mentally disturbed may simply be due to the logical
consequences of such thinking; because young children were not
reasonable, they could hardly suffer from diseases that manifested
themselves in unreasonable thoughts and actions.[97] Proverbs and
sayings equating children, animals, lunatics, and fools came easily
to English lips. Lewis Bayly, in an immensely popular devotional
handbook, asked: "What wast thou, being an infant, but a brute
having the shape of a man?"[98] Although other writers warned
that children, like fools and melancholics, were easy prey for Satan's delusion, proverbial wisdom held that they were spared
emotional anguish. "Children and fools have merry lives" ran one
version of a popular saw.[99] The legal procedures of the Court of

Wards presumed that minors, like lunatics and idiots, could not manage their affairs responsibly.[100] The rites of the church that celebrated the child's attainment of the "years of discretion," confirmation and first communion, were postponed till the early teens.[101] John Earle crafted this character of a child: "He plays yet like a young prentice the first day, and is not come to his talk of melancholy."[102] Popular beliefs about children's mental development were perhaps the cause of the extreme rarity of child maniacs and melancholics in Napier's practice.

Seventeenth-century physicians thought that the aged were exceptionally vulnerable to gloom and unhappiness. "Distress of mind," wrote one London doctor named John Smith, "is the passion that is most incident to age."[103] Every reader of *King Lear* knows that common opinion expected that the physiological decay that beset the elderly would make them sad and doting: "The best and soundest of his time hath been but rash; then must we look to his age to receive . . . the unruly waywardness that infirm and choleric years bring with them."[104] Goneril's harsh judgment was undutiful, but it was based on accepted scientific lore. According to Burton's summary of medical opinion, old age was one of the outward natural causes of melancholy, "which no man living can avoid." Old age is "cold and dry and of the same quality as melancholy is, must needs cause it, by diminution of spirits and substance, and increasing of adust humours." Authorities as profound as Melanchthon and Aristotle therefore declare that "old men familiarly dote . . . for black choler, which is then superabundant in them." There is, Burton continues, other evidence that the aged suffer more from mental disease:

After seventy years (as the Psalmist saith) "all is trouble and sorrow"; and common experience confirms the truth of it in weak and old persons . . . They are overcome with melancholy in an instant, or . . . they dote at last . . . and are not able to manage their estates through common infirmities incident in their age; . . . full of ache, sorrow, and grief, children again, dizzards, they carle many times as they sit, and talk to themselves, they are angry, waspish, displeased with everything, "suspicious of all, wayward, covetous, hard" (saith Tully).[105]

Although the elderly left behind some of the disturbing turmoil of youth and middle life, their physical decline was commonly thought to be the harbinger of emotional anguish and intellectual incompetence.

The widespread repetition of such beliefs in proverbs, plays, doctors' writings, and philosophy makes one wonder why old people were not more common among the mentally disturbed in Napier's practice. Although in Gregory King's estimates for England in 1695 about one in five adults was over sixty, only 7.8% of the disturbed adults Napier treated were so old (Table 2.2). Very few of these patients suffered from the kind of mental decay that impatient children and pessimistic scientists declared to be the inevitable condition of old age. "Old Master John Booth," a kinsman of the future Lord Delamere, conceived a melancholy terror that the episodes of aphasia and amnesia he experienced would end in permanent oblivion: "Melancholy by a sudden frighting; feareth loss of memories and senses because that he hath been often taken therewith."[106] Goody Foukes (sixty-eight) and Mary Whitlock (seventy-two) uttered mad suspicions that they were bewitched, and Richard Dichmoc (eighty), Sir Paxall Broket (sixty-eight), and Old Lady Booth (eighty) raged like perfect Lears, wrangling with their children about the division of their goods. Even in these cases, however, Napier did not think that all these ancients suffered from irreversible senility. He predicted that two of the oldest and maddest among them would recover their wits before they died; and if he was not optimistic about the most hostile and vexing of them all, Old Lady Booth, perhaps that was because her faithless husband had long ago infected her with syphilis.[107] Napier himself was an old man when he treated these patients, and he may have been reluctant to believe that aging alone corroded the memory and sanity of people like himself, but his own prejudices cannot explain why so few elderly patients sought medical advice from him. The fact that people who were sixty years old or more are found among his physically ill patients only about half as often as one would expect from King's figures is important. The aged were obviously more often afflicted by life-threatening illnesses than adults in their prime. If they were sending to Great Linford for treatment at the same rate as their juniors did, the elderly physician would have had many more patients as old or older than himself.[108]

The favorite Elizabethan phrase that old age is but a second childhood seems ironically true. The elderly, like little children, were especially likely to perish from their sicknesses, and the sight of old men and women ill and dying must have been very familiar. The barbarous and debilitating medical routines that purged and bled the sick certainly cannot have helped most aged patients, and perhaps their maladies were regarded with the same resignation that parents felt when their infants fell ill. Even in a gerontocratic society, Keith Thomas has recently reminded us, the plight of old people too weak or poor to work was dire.[109] They were often as dependent economically as children and even less valued if the stories and sayings of the period echo common thought. A preacher named Thomas Granger declared in 1621: "Mothers and nurses have pleasure in infants, but old people are burdensome to all; neither their talk nor company is acceptable."[110] Some of the old people Napier treated struggled to avoid becoming dependent upon their children by retaining control of their estates, so that their hopeful heirs were forced to attend to their needs and wishes. The vexatious Lady Booth waged economic war against her family, especially her oldest son, to keep them from enjoying her riches or distributing them as they pleased: "Putteth her money out into other men's hands, lest [she] dying, her son should get the administration and get away all her money from her children. Careth not much for her own children, nor will trust them or have any about her."[111] It was not only the rich who played this game. Anthony and Alice Write were given a place in her father's house when they married in return for keeping Alice's idiot brother. But the old man could not endure the arrangement. He quarreled with his own wife and abused the children, declaring to his son-in-law that "he will [be] rid of him and his wife."[112] There were good reasons for old people's reluctance to relinquish control of their property. An elderly man or woman who had not reserved some part of his estate to himself had to rely upon his children's concern and willingness to pay all of his expenses, including the charges to obtain medical treatment. The fact that mortal sickness and mental decay were considered the natural companions of old age may have made the younger persons who controlled the purse reluctant to part with their money. Young people's familiarity with their elders' illnesses and low regard for their mental powers accounts more plausibly for the rarity of the aged in Napier's practice than

Table 2.3. *Marital status of Napier's mentally disturbed patients* (N = 2,039)

Sex	Single	Widow	Married	Remarried	Has child	Unknown
Male	133	13	116	2	22	462
Female	161	60	340	16	198	511
Unknown	0	0	0	0	0	5
Totals	294	73	456	18	220	978

the alternative speculation that they were proof against the afflictions of the mind.

Marital status

Marriage, according to modern students of mental disorder, is a paradise for husbands and a purgatory for wives. The highest rates of reported psychological illness in England and America are found among married women and single men, the lowest rates among married men and single women.[113] Most students of this phenomenon think that some combination of economic and social factors affecting the readiness of health services to brand women insane and the stress and limitations of family life adding to the anxiety and isolation of wives accounts for the preponderance of married women among the ranks of the mentally disturbed. As we shall see in a subsequent chapter, many of Napier's female patients blamed their psychological distress on marital problems, and popular works such as the homily on marriage admitted that women suffered from the tribulations of marriage more than men because they relinquished their liberty when they wed.[114] We would therefore expect that the distribution of marital status among Napier's disturbed patients would closely resemble the patterns found today.

Unfortunately, the astrologer was lax about recording his clients' marital status, and so no statistically significant figures can be tabulated from his notes. Even so, a glance at Table 2.3 shows that married women are the largest group of patients for whom we have evidence and that if the disturbed clients who were remarried or had children at the time of consultation are added to those wives, the number of female patients who were probably married swells to 554, 52% of the known marrieds and unmarrieds, 27% of the whole pool of disturbed clients. Husbands, verified and probable, account for only about half as many cases of disorder, 140, or 13%, of those for whom marital status can be determined and 7% of the whole group. There were also more men definitely known to have been single and widowed among the disturbed than there were married men. Even though information is lacking in so many cases, these figures are nevertheless consistent with the hypothesis that marriage had the same dolorous effects on the mental health of women in the seventeenth century as it has today.

Social status

Napier's patients were drawn from the entire range of the social hierarchy. Few were very rich; few were very poor. As his reputation grew, so did the numbers of his clients who were men and women of breeding and fashion, but even at the peak of his renown in aristocratic circles the bulk of his patients were still humble farmers and artisans. It is relatively easy to recapture the precise status of the aristocrats and gentry Napier treated and to list the occupations he recorded for some of his patients who were neither exalted nor rich. But the most complete and interesting picture of the role that social rank played in his practice can be sketched from the titles of honor he attached to his patients' names. When Napier paused to write down the appellation of status that his patient seemed to deserve, he was making a record of the social relationship between himself and his client. No historian who is interested in how social status affected the perception and management of mental disorder could ask for better evidence than the diagnostician's own record of the prestige of his clients. These judgments of social standing by a single man are more revealing than pedigrees and lists of occupations, because they were made in the context of assessing the nature of the client's problems. Class, as E. P. Thompson reminds us, is something that happens in human relationships, and to be understood fully, it must be "embodied in real people and in a real context."[115] That is precisely what Napier's records permit us to do.

Napier used three sets of titles to describe his judgment of his patients' status. He scrupulously referred to the aristocracy by their titles or called them Lord or Lady. He called a larger number of his clients Master or Mistress. These people included members of the local gentry, university graduates, fellow clergymen, merchants, and important local craftsmen – the kind of men and women whom the physician regarded as his social equals. He omitted titles of honor from the names of patients who were his social inferiors, calling them Goodman or Goody when he did not know their first names.[116] When one examines the occupations he sometimes recorded for these people it is plain that they comprised a cross section of the farming and artisanal community of the region. Farmers, servants, small craftsmen, and agricultural laborers were most common among these untitled folk (Table 2.4).

During the first dozen years that he practiced medicine, Napier treated his parishioners and the farmers, servants, and laborers from the surrounding countryside. His most prestigious clients were members of the local "parish gentry" – his friends the Uvedales and Blundells – and the troubled womenfolk of Sir John Manners and Sir Francis Fortescue, Buckinghamshire notables, and the wife of Sir Oliver Luke, a Bedfordshire M.P. The elevation of Robert Napier to the aristocracy as a baronet in 1612 and his insinuation into court circles transformed the relationships Napier had with his social superiors. During the middle of the second decade of the century he acquired a nucleus of noble patients from the Midlands who became his friends. He was an intimate of the young Sir Kenelm Digby and a familiar of the recusant clans in the area, the Digbys, Mordaunts, Dormers, and Treshams. Those whom he thought of as his neighbors now included especially the Tyrringhams and the Throckmortons, who had not noticed him before. Their enthusiasm and Sir Robert's connections brought still more esteemed personages to Great Linford: the Earl of Cleveland and his family, the Earl of Rutland's clan, and Sir Robert Spencer, the richest man in England. The Earl of Kent honored him with his friendship. Aristocratic swans came in flocks during the last fifteen years of Napier's life. He counted as his friends Sir Thomas Myddleton's family and the relatives of Thomas Egerton, Lord Ellesmere, into whose midst Sir Robert's children had married. He treated the Duke of Buckingham's brother and mother and consoled her melancholy husband, Thomas, Lord Compton. The Earl of Northampton, Dudley,

Table 2.4. *Occupations of Napier's patients*[a]

I: Disturbed patients

Servants 44 (27 women, 17 men)	Butcher
Apprentices 2	Mercers 3
Butlers 2	Tailors 2
Page	Candlemaker
Gentlewomen in waiting 2	Millers 2
Gardener	Draper
Fowler	Baker
Steward	Artisans 2[b]
Gamekeeper	Shopwife
Schoolmasters 3	Merchant
University dons 4	Husbandmen 7
University students 6	Shepherds 3
Clergy 13	Farmer
Lawyers 4	Laborers 6
Student at the Inns of Court	Woolwinder
Tilemaker	Beggars or "Poor" 7

II: Patients consulting Napier for all maladies in 1610 and 1620

Servants 104	Yeoman	Cooks 2
Retainers 2	Husbandmen 7	Baker
Attendants 2	Shepherds 4	Butcher
Woman in waiting	Laborers 3	Shoemakers 2
Butlers 2	Apprentice	Saddler
Coachmen 2	Millwright	Glover
Gameskeeper	Weavers 2	Parchment maker
Schoolmasters 2	Tailors 3	Soldier
Clergy 10	Carpenter	Ratcatcher
Lawyer	Mason	

---

[a]These lists contain only those occupations Napier recorded among the information that identified the patient. His notes imply that many of his female patients were occupied in the home and that many of his male clients farmed. I have not tried to tabulate these or other implicit occupational references.
[b]One of these artisans may have been a carpenter; about the other we know only that he was an apprentice and then set up his own shop.

Lord North, the Earl of Sunderland and his family, the Earl of Bedford and his wife, the scandalous Earl and Countess of Sussex, and Sir Walter Raleigh's widow (who had suffered "many griefs") all consulted him for their physical or mental afflictions.[117]

Although he became familiar with many of the important political and social figures of his day, Napier remained uniquely inde-

pendent. Unlike many other physicians he did not become a creature of the rich, a servant dependent upon their wealth and favor.
He continued to treat people of middling and humble means in
large numbers and preferred not to leave his home at Great Linford to attend the nobility personally. In 1610 and 1620 the number of peers and knights (including their wives) among his patients
accounted for just 2.7% and 1.9% of his clients, respectively (Table 2.5). The proportion of such nobility among the mentally disturbed never exceeded 5%. Indeed, if one examines the changing
proportions of disturbed patients whom Napier thought worthy
of titles of distinction, it becomes apparent that the only substan-
tial change during the years he practiced medicine was the gradual
expansion of the group he styled Master or Mistress. Between
1621 and 1635 they came to account for about 20% of his disturbed clients, so that in those later years about 75% of the disturbed people he treated were untitled.

In spite of his greater familiarity with gentlemen and gentlewomen, Napier's practice never became overburdened with noble
ladies and courtiers (Figures 2.1 and 2.2). His fees were comparatively small, typically about 12d. in the early years of the seventeenth century.[118] A consultation with him would have put a la-
borer out of pocket about one day's wages.[119] The smattering of
occupational labels he tagged to his clients show that many servants and humble artisans could pay his charges, and he no doubt
continued to forgive them for those who could not afford to pay.
Nevertheless, the knowledge that he charged a fee, any fee, must
have deterred some of the very poor in the area from seeking his
help. And there were plenty of impoverished laborers living
nearby. The forest villages of Northamptonshire filled up with the
human flotsam and jetsam set adrift by a late wave of enclosure in
the Midlands during the seventeenth century. A Digger broadside
that claimed there were 1,169 people on the dole in Wellingbor-
ough alone in 1650 must have exaggerated, but it is plain that the
problem of poverty was acute.[120] A meticulous scholar has discovered that in the late seventeenth century 44% of the inhabitants
of forest villages and 35% of non-forest villages in Northamptonshire were excused from the hearth tax.[121] Some of these people
would probably have been among the groups Napier treated – the
very small farmers and craftsmen – and he also counseled servants who would not have been among the taxable population.

Table 2.5. *Social status of Napier's disturbed patients by five-year periods*[a]

Title	1597–1600	1601–05	1606–10	1611–15	1616–20	1621–25
Peers and knights	0	3(1.8)	11(4.2)	4(2.1)	9(2.7)	11(3.4)
Mr. and Mrs.	9(12.5)	14(8.2)	30(11.5)	26(13.3)	57(17.3)	71(20.0)
No title	63(87.5)	154(90.0)	221(84.3)	165(84.6)	264(80.0)	272(76.6)
Totals	72(100.0)	171(100.0)	262(100.0)	195(100.0)	330(100.0)	354(100.0)

Title	1626–30	1631–35	1636–46	Unknown	Totals
Peers and knights	18(4.8)	6(2.2)	0	0	62(3.0)
Mr. and Mrs.	71(18.9)	53(19.7)	0	0	334(16.4)
No title	287(76.3)	210(78.1)	1	3	1,643(80.6)
Totals	376(100.0)	269(100.0)	1	3	2,039(100.0)

[a]Figures in parentheses are percentages.

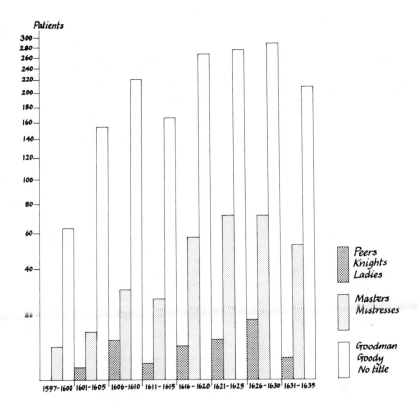

Figure 2.1   Social status of disturbed patients

The evidence suggests, but certainly does not prove, that perhaps a quarter or a third of the natives of the area were so poor that they rarely if ever could have sought his medical advice.

If the disturbed patients he ministered to were drawn largely from the upper two-thirds or three-quarters of the social hierarchy, which is plausible, then Napier's growing familiarity with people exalted enough to style themselves Master or Mistress does not signalize a large shift in the social composition of his practice. In the early seventeenth century there was a general inflation of honors as the crown hawked peerages and knighthoods and prosperous farmers bought their way into the gentry in increasing numbers. The explosive debate about this scramble for social prestige and its true dimensions, notwithstanding, one thing is clear: The area of Napier's practice is one of the places where the infla-

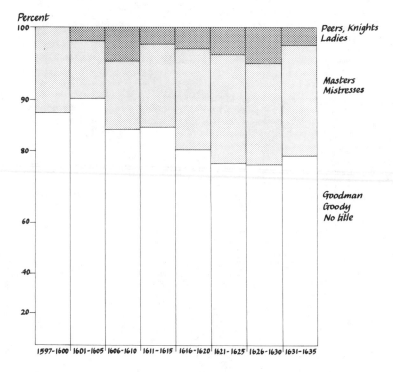

Figure 2.2   Social status of disturbed patients (percentages)

tion of honors and rise of the gentry really did exist. The Northamptonshire and Buckinghamshire elites were full of new
men.[122] The gentle expansion of the group of lesser gentry among
Napier's clients must reflect this wider social change as well as the
attitudes of the astrologer and his prospective patients. All of this
strongly suggests, but (again) does not prove, that Napier's mad
and troubled clients represent a faithful cross section of the social
composition of the top two-thirds or so of rural society and that
throughout the four decades that he practiced medicine his services were available to all save for an indigent minority.

The geography of desperation

A map showing the homes of mental patients who consulted Napier is a static and two-dimensional sketch of a dynamic movement too complex to be captured by that means. Such a map represents choices and opportunities, obstacles and compulsions. The

motives of the living people represented on it merely as points, parishes, hundreds or counties, cannot be reconstructed with certainty. Nor are the changes in their collective mentality – the reputation of the physician in the minds of his potential clients – easily displayed. But by studying the distribution of Napier's disturbed patients among the settlements in the region and by finding out what is at present known about the communities they came from, we can make some informed speculations about the effects of geography, reputation, and competition on medical practice and gain some tentative insights into the ecology of insanity and misery.

Modern studies of the epidemiology and ecology of mental disorders are perplexing. Ecological studies in particular seem to be sapped of most of their significance by a persistent failure to agree on the definition of the maladies and variables they seek to explain. The idea that underlies most investigations is that communities that are hostile, divided, poor, squalid, ridden with disease, and highly mobile should make more people mad than communities that are harmonious, cohesive, prosperous, clean, healthy, and stable. Amazingly, it seems that nobody has been able to prove that this assumption is valid or even to explain convincingly the data that seem to support it.[123] Given the imprecision of Napier's diagnostic methods and the scanty evidence available about actual conditions in the villages near his home at Great Linford, this study naturally cannot succeed where able social scientists working with modern data have failed. What it can and does try to do is suggest how the factors of geography, population distribution, and reputation affected Napier's clientele, to demonstrate that mental anguish was widespread and known even in the tiniest hamlets, and to speculate about how the impact of economic change and religious strife might have made some communities particularly dolorous places to live.

The distribution of the homes of Napier's mad and anxious patients reveals more about the availability and attractiveness of his services than it does about how social conditions affected mental health. Napier seldom attended his clients, and the chief considerations that appear to have determined how many people resorted to him from a particular village were the length of the journey to Great Linford, the size of the community from which the patient came, and its proximity to a major thoroughfare. When one maps the settlements his clients lived in over time, one can display the effect his expanding reputation had on his practice and locate communities that had a special tie to this healer because of his friendship with their leading families.

The number of disturbed patients Napier treated was inversely proportional to the distance they had to travel to reach his home. Great Linford is near the tip of a projection of northern Buckinghamshire that is bordered on the north and west by Northamptonshire and on the northeast and east by Bedfordshire. Nearly 80% of mentally disturbed patients were from these three counties: 37.5% of all locatable cases were from Buckinghamshire, 21.2% from Bedfordshire, and 19.4% from Northamptonshire (Map 1).[124] The dispersion of cases in the hundreds of these counties illustrates the significance of distance even more plainly (Map 2). Patients in almost one-fourth of all the cases of mental disorder came from the hundred in which Great Linford was, Newport Hundred. The neighboring hundreds also contributed heavily to the population of disturbed patients. Over 60% of them lived in the eighteen hundreds within a fifteen-mile radius of Napier's village; and over 50% were from hundreds within ten miles of his home.[125] And even within these hundreds, patients tended to come from the nearest villages. Just over 20% lived in villages fewer than five miles from Great Linford. Beyond that radius, towns contributing 10 or more disturbed patients to the practice lay along the main roads or had easy access to them (Map 3). These towns included Ivinghoe and Wing in Buckinghamshire; Cranfield, Kempston, Bedford, Stagsden, Turvey, Dunstable, Bolnhurst, and Luton in Bedfordshire; and Cogenhoe and Higham Ferrers in Northamptonshire.

Travel was not easy during the seventeenth century, and the distribution of disturbed patients spread out beyond the immediate area along the main roads and waterways. Great Linford was near the intersection of Watling Street and the Oxford-to-Cambridge road. Small numbers of patients journeyed up Watling Street from Hertfordshire and London to consult Napier, and others traveled to him from Oxfordshire and Cambridgeshire and up the river Ouse from Huntingshire: About 17% of his disturbed patients came from those counties (Table 2.6). Very few lived in more distant shires: 19 were from Warwickshire, 15 from

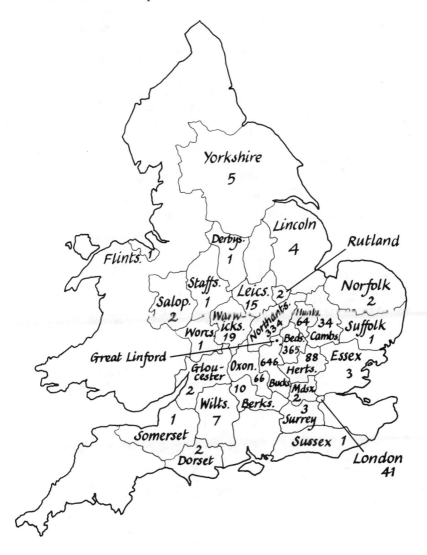

Map 1   Home counties of Napier's disturbed patients

Leicestershire, and 10 from Berkshire. The rest of England contributed only 41 cases, just over 2% of the total.

Besides the ease with which patients could travel to Napier's
home, the most important factor in determining how many disturbed persons consulted Napier from a particular village was its
size. When Buckinghamshire and Bedfordshire parishes are

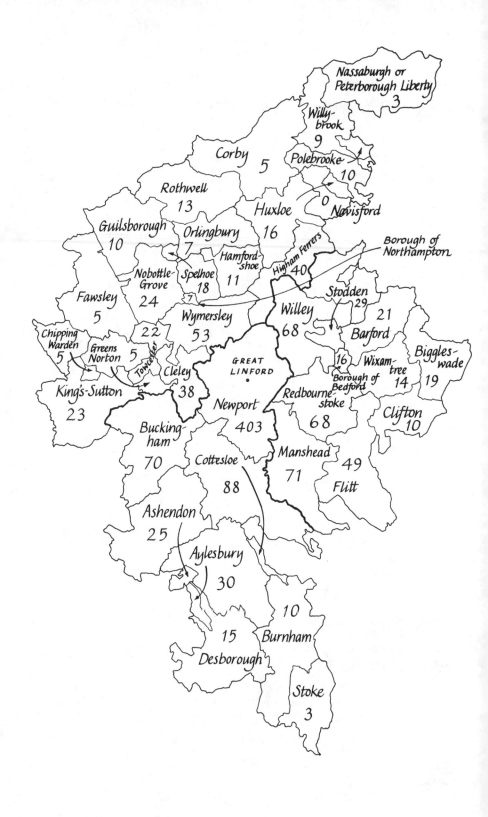

Nassaburgh or
Peterborough Liberty
3

Willy-
brook
9

Corby
5

Polebrooke
10

Rothwell
13

Huxloe
16

Navisford
0

Guilsborough
10

Orlingbury
7

Hamford-
shoe

Higham Ferrers
40

Borough of
Northampton

Nobottle-
Grove
24

Spelhoe
18

11

7

Stodden
29

21

Fawsley
5

Wymersley
53

Willey
68

Barford

Chipping
Warden
5

Greens
Norton

22

Towcester

5

Cleley
38

GREAT
LINFORD

16

Wixam-
tree
14

Borough of
Bedford

Biggles-
wade
19

King's-Sutton
23

Newport
403

Redbourne-
stoke
68

Clifton
10

Bucking-
ham
70

Cottesloe
88

Manshead
71

49

Flitt

Ashendon
25

Aylesbury
30

10

15

Burnham

Desborough

Stoke
3

ranked according to the number of communicants in them in 1603 (the best guide to relative population readily available), it is easy to see that there is a strong association between a village's size and the number of patients it supplied (Table 2.7). No Northamptonshire village produced many cases of disorder in this practice: Only four settlements supplied 10 cases or more. Two sets of rapidly expanding forest villages, which had fused into single settlements, Passenham and Densanger and Potterspury and Yardley Gobion, produced 12 and 11 cases.[126] A busy little market town, Higham Ferrers, was the source of 10 cases of disorder; and the tiny town of Cogenhoe, whose population ranged from 150 to 187 between 1616 and 1628, also supplied 10 cases.[127]

The knowledge that help was available was obviously another factor affecting the number of patients who consulted Napier. As his reputation grew, so did the size of his practice and the distance his clients traveled to reach him; and this is reflected in the dispersion of mentally disturbed patients. The number of persons he treated for mental disorder yearly rose from an average of about 38 during the decade from 1600 to 1609, to about 53 during the next decade, to about 76 during the twenties, and finally to about 81 during the first years of the thirties (Maps 4 and 5).[128] As one can see in Figure 2.3, this growth in the number of mentally disturbed patients was very closely tied to the expansion of the practice as a whole, especially after 1614.[129] The proportion of the disturbed who came from homes beyond the three principal counties in the practice also increased: Between 1601 and 1610 1 out of 5 cases was from an outlying county; by the 1620s one-third of them were.

Napier had special connections with the leading families of some towns, and the rather numerous cases of disorder that they produced probably reflects the confidence they had in him. Gayhurst and Wing in Buckinghamshire were tiny settlements, but patients suffering from 15 and 10 cases of mental disorder, respectively, lived in them. Gayhurst was the home of the Digbys, a prominent recusant family whose most dashing member, Sir Kenelm Digby, received instruction on astrology and alchemy from Napier. Wing was dominated by the Dormers, who often

Map 2 Disturbed patients from hundreds in Buckinghamshire, Bedfordshire, and Northamptonshire

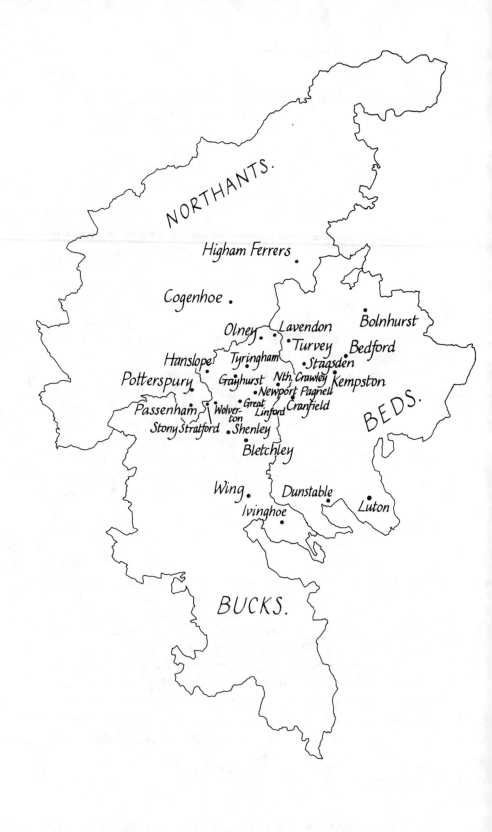

NORTHANTS.

Higham Ferrers •

Cogenhoe •

Olney • Lavendon • • Bolnhurst

Hanslope • Tyringham • Turvey Bedford

Potterspury • Gayhurst • Nth. Crawley • Kempston
Stagsden •
Passenham • Newport Pagnell
Wolver- • Great • Cranfield
ton Linford
Stony Stratford • Shenley

BEDS.

Bletchley

Wing • Dunstable

Ivinghoe • Luton •

BUCKS.

sought his advice about medical and astrological matters. Both families seem to have encouraged their servants and dependents to consult him as well. Twenty-two disturbed clients came from Luton, a Bedfordshire village seventeen miles from Great Linford. Napier's brother, Sir Robert, had his country home there, and messengers shuttled back and forth between the two places regularly.[130]

The number of psychiatrically disturbed patients from a particular village who consulted Napier was therefore largely determined by factors affecting all of the patients in the practice: the ease with which they could reach Great Linford, the number of potential clients in the village, and knowledge of Napier's reputation. In a few instances, however, social and intellectual factors may have increased the number of villagers who suffered from mental disorders. The tempo of economic change was very brisk in Napier's region. London grew even more rapacious during the seventeenth century, and grain farming, beef and sheep raising, and the transportation and marketing networks became more specialized. Two kinds of geographical mobility were stimulated by these developments: the ordinary movements of men engaged in trade and the extraordinary displacement of villagers squeezed out by enclosure.[131] Stony Stratford and Fenny Stratford were local centers of marketing and transport, and they had large populations of transients. Twenty-eight and thirty cases of mental disorder originated in them. Both were important stops along Watling Street, a main avenue between the counties of the Northwest and Midlands and the London market; and both appear to have had similar social characters and problems. Plague, a disease that followed poverty and overcrowding, struck hard at both towns during the earlier seventeenth century, and this suggests the possibility that commercial bustle had created in both villages slum conditions usually associated with much larger cities.[132]

Enclosure was a more serious threat to psychological security, because it inevitably displaced some people and angered others unable to find cheap leases. Midlands farmers responded to stagnating grain prices in the seventeenth century by enclosing their lands to facilitate convertible husbandry, and Northamptonshire and northern Buckinghamshire were among the areas most dra-

Map 3 Villages producing ten or more mentally disturbed patients

Table 2.6. *Geographical origins of Napier's mentally disturbed patients (N = 2,039)*

County	1597–1600	1601–05	1606–10	1611–15	1616–20	1621–25	1626–30	1631–42	Totals
Buckinghamshire	42	80	104	85	108	83	93	51	646
Bedfordshire	6	40	56	36	72	61	56	38	365
Northamptonshire	6	23	32	22	57	73	68	53	334
Hertfordshire	0	5	9	7	19	16	16	16	88
Oxfordshire	1	2	3	7	10	20	17	6	66
Huntingdonshire	0	2	4	9	7	15	10	17	64
London	1	3	7	0	4	9	7	10	41
Cambridgeshire	0	1	3	1	1	6	11	11	34
Warwickshire	0	0	1	0	1	4	6	7	19
Leicestershire	0	0	1	0	1	3	5	5	15
Berkshire	0	0	0	0	4	3	1	2	10
Wiltshire	0	0	2	0	0	2	1	2	7
Yorkshire	0	0	0	0	0	1	2	2	5
Other counties	1	1	2	0	3	4	10	8	29
Unknown/not locatable	15	14	38	29	42	57	73	48	316
Totals	72	171	262	196	329	357	376	276	2,039

Note: Counties contributing fewer than 5 cases of mental disorder to Napier's practice include Lincolnshire, 4; Essex, Surrey, 3; Rutland, Dorset, Gloucester, Norfolk, Shropshire, Middlesex, 2; Somerset, Derby, Flintshire, Staffordshire, Sussex, Suffolk, Worcestershire, 1.

Table 2.7. Parishes producing ten or more cases of mental disorder

Buckinghamshire		Bedfordshire	
Ranked by number of communicants, 1603	Ranked by cases of mental disorder	Ranked by number of communicants, 1603	Ranked by cases of mental disorder
Newport Pagnell (806)	Newport Pagnell (58)	Luton (1,200)	Luton (22)
Ivinghoe (563)	Hanslope (30)	Bedford (1,033)	Kempston (18)
Stony Stratford (540)	Fenny Stratford/Bletchley (29)	Dunstable (est. 500)	Dunstable (17)
Onley (525)	Stony Stratford (28)	Kempston (454)	Bedford (16)
Hanslope (500)[a]	Great Linford (28)	Turvey (140)	Turvey (12)
Fenny Stratford/Bletchley (462)[b]	North Crawley (19)	Stagsden (140)	Stagsden (11)
Wing (421)	Shenley (15)	Bolnhurst (120)	Bolnhurst (10)
North Crawley (290)	Woulverton (15)	Cranfield (50)	Cranfield (10)
Shenley (260)	Gayhurst (15)		
Grant Linford (220)	Olney (13)		
Woulverton (120)	Ivinghoe (12)		
Tyrringham (110)	Tyrringham (12)		
Lavendon (99)	Lavendon (11)		
Gayhurst (71)	Wing (10)		

[a]Includes Castle Thorpe.   [b]Includes Simpson, Water Eaton.
Source for number of communicants: "Liber Cleri, A.D. 1603," in C. W. Foster, ed., The State of the Church in the Reigns of Elizabeth and James I (Lincoln Record Society, 23, 1926), pp. 253–75.

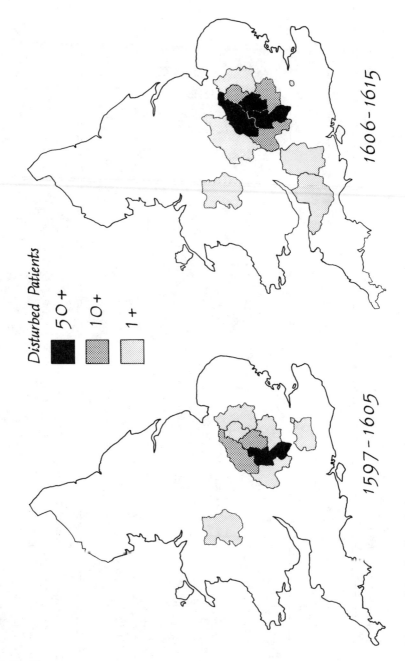

Disturbed Patients

50+

10+

1+

1606-1615

1597-1605

Map 4   Growth of Napier's practice, 1597-1615

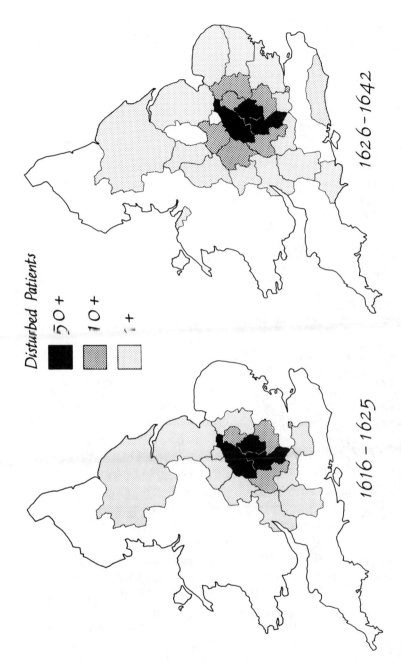

Disturbed Patients

50 +

10 +

1 +

1626 – 1642

1616 – 1625

Map 5 Growth of Napier's practice, 1616–1642

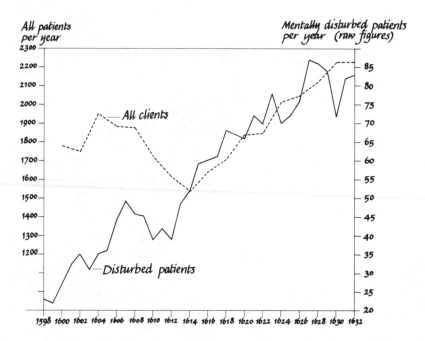

Figure 2.3   Estimated case loads in Napier's practice (three-year moving averages)

matically affected by these changes.[133] The laboring population
was redistributed; the open villages of the Northamptonshire forests expanded rapidly.[134] The revolt of 1607 and a barrage of pamphlets in the 1650s are evidence of the anger and distress enclosure
caused in the region.[135] In spite of the collective hostility enclosing
landlords aroused among the tenants in the region, very few of
Napier's clients blamed their anxieties on poor relationships with
their landlords. One of them was certainly a victim of the capital-
ist spirit, and at the hands of a Puritan gentleman at that. Edward
Iust told Napier that he felt "much sorrow and grief, for that the
Lord Russell hath taken his lease from him and let it to another for
more money.[136] Alice Stonell's parents received pitiless treatment.
Their landlord dispossessed the old couple, probably because their
tenure had expired: "Her landlord did turn her old father and
mother of ninety years old apiece out of their house; and this old
man goeth to plough and was never sick in his life."[137] Even when
landlords behaved ruthlessly, however, they were not always hostile or indifferent toward their tenants. Explaining the cause of

Robert Deanes's distress, Napier wrote: "Hath a copyhold, but his landlord, although he love him exceedingly well, yet will not let him change young people's lives for the older" to extend his tenure.[138] Too few people complained to Napier about their landlords to show how the social and economic changes in the region may have altered the blend of self-interest and paternalism that typified landlords' attitudes. The immediate problem for people who lost their holdings was to find a new place to live and work, and few of them paused for medical treatment and consolation, even if they could afford it. Many families seem to have immigrated to the nearby forest villages. These settlements did produce more than their share of mentally disturbed patients in Napier's practice, but because they were larger than non-forest villages, it would be rash to conclude that economic changes and dislocation were responsible. Nevertheless, it is possible that there was a connection.[139]

The traditional hazards of economic life caused a great deal of reported distress among Napier's patients. Of the 767 disturbed people who described their problems to him, 99 complained about economic misfortunes. More than half of them were troubled by losses or indebtedness that threatened to plunge them into ruin. Debt was by far the greatest single source of anxiety. John Sceavington, for example, was so "crossed with debts that it broke his wits and senses," and Robert Bell grew mopish and fearful, lamenting "that they will take away his goods and he shall be undone."[140] Everyone of any substance in Tudor and Stuart England was in debt. The pages of Napier's casebooks record small, interest-free loans to hundreds of his neighbors; probate inventories show that it was not unusual for people to be creditors and debtors simultaneously.[141] English villages were bound together by bewilderingly complex networks of credit and debt. In economic terms, people lent money because there were no banks, and it was safer to lend cash than to hoard it. The borrower had to return the money on an agreed date or lose his security. People borrowed to meet their need for cash between harvests or when their rents were due. In social terms, villagers lent because it strengthened their relations with their kinsmen and neighbors. As Alan Everitt has remarked, credit was essentially personal, a tangible manifestation of one's standing in his community, and to build credit one extended loans to other people when they needed them. This fusion of economic and personal advantages helps to explain why villagers who could not repay their debts were so anxious. A ruined reputation was not just an economic catastrophe, it was also a social disaster.[142] We shall see in the next chapter that the bonds between ordinary men and women and people outside the circle of the nuclear family were loose, but important. Bad debts threatened to break those ties. People were understandably dismayed when their failure to fulfill their responsibilities became public knowledge. Thus John Holman was grieved by his neighbor's mere threat to sue him, and Samuel Houston suffered a nervous collapse when his creditors came and drove his cattle away.[143] Blanche Bonfield complained that because her brother had not repaid 20s. he owed, her husband had been arrested for failure to satisfy his own creditors.[144] Some people rushed headlong into ruin; others met it unexpectedly. A man who overreached himself by taking on too much land or gambling his substance in buying and selling had only himself to blame. But the most common sources of economic misfortune were beyond anybody's control. Napier's clients fell into debt because of animal diseases, fires, sickness, and the deaths of their husbands or fathers.[145] Keith Thomas has emphasized that Englishmen were extremely vulnerable to the hazards of the environment in the seventeenth century, because there were few well-developed social and economic institutions to help them when misfortune struck, and that many people sought solace in religion and magical practices.[146] The evidence in Napier's practice books suggests that he is right.

Sociologists, at least since Durkheim, have thought that religiously united communities produce less harmful deviance – suicide, crime, insanity – than divided or secularized communities.[147] But the fact that a religious group is obviously a social rather than a geographical entity (two or more strongly integrated congregations could exist in one town) makes it difficult to measure the significance of religion spatially. Religious divisiveness and its complement, political competition, were the most important problems of the seventeenth century in the eyes of contemporaries, and religious issues moved men to extremes of passion. Several villages that produced numerous cases of mental disorder contained Puritan or Catholic recusants. Puritans were very active in Stony Stratford, Hanslope, Sherington, Newport Pagnell, and Ivinghoe in Buckinghamshire, the last being "something of a cen-

ter of Brownist activity."[148] Dunstable was among the Bedfordshire towns with a Puritan lectureship.[149] Puritans from several
Northamptonshire villages came to the attention of zealous authorities: These included Northampton, Daventry, Oundle,
Rothwell, Brackley, Towcester, Denford, Cogenhoe, and
Higham Ferrers.[150] Cogenhoe and Higham Ferrers are interesting.
Both of them were small, Cogenhoe very small, but each produced 10 cases of disorder. Cogenhoe had a Puritan rector around
the turn of the century, but by 1640 a Laudian had been placed in
his stead and there is reason to believe that the town was divided
religiously. The 1640 election at Higham Ferrers revealed that the
town's leading citizens were split into politically competitive
camps, one definitely Laudian, the other probably Puritan.[151]

Many of Napier's aristocratic clients were Catholics. The Mordaunts, the Digbys, and the Dormers consulted him often and
their home villages, Turvey, Gayhurst, and Wing, supplied more
troubled patients than one might have expected, gauging their distance from Great Linford and their sizes.[152] It was surely Napier's
friendships with these families that brought their troubled neighbors to his consulting room, not anxiety about religious schism.
Gayhurst indeed was so tiny that it is hard to believe that any of its
seventy or so adult inhabitants failed to embrace their master's
creed, and yet it dispatched 15 disturbed men and women to the
astrologer during his years of practice. The mere existence of religious diversity in the parishes in Napier's region does matter,
however, even though no satisfying links can be made between
hotbeds of doctrinal strife and rampant mental disease. As we shall
see in a later chapter, religious imagery suffused ordinary people's
ideas about their feelings and urges, and many of them were
deeply fearful about sin and damnation. Religious controversy amplified and transformed contemporary interpretations of anxiety
and despair, and it is plain that this was an area in which villagers
were exposed to the full range of competing beliefs, from recu-
sancy to separatism.

The most significant feature of the geographical distribution of
Napier's mentally disturbed patients is their dispersion. The vast
majority of the villages surrounding Great Linford must have produced at least a few cases of mental disorder during the earlier
seventeenth century. Napier treated disturbed clients from 291 of
the 493 settlements in hundreds within fifteen miles of Great Lin-

ford. In other words, about 60% of the villages within a long day's walk of Napier's home produced a case of mental disorder in his practice. There were certainly many more cases of mental disturbance in the region than those that he treated. Some must not have sought medical care at all, turning to clergymen or local wizards for help. Even among physicians, competition in the area was keen. During the first four decades of the century there were fifteen licensed practitioners in Northamptonshire, eleven in Bedfordshire, and twelve in Buckinghamshire, not counting Napier and the assistants whom he trained to practice medicine.[153] The effects of competition for disturbed patients can be seen in the distribution of Napier's patients: He treated just 7 cases from the large, nearby town of Northampton, and we know that there were three physicians licensed to practice there at the same time. One of them was John Cotta, whose books about quacks and witches were contrived as oblique attacks on Napier, according to William Lilly.[154]

The sprawling dispersion of cases of mental disorder in Napier's practice is important because it shows that such afflictions were an ordinary feature of rural life. No sort of community was entirely free from psychiatric disorder: Napier treated disturbed patients from large towns and small hamlets, from enclosed and unenclosed villages, from forest and non-forest settlements, from marketing centers and clusters of cottages too small to have been actual villages. Rural areas today apparently produce just as much mental disturbance as cities, despite intuitions to the contrary.[155] Still, the crude notion persists that agrarian preindustrial communities were safe and secure, their inhabitants relatively free from stress and anxiety. The evidence from Napier's practice shows that if such communities ever actually existed, they were certainly absent from the English countryside in the early seventeenth century.

One other effect of the widespread dispersion of mental disorder is important. Because insanity and emotional distress were regular features of village life, many villagers had the opportunity to observe the behavior of lunatics and learn about emotional instability firsthand. Sociologists have pointed out that laymen are the first to recognize mental disorder, and this was certainly true in Napier's practice. Some of his patients, for instance, did not consult him personally but were represented by members of their families or by friends. To decide that somebody was mad or emotionally disturbed, laymen had to know what these conditions were like. They learned the stereotypes of thought and action that defined these conditions from literature, drama, reports of notorious cases, firsthand observation, and the oral tradition of proverbs and commonplaces. The examination in the following chapters of these stereotypes and the ways they were used to recognize mental disorder will give us some insights into contemporary ideas about the limits of normal thought and action.[156]

3

Stress, anxiety, and family life

MISFORTUNE AND MENTAL DISORDER

Material life has improved vastly since the Middle Ages. Modern industrial societies offer ordinary men and women far more freedom to pursue the kinds of work and play that make them comfortable and amused than medieval peasants enjoyed. And yet many people are unhappy, and intellectuals frequently wonder if our ancestors were not more contented when technology, economic institutions, and social structures were simpler and more personal. Our media agree: The turbulence and complexity of modern life are ruining our health, dividing generations, shattering marriages, and destroying our serenity. Some eminent historians and social scientists are persuaded that the psychological environment of Western Europe deteriorated during the sixteenth and seventeenth centuries. They have called attention to macabre events and tormented individuals, arguing that these are tokens of social stress.[1] English historians have examined witchcraft, the proliferation of bastards, suicides and criminals, the outbreaks of riot and rebellion during the period; and they have attempted to connect them with the profound social and intellectual changes England experienced.[2] In this chapter I shall discuss the psychological environment from a different point of view. Instead of asking how much misery and alienation Shakespeare's contemporaries endured, I shall examine the problems that ordinary men and women believed to be causes of anxiety and insanity.

Seventeenth-century people were as convinced as we are that social and psychological stress disturbed the minds and corroded the health of its victims. A contemporary proverb proclaimed that "oppression makes the wise man mad,"[3] and writers of all kinds warned that fear and grief, especially when they were sudden and intense, sometimes caused madness and even death. Doctors, astrologers, preachers, and philosophers drew up almost identical lists of commonplace misfortunes that imperiled the sanity of ordinary people. The physician and demonologist William Drage printed this catalogue of typical disturbing experiences: "Sadness, fears, and scares, jealousy, discontents betwixt man and wife (the most lacerating of all grief), . . . loss of love, and disappointment in a marriage, destiny of friends and loss of estates."[4] (Drage, incidentally, was using the word *friends* in its seventeenth-century sense to mean members of one's immediate family and important well-wishers, rather than one's comrades.) The conventional warnings of popular writers like Drage precisely echoed the sentiments of autobiographers and of Napier's mentally disturbed patients. Over 800 of the troubled people Napier treated had suffered some terrifying or distressing experience. The astrologer briefly described the stresses reported by his clients and their relatives in 767 cases, and when these short tales are assembled into groups with common themes, they illustrate the everyday anxieties of villagers of middling and humble status. Frustration is the mirror of expectation. If we can make out the most familiar sources of anxiety and gloom these ordinary men and women complained about, then we shall be able to glimpse an image of the satisfactions they experienced and to explore a part of the emotional lives of those whose thoughts are normally obscured by the darkness of illiteracy.

Neither the patients who endured unbearable stresses nor their experiences were bizarre or unusual. As a social group these men and women were very like the rest of Napier's mentally disturbed clients, except that the group contained even more women than the larger category of which it was a part. People of every social rank reported stressful experiences, and their distribution along the spectrum of status closely matches the ranks of Napier's other patients, both those physically and mentally ill. The vast majority of them, more than four out of five, were too mean to warrant a title but too respectable to be classed as paupers (Table 3.1).

Women outnumbered men among the ranks of distressed patients by a ratio of almost 2:1. Of the 767 cases, 503 involved women, 263 concerned men, and the sex of one patient could not be determined from the case notes. Translating these figures into the same sort of sex ratios that we calculated in the last chapter,

Table 3.1. *Social status of patients reporting stress (in percent)*

Social rank	Stressed (N = 767)	Disturbed (N = 2,039)	1610[a] (N = 1,313)	1620[a] (N = 1,365)
Peers and knights	2.5	3.0	2.7	1.9
Mr. and Mrs.	16.0	16.4	14.6	21.2
No title	81.5	80.6	82.7	76.9
Totals	100.0	100.0	100.0	100.0

[a]Calculations include all patients, regardless of the nature of their illness.

one finds that the sex ratio among distressed patients was 52.3. That is a very low figure, lower than the ratio among all mentally disturbed patients (about 58), lower than the ratio among all of Napier's clients (about 70 or 80), and lower than the lowest ratios estimated for seventeenth-century cities.[5]

The part that psychological stress plays in causing mental and physical disorders is disputed, but it is evident that the difference between disturbed people and mentally robust ones lies not in their experiences but in their reactions to them. Most stressful events are everyday disasters, experienced by the sane and insane alike. Here are the examples one psychologist gives: "bereavement, imprisonment, or life-threatening illness."[6] The frustrations that troubled Napier's humble clients reflect the expectations of ordinary men and women, but they naturally tell us more about the vexations endured by wives and daughters than about the difficulties of husbands and sons. They show again the anguish that morbid and incurable gynecological maladies and obstetrical disasters inflicted on women. One need only recall the protracted sufferings of Samuel Pepys's wife to imagine how women's maladies could interfere with the social and sexual satisfactions of everyday life.[7] But the most common stresses Napier's clients experienced were conflicts with their families, lovers, and neighbors, the loss of their loved ones slain by disease, and fear of poverty and want. Even these social frustrations caused women more psychological illness than their husbands reported, probably because patriarchal customs and values prevented them from taking direct action to remedy intolerable situations and made the widow's lot especially dire. Thomas Wright attributed the emotionality of

Table 3.2. *The four most common categories of stress reported by Napier's patients (N = 767)*

	Males	Females	Totals	%
Troubled courtships	63	118	181	23.6
Marital problems	21	114	135	17.6
Bereavements	22	112	134	17.5
Economic problems	48	50	99[a]	12.9

[a] The sex of one patient could not be determined.

women to their "unableness to resist adversities or any other injury offered," and this explanation for their inclination to mercy and pity is also the best explanation for vulnerability to anxiety and gloom.[8]

The complaints described in Napier's brief notes can be divided into commonly repeated tales. Love and marriage, death and money are their principal themes, and the events themselves are usually unremarkable. The most familiar problems may be paralleled with stories found in diaries, drama, sermons, and treatises, and were also cited to explain the illnesses of people who were psychologically robust. The kinds of situations Napier's distressed clients described most often are shown in Table 3.2. Because most of Napier's clients were neither very rich nor very poor, their complaints are a good guide to the stresses ordinary people experienced; because most of them were wives and daughters, their problems illuminate especially vividly the significance of the family in their lives.

THE EMOTIONAL SIGNIFICANCE OF THE FAMILY

Many social historians believe that the physical environment of preindustrial England was so dangerous that it inhibited the formation of close emotional ties between family members, even though households were normally small, containing a married couple and their young children, servants and apprentices if the family was rich enough to afford them and elderly parents if they were too old to work and live by themselves.[9] Contemporaries were keenly aware of the perils of emotional intimacy; life's fragility was a favorite theme for writers and preachers. Elaborating on verses from the Bible, Thomas Becon wrote: "'All flesh is grass and, all the glory thereof is as the flower of the field. The grass is withered, the flower falleth away: even so is the people as grass, when the breath of the Lord bloweth upon them.' Thus we see the misery, vanity, and shortness of our mortal time painted out before our eyes; and that these things are true daily experience proveth."[10] Books like Becon's, which were meant to help the sick endure their afflictions piously and to prepare themselves for death, were a staple product in the book trade of the sixteenth and seventeenth centuries. Their message was common wisdom methodized; the familiar danger of dying suddenly of diseases and injuries that physicians were helpless to cure was palliated with theology and piety. A Cambridgeshire yeoman invoked the same theme in the preamble to his will, written in 1649: "Considering the frailty of this life, although there is nothing more certain than death, yet there is nothing more uncertain than the time of the coming thereof."[11] Diarists and astrologers' clients reported terrifying accidents and wonderful recoveries with the same astonished piety that marked their medieval ancestors' accounts of healing miracles. Godly Protestants fastened on to the popular awareness of death's imminence, and they taught converts to consider narrow escapes as tokens of God's providential care.[12]

The pious did not exaggerate the dangers they experienced or witnessed; they sought merely to find some comfort in the everyday spectacle of accident and disease, which slaughtered indiscriminately the good and the evil, the loved and the hated, intimates and strangers.[13] Seventeenth-century Englishmen were death's familiars, for epidemics, consumption, parasites and dysentery, accidents, infections, and botched childbirths killed children and adults, family and friends, earlier and more suddenly than the diseases we dread today. Everybody had seen someone die; villagers young and old attended the last illnesses and deaths of relatives and neighbors. Most people died of infectious diseases: consumption, fevers, and contagions, illnesses that killed suddenly and whose victims might be any age.[14] Here are the misfortunes of one of Napier's clients, William Stoe: "Much grief from time to time. Had a wife long sick who died after much physic. Lost much cattle which died. Had the plague in his house; two children died [and he] himself had it . . . Never well since."[15]

Clergymen and physicians cautioned against excessive mourning, and even advised their congregations and clients to moderate their affection for their intimates to protect themselves against unbearable pain when they perished. Richard Baxter returned to this topic several times, always stressing that excessive grief was the harvest of excessive affection.[16] A minister warned Adam Martindale to moderate his affection for his eight-year-old son with the pessimistic observation that the boy was "too forward to live."[17] When Thomas Fuller depicted the ideal widow, he drew a portrait of restrained sorrow:

The good widow . . . is a woman whose head hath been quite cut off, and yet she still liveth . . . Her grief for her husband, though real, is moderate. Excessive was the sorrow of King Richard the Second, beseeming him neither as a king, man or Christian . . . But our widow's sorrow is no storm, but a still rain. Indeed some foolishly discharge a surplusage of their passions on themselves tearing their hair, so that their friends coming to the funeral know not which most to bemoan, the dead husband, or the dying widow. Yet commonly it comes to pass, that such widows' grief is quickly emptied, which streameth out at so large a rent; whilst their tears that drop will hold running a long time.[18]

Napier's remarks about one of his clients echo the same theme: "Much grief for the death of two children . . . Not altogether so much for the latter as for the first, but too much."[19]

What was familiar was not always easily borne, and in spite of the awful risk of disappointment and the caution of clergymen, many men and women formed intimate attachments and were inconsolable when their loved ones died. Bereavement was a common explanation for madness and despair, and the sufferings of the survivors reveal something of the intensity of the emotional bonds within the family. Robert Burton insisted that although the extrinsic causes of melancholy were "so numerous that they seem to multiply as they are discovered, . . . loss and death of friends may challenge a first place." Nobody, not even the most stolid soul, could endure the death of a father, a husband, a son, a mother, a wife, a daughter without a fit of grieving madness.[20] The stories Napier's patients and their worried relatives told him reflect the same belief that the loss of family members was so hard to bear that it made some people insane. Bereavement was the third most common stress revealed to him; it is mentioned in

Table 3.3. *Bereavement (N = 767)*

Patients	Males	Females	Totals
Deaths of			
child	7	51	58
parent	4	18	22
spouse	9	33	42
others	4	15	19
Totals[a]	22	112	134

[a] Patients who lost loved ones in more than one category are counted only once in the totals.

17.5% of the cases occasioned by a personal problem. Its victims grieved for their dead parents, children, husbands and wives; only 19 of the 134 people disturbed by grief mourned the death of a more distant relation, and nobody's anguish was explained as the consequence of the passing of a companion or neighbor (Table 3.3).

The concern Napier's clients expressed about their loved ones' illnesses shows the same intense attachment to members of their immediate families, the same emotional remoteness from distant kin and neighbors. Most of his clients were naturally frightened by their own diseases, but such fears were seldom unusual enough to be counted as a cause of mental disorder. Among those, however, whose anxieties were acutely noticeable, 54 were terrified that they would die themselves, 11 were upset because their spouses were ill, 9 worried about sick children, and 6 were concerned about other relatives and friends. A more ample measure of apprehension about the illnesses of intimates is the identity of the messengers who consulted Napier on behalf of men and women who were too sick to come to Great Linford themselves. Three out of four of these concerned people were the parents, spouses, siblings, or children of the afflicted person; just 4% were other relatives, and 19% were apparently unrelated to the sufferer (Table 3.4).

Ordinary men and women responded to danger and death in different ways. Some faced peril and loss coolly and fatalistically, fulfilling the preachers' advice to spurn worldy attachments;

Table 3.4. *Relationships of intermediaries to mentally disturbed patients (N = 198)*

	Relationships	%	Totals	%
Immediate family			152	76.8
Parents	56	28.3		
Spouses	48	24.2		
Children	10	5.0		
Siblings	38	19.2		
Other kin	8	4.0	8	4.0
Apparently unrelated	38	19.2	38	19.2
Totals	198	100.0	198	100.0

others found anxiety and grief unendurable, falling into gloom or even madness. Neither response was the only normal and correct way to behave. The quality of the emotional ties Tudor and Stuart Englishmen formed with the members of their families was influenced by other forces besides peril and pessimism. Chief among these were the country's peculiar family structure, its high geographic mobility, and the increasing interest that divines and philosophers were taking in personality and the cultivation of sentiments, pious and profane.[21] Each of these factors influenced rich and poor, honored and humble, rustic and urban, Protestant and Catholic, variously and at different rates. The result was an untidy congeries of values and injunctions, which were often contradictory. The prevailing movement of social and intellectual change nevertheless can be said to have enhanced the psychological significance of the nuclear family.

The households of the poor had always been tiny, seldom sheltering any kin other than a pair of adults and their children. The changing pattern of geographical mobility and the diffusion of Puritan ideals encouraged the rich to reduce the sizes of their families as well and further isolated most people from their distant relatives and even from parents and siblings.[22] Almost a decade ago Alan Macfarlane argued that mobility, a late age of marriage, and contemporary inheritance customs conspired to reduce the significance of extended kinship ties and enhance the importance of the nuclear group, and all the evidence about the lives of ordinary people gathered since, including this analysis of Napier's anxious and grieving clients, suggests that he was right.[23] Emotional austerity and indifference to members of the immediate family seem to have prevailed only among the aristocracy and landed gentry, and even these groups, preoccupied as they were with property and lineage, grew more attentive to the feelings and needs of their spouses and children during the seventeenth century. Contemporaries, of course, knew intuitively what we are still laboring to prove. Discoursing on the Devil's protean guile, Thomas Nashe addressed his readers with this observation:

> It will be demanded why in the likeness of one's father or mother, or kinfolks, he oftentimes presents himself unto us. No other reason can be given of it but this, that in those shapes which he supposeth most familiar unto us, and that we are inclined to with a natural kind of love, we will sooner harken to him than otherwise.[24]

PARENTS AND THEIR CHILDREN

Using a mixture of scattered references and relentless logic, pessimistic historians have recently made seventeenth-century parents appear as demons to their children. It has become a commonplace to argue that they were indifferent to their infants' individuality, negligent in caring for them, and untroubled by their children's deaths.[25] Philippe Ariès originally proposed that paternal austerity was a psychological defense against the insupportable grief that terrible rates of infant mortality would otherwise have caused.[26] Edward Shorter is not content with this reasoning and indicts peasant mothers for murder, declaring that at least until the eighteenth century they were so careless of the health and safety of their infants that they were themselves responsible for the slaughter of the innocents.[27] Lawrence Stone embraces both arguments, claiming that mortality bred austerity, that austerity bred neglect, and neglect, in turn, bred mortality. He carries the case against parents in the era of this study still further. The Puritan doctrine of original sin taught mothers and fathers that it was necessary to break the child's will to make him tractable as a domestic beast; the brutality schoolmasters routinely inflicted on sluggish students was, by this account, consistent with the harsh attitudes of parents themselves.[28]

The Tudor and Stuart family was certainly not "child-centered" and there is plenty of evidence that some parents and especially aristocratic fathers were very aloof from their young children. Many adults shared the views of popular psychologists, who taught that children were unreasoning creatures incapable of controlling their passions. Thomas Wright, for example, declared that children "lack the use of reason and are guided by an internal imagination, following nothing else but that pleaseth their senses, even after the same manner as brute beasts do, for as we see beasts hate, love, fear and hope, so do children."[29] Legal thought and popular wisdom routinely equated children, madmen, and fools, as we have already seen. Parents were also fatalistic about childhood diseases and did not consult physicians about treating them as often as they resorted to doctors for themselves.[30] But against these signs of aloofness and the other evidence marshaled by Shorter and Stone must be set the "natural kind of love" Nashe declares to be the Devil's cloak. In the seventeenth century there were repeated injunctions to parents, especially mothers, to take special care of their children, and several kinds of evidence suggest that although fathers might have remained rather indifferent toward their very young offspring, mothers commonly formed deep attachments to their babies and children.

Women were prevented from achieving success in any endeavor that was not centered on the hearth, and however varied the social and economic functions they fulfilled in the home, their first duty was to bear and nurture children. The Swiss reformer Bullinger, whose translated works were the pattern of other contemporary conduct books, wrote that a woman pleases God when she "doth love her husband, while she doth bring forth children with grief and pain, and, when they are brought forth, doth diligently nourish them and labour to bring them up."[31] Thomas Becon voiced the same values in his *Catechism*. Recommending that mothers nurse their own babies, Becon wrote that "in so doing she shall greatly please God and satisfy the office of a true and natural mother." And while their children are still nurslings, parents "must provide, that no bodily harm chance to the children, either by fire, water, overlaying, or otherwise; but that they be kept warely and diligently both by night and day. But this is chiefly the office of the mother, which ought principally to attend young ones in their infancy."[32] Writing to a grieving mother in the

1650s, John Janeway presumed that all mothers loved their children and suffered their loss deeply: "It hath pleased the Lord to make a breach in your family, there where the knot is fastest tied . . . The strength of mothers' affection, I believe, none but mothers know; and the greatest affections when they are disturbed breed the greatest grief."[33] Janeway's sentiment was conventional. Almost eighty years before, the Marquis of Winchester had included this aphorism in his book of platitudes: "The love of the mother is so strong, though the child be dead and laid in the grave, yet always she hath him quick in her heart."[34]

The searing grief experienced by bereaved mothers among Napier's patients and the desperation of the childless show that the idea that intimate relationships should and did exist between mothers and children was not merely a literary artifact. Of the 134 cases of disturbing grief, 58 were attributed to children's deaths, and 51, or 88%, of these sufferers were mothers. Unfortunately, the ages of the children they mourned were recorded in only a few case notes. Mistress Judith Gostick "took grief" when her four-year-old died of the pox, and her misery was worsened when an accidental gunshot killed another child.[35] The mistress of the Red Lion Inn was "ever leaden with grief" because she believed that a careless neighbor had killed her child of four, and she found no consolation in the infant she was nursing.[36] After the burial of a three-month-old baby Mistress Elizabeth Foster was terrified by an owl's cry, trembled and said she had a sinking heart.[37] Nor did Napier think that grieving the death of a child was itself a sign of mental instability; it was instead a source of profound distress, which might cause emotional disturbances or physical illnesses. Sir James Wynfield's wife contracted a tertian ague (a fever) after she "took grief for her daughter dying of consumption." At the other end of the social scale, Ellen Craftes "took a fright and grief that a door fell upon her child and slew it. Presently head, heart and stomach ill; eyes dimmed with grief that she cannot see well." Lyddye Ellis came down with fainting spells and headaches because her five-year-old was nearly killed in an accident. None of these women was counted melancholy or insane.[38]

There is other evidence that women took the injunction to bear and care for children to heart. Napier's consulting room was visited by women who were in despair because they were barren or could have no more children. Abigail Browne's fears were typical. Her infant died, and she sought help and reassurance from the astrologer, who wrote: "Feareth and grieveth that she shall have no child more because that she hath been troubled with her terms so much."[39] Two of his patients complained that they had been slandered as barren women. Mothers who abused or neglected their children were tormented with grief and thought by others to be insane. Still despairing a year after her child's death, Agnys Nueman "took great grief that she did not tend it well." Joan Plotte fell into a suicidal gloom because she had said of her dying child, "if he die, let him die": "This thought troubleth her mind; careth not for her husband nor child but goeth into a corner to weep."[40] Sara Crawley was "grieved that she could not nurse her child" and suffered from melancholy and fearfulness.[41] Matthew Rowly was distraught because her child smothered in bed and neighbors apparently rumored that the death was deliberate.[42]

The two women among Napier's patients who actually did commit infanticide were considered acutely disturbed. He diagnosed Alice Goodcheap as a "light-headed" (delirious) person because she savagely murdered her newborn baby, and the mental condition of Agnys Morton who helped her maid dispose of an illegitimate child was described like this: "This woman is distracted of her wits . . . This old woman went to make herself away, being tempted as she sayeth thereunto by the Tempter. Will not in any case say her prayers . . . Very ravenous and greedy, and will say the foul Fiend lyeth at her heart, that she cannot feed him fast enough."[43] Indeed, mothers who wanted to kill their children frequently found the thought so troubling that they believed it had been implanted into them by the Devil or by witchcraft.[44] The most careful study of infanticide in this era, an essay by Keith Wrightson, confirms the impression that one gathers from reading coroners' inquests and calendars of assize records; the crime appears to have been rare and few suspicious deaths passed unnoticed. There is no persuasive evidence that Englishwomen commonly killed their children with neglect or murdered them deliberately in the seventeenth century.[45]

Napier thought that a woman's failure to love her children was a sign of mental disorder. Here is his list of Elisabeth Clark's symptoms: "Careth not for her children; can take no joy of her children; tempted to hang herself."[46] And among the indications of Jane Faldoe's mental abnormality was that she experienced "no joy of herself nor her children."[47] Indeed, some mothers were so strongly attached to their children that when they became depressed and suicidal they thought of their youngsters as extensions of the identity they wished to exterminate. Twenty women were tormented by urges to kill themselves *or* their children: Margaret Koburne, who was "tempted by Satan to kill herself or her child," is typical of these mothers.[48] Recounting Alice Savil's attempts to kill herself (which eventually succeeded), Napier wrote that just before her death she had been "desperate to drown herself, . . . desirous to have her child to go into the water with her"; twelve other women he treated also wanted their children to die with them.[49] Thus, even the hostility disturbed women expressed toward their children betrays their involvement with them.

Nor were men always uncaring and indifferent toward their sons and daughters, particularly after they were old enough to detach themselves from the maternal presence that dominated their early lives. The Puritan diarists Adam Martindale, Sir Simonds D'Ewes, and Ralph Josselin all wrote moving accounts of the deaths of children they loved.[50] When the clerical astrologer William Breden failed to complete on time some nativities he was casting for Sir Richard Napier, he wrote explaining that the deaths of two of his daughters had made it impossible to work.[51] A friend of Napier's wrote anxiously to him about his young son's perilous affliction: "Concerning his disease I much fear him. And much grieved I shall be to lose him." He was especially fond of the boy "by reason of his forwardness in learning."[52] When Sir Robert Napier's son was ill he wrote a similar letter to the physician, and when he lost two children he and his family visited Napier for a week to be consoled.[53] Nevertheless, men appear to have found it easier to protect themselves from unbearable sorrow by remaining emotionally aloof from their children, and the attitudes historians have emphasized were in fact masculine feelings. Paternal severity among the upper classes is notorious.[54] And men in general were sufficiently remote from their sons and daughters to be, for example, seldom troubled by urges to murder them: Of the 60 persons contemplating child killing among Napier's clients, only 9 were men, and in prosecuted cases of infanticide the slayer was invariably female.[55]

Women in seventeenth-century England were subjected to contradictory advice and antithetical passions. Moralists and divines
urged them to form intimate attachments to their children and to
measure their self-worth by their success in bearing and rearing
sons and daughters; at the same time they were cautioned not to
become too involved emotionally with their perishable infants and
not to grieve excessively when they died. The danger and pain of
childbirth, the physical needs and responsiveness of nursing infants, the simple work of feeding and governing young children,
all enhanced the identification of mother and child; the custom of
swaddling, Calvinist beliefs about the depravity of infants, and the
expectation that children should be harshly disciplined all inhibited sentimentality about the young. None of these customs and
attitudes helped women to bear the routine deaths of their babies
sanguinely, and the increasing emphasis by religious writers on
the individuality and preciousness of infants during the seventeenth and eighteenth centuries must have sharpened the dilemma
many of them faced. These intellectual trends ultimately resulted
in more effective kinds of child care, but before that benefit appeared in the second half of the eighteenth century, village women
nevertheless formed deep and enduring bonds with their children
and were forced to suffer again and again as disease slew one child
after another.[56]

MASTERS AND SERVANTS

Many households in early modern England harbored a Caliban, a
"servant-monster," partly adult, partly child, partly domestic
beast of burden. Between the time they achieved puberty and the
time they married, a period that averaged ten years or more,
young men and women served; all but the poorest households had
servants or apprentices to perform the distasteful and menial
chores of domestic life.[57] To be fully an adult, sexually active, and
financially independent, it was necessary to be married. Servants
and apprentices were normally compelled to remain at the outer
valence of the household, continent and subordinate to the master
of the house. "All servants, labourers and others not married,"
observed Sir Thomas Smith, "must serve by the year . . . And if
any young man unmarried be without service, he shall be compelled to get him a master whom he must serve for that year."[58] As

Smith's equation of servants and laborers implies, the position of young, unmarried adults on the ladder of social prestige was usually near the very lowest rungs, however varied the ranks of their parents.[59] Their standing within the households they served depended entirely upon their masters and mistresses. There were good masters and bad; and servants were treated as well as loved children or as badly as domestic beasts.

The relationship between masters and servants or apprentices was in many ways like that between parents and their children and quite unlike the limited and impersonal ties between employers and employees that are normal today.[60] John Bunyan declared that his guide to moral behavior taught "the fruits of true Christianity, shewing the ground from whence they flow, in their Godlike order in the duty of relations, as husbands, wives, parents, children, masters, servants, etc."[61] There was nothing unusual about including the roles of master and servant in a discussion of the ideals of conduct within the family. The chief responsibilities of masters toward their servants were the same as those of parents toward children, to provide them with the necessities of life and teach them the skills, manners, and morals appropriate to their callings and stations in life. Nor were the duties of servants different from those of children. They were to be deferential and obedient, submissive always to the authority of their elders.[62]

The authority of a young person's parents over matters concerning his future, such as marriage, was certainly not abrogated when he entered into service. Because masters and mistresses were at hand when parents were not, however, they frequently acted precisely as parents might. The employers of three of Napier's patients, for instance, intervened to prevent undesirable marriages.[63] The fact that service was a childlike, dependent status, which deprived adults of their dignity and autonomy, is illustrated by one of these cases. Henry Fisher, a forty-year old servant in the household of Lord Harrington, was, in Napier's words, "in love with a maiden of the house which his mistress would not let him marry, but broke it off and put him away." At one stroke he was deprived of his lover and his livelihood.[64] When his own servingmaid was impregnated by her sweetheart, Napier straightaway betrothed them, without pausing to ask their families' consent or to consider their own wishes. The guilty man had neither the money nor the inclination to marry, and he quickly absconded, turning up some time later pathetically imprisoned in the Bedford jail, charged with theft and pleading for Napier's help.[65] Neither Fisher's mistress nor Napier exceeded the customary authority of masters in interfering in their servants' love affairs.

Servants and apprentices were not their masters' children, though, and there were important differences between the master and servant relationship and the parent and child connection. Most important, masters and servants were bound together by contract and not by sentiment. Indoctrinating children in the mysteries of a craft and the manners suitable to their station could best be accomplished by imposing a savage discipline on them – or so many adults believed.[66] Affection might make parents more sparing with the cudgel, but a master's hand was loosely restrained by law and custom. Complaints of apprentices and servants who had been beaten by their masters were a staple item of business in municipal courts and Quarter Sessions.[67] A few of Napier's patients also blamed their masters' ill treatment for their distress. Richard Osburne grew mopish and lost his "special gift in prayer" after a wild fracas with his master: "His master broke his pate, and he threw him down. And his master cast him into prison, and there [he] remained eight or ten days. Took a grief; never well since."[68] Thomas Cardwell's master also availed himself of an official institution that provided no means of protecting the rights of social inferiors: He had the young man cast into Bedlam where his unhappiness quickly deteriorated into outright insanity.[69] Young women were vulnerable to rape or seduction, and many servants fell prey to their masters' lust. Napier was disturbed to learn that his friend and kinsman William Marsh had raped his servant, an incident that came to light only after the man's death. For three years, Agnys Burton confessed, she had been anxious and guilty: "Did dwell with my Cosen March (that dead is) and he did overcome her and abused her; yet had no child. Ever since ill . . . and can take no rest nor sleep."[70] Agnys Fenkes's master fell in love with her, and when he found out that she was already in love he "turned [her] out of doors. And she lay out of doors two days and cried 'he cometh, he cometh.' "[71] Another master employed his social and economic power more cunningly: He impregnated his servant and then married her to a bitter and resentful tenant whom he coerced into agreeing to the match.[72]

The law did little to limit the power and status that masters enjoyed, and in fact it was designed primarily to reinforce their authority. Servants who were beaten, raped, or ejected from their jobs before the end of their contracts could appeal to local authorities for redress; because corporal punishment was condoned, however, proving physical abuse must have been difficult, as the severity of the cases in court records suggests. Similarly, a young woman who had been sexually abused had to choose between the disgrace of admitting that she had lost her virginity and her desire for revenge: Many of those who were lucky enough not to become pregnant must have preferred silence.[73] Only one of the eight young women whose masters were reported to have abused them is known to have prosecuted her employer.[74]

The laws that assisted masters in maintaining their authority, on the other hand, were savage. Maximum, not minimum, wages were established by law. A servant who struck or killed his master was liable to be prosecuted for petty treason, not simple assault or murder. Servants and apprentices who ran away from their masters were tracked down; and if they were caught they might be branded or (for a brief period during the sixteenth century) sold into slavery. Custom and simple decency, however, assured that most apprentices and servants were not treated savagely.[75] The universality of the custom of service also helped make it supportable, however exploitative and repugnant the practice appeared to the minds of foreign visitors or seems to modern historians. When John Smyth's father decided to keep his son at home rather than apprenticing him to another to learn his craft, the lad was, in Napier's words, "grieved that he can have no service, and that his father would have him bound with him."[76] Service and apprenticeship were experienced by almost every adolescent, and their emotional consequences cannot easily be typified. A servant might be treated as brutally as Caliban or as lovingly as Ariel, but the bond of sentiment between him and his master was looser than that with his parents.

THE PERILS OF COURTSHIP

About 40% of the men and women who described their anxieties and dilemmas to Napier complained about the frustrations of courtship and married life. Their tales make nonsense of histo-

Table 3.5. *Courtship stresses by sex (N = 767)*

Nature of complaint	Males	Females	Totals
All courtship	63	118	181
Lovers' problems	51	90	141
Patients in love	35	37	72
Lovers' quarrels	15	44	59
Jilted lovers	3	20	23
Seduced and betrayed	0	4	4
Other premarital sex	8	5	13
Marriage broken off	17	42	59
No culprit/lovers blamed	7	12	19
Parents object	6	15	21
"Friends" object	3	14	17
Master/Mistress objects	1	2	3

Note: Because some cases included more than one stress, they have been counted only once in the totals.

rians' confident assertions that romantic love was rare in seventeenth-century England or that it was unimportant in choosing marital partners.[77] Passionate attachments were very common among the astrologer's clients. Lover's quarrels, unrequited love, and double-dealing accounted for the emotional turmoil of 141 persons, about two-thirds of whom were young women (Table 3.5); another 40 patients mentioned that they had been in love before they were married. These young people suffered the unmistakable pangs of romantic love. Consider Jane Travell's extravagant unhappiness: "Sayeth that nobody can tell the sorrow that she endureth . . . Sometimes will sigh three hours until as sad as can [be] . . . Should have married one, and they were at words as if she would not have him. And then bidding him to marry elsewhere she fell into this passion. She knoweth that she will never have him."[78] Thomas May swore that he would kill himself if he could not marry his sweetheart: "Grief taken for a wench he loves," wrote the physician; "he sayeth if he may not have her he will hang himself."[79]

Dejected lovers like Jane Travell and Thomas May were stock characters in poems and plays, the lovesick youth who gave Shakespeare the opportunity for his best comic satire. Rosalind chides

Orlando in *As You Like It* for saying, with Thomas May, that he will die if he may not have his beloved:

"The poor world is almost six thousand years old, and in all this time there was not one man died in his own person, *videlicet*, in a love cause . . . Men have died from time to time and worms have eaten them, but not for love."[80]

But Rosalind was wrong. Men (and women too) did die for love from time to time – or at least they were thought to have done so. Aubrey believed that Viscount Falkland threw away his life in battle because his mistress had perished; and at the other end of the social scale Robert Malins, a mere husbandman's son, "died poisoning himself for that he could not marry a maid that . . . he loved extremely, as some suppose."[81]

Preachers, poets, and medical writers all warned young people that carnal love was a pernicious emotion. According to Robert Burton, it turned its victims into "very slaves, drudges for the time, madmen, fools, dizzards, *atrabilarii*, besides themselves, and blind as beetles."[82] Neither the *Catechism*'s stern denunciation of "blind judgment, foolish fancy, carnal appetite, sensual pleasure, etc.,"[83] nor the extravagant suffering of poetic lovers, nor the frightful catalogues of loves' pathological effects compiled by Burton and his medical colleagues prevented ordinary young people from falling in love. Although they sometimes scrutinized the economic and social qualifications of their suitors with a calculating gaze, Napier's clients placed a high value on their affection and hoped to marry their heart's choice if they could. Mary Fossy's fiancé, for example, agreed to release her from her vows if she could not love him: "Is betrothed to this man who intensely loveth her," Napier wrote, "and [he] would release her if she would leave him, because her heart grudgeth against him, as lately she revealeth and thinketh it will never be otherwise."[84] When Ann Winch's father was satisfied that the man she wanted to marry had enough money to maintain her, he permitted her to live with him in his house for five weeks while she made a tormented attempt to decide whether she really loved him: "Hath been five weeks with him and by fits careth much for him and sometimes will not have him."[85] Thomas Knight, like Mary Fossy's fiancé, broke off his engagement to Frances Knox when he discovered that she did not love him: "Hath taken a grief touching a maiden he very lately should have married or was betrothed unto by her friends' means. And it seemeth she cared not much for him before, for she cared not to come to him . . . Because he perceived her mind unsteadfast, [he] shook her off as he himself told me."[86] A young man of higher status than these lovers, Master John Faldo, was content to bide his time, looking for just the right woman regardless of money or prestige. "Might have had a knight's daughter," Napier related, "but [he] would not, and many other matches but still refuseth either because they be not fair enough or else not so virtuous as he would have them."[87]

There are other indications that romantic love was common among youth of low and middling parentage. Archbishop Sandys complained in 1585 that "there is a great fault in many at this day that . . . they dispose themselves in marriage as they list, without consent of their parents."[88] Numerous shotgun weddings and cases of couples who defended themselves against bastardy charges by asserting that they had secretly pledged marriage suggest that he was right. Secret promises of marriage were a favorite gambit of predatory males trying to get country girls into bed; and the ploy would not have worked if such vows had not been familiar enough to be taken seriously.[89] Jilted lovers like Ann Walker often complained that suitors had deceived them with promises to marry: "Loved a fellow that pretended marriage and denieth to have her or that he ever intended any such matter."[90] Rustic couples normally began sleeping together as soon as they were fastly engaged and their marriages seemed assured, a relaxation of customary sanctions against premarital sex that was tolerated because a hasty wedding could easily be arranged if the bride became pregnant. But in times of economic hardship like the 1590s, peasant customs and scarcity clashed and illegitimacy rates soared. Guilty couples dragged into the ecclesiastical courts or arraigned before the local magistrates often defended themselves by explaining that they had agreed to marry.[91]

The propertied classes hated the sordid freedom enjoyed by the poor to mate without prudent regard for their social and economic circumstances. They denounced the peasant's passions as animal lusts and complained that vagabonds and knockabouts were "generally given to horrible uncleanness. They have not particular wives, neither do they range themselves into families, but consort together as beasts."[92] Puritan justices strove to curb bridal pregnancy and illegitimacy, and recent research by David Levine and Keith Wrightson shows that they had some success in Essex – all the more remarkable because young people of middling status were beginning to expect the same liberty to marry for love that had always been the prerogative of abject and vagrant poverty.[93] The hostile comments of gentlemen and doctors should not lead us to believe that the aristocratic passions celebrated by the great lyricists of the age were romantic love when the affections of the rabble were not. Writing about lovesickness in 1665, the physician William Drage penned this aphorism: "Some call it [love] the nobleman's madness, but poor are struck with Cupid's dart as well as rich."[94] The tales lovesick youths told Napier show that Drage was right.

Traditionalists condemned romantic love and sexual desire because they corroded parental authority, not because heated passions cooked lovers' humors to the boiling point and spoiled their reason. The ideal of parental despotism was repeated incessantly in sermons, conduct books, and in tracts of advice to sons and daughters. From Thomas Becon to Lord Halifax, from the reign of Henry VIII to the Glorious Revolution, clergymen and aristocrats admonished youth to defer to their elders' wisdom when selecting marital partners. And throughout the period some parents continued to arrange marriages for their children. This practice was most widespread and enduring among the rich, who were concerned to preserve the landed estate and social standing of their families. Aristocratic parents regarded their children's marriages as opportunities to enhance their wealth, prestige, and even their political power; and they could be appallingly insensitive toward the emotional consequences of forcing their sons and daughters to marry suitors they detested. Sir Edward Coke's brutal and effective efforts to make his stepdaughter marry Viscount Purbeck, part of the great jurist's ploy to regain favor at court, ended in a notorious scandal. Soon after the wedding the groom went mad and the bride bolted to the side of her lover, Sir Robert Howard. Napier labored in vain to restore Purbeck's sanity; the Duke of Buckingham and Archbishop Laud strove unsuccessfully for almost fifteen years to force a reconciliation between the couple.[95] The very public enmity between Lord and Lady Purbeck was uncommon only in its vehemence and duration. Lawrence Stone estimates that as many as one-third of the peerage were estranged from their wives in the period between 1595 and 1620.[96] Examples of arranged marriages that were emotional failures may occasionally be found in documents about people who were neither rich nor prestigious by aristocratic standards. Ann Myles's father matched her with a "sullen, dogged, jealous man" whose comfortable means did not compensate for her "much sorrow and grief."[97] Another of Napier's patients was engaged to a cobbler although at first she did not want to marry him: "Her friends father and mother, liking of a stranger, would persuade her to marry him, but she fancied him not. Yet her friends were very willing thereunto, and it was concluded in a week." When the parents discovered the shoemaker was a debtor, they broke the engagement with equal indifference to the wishes of their daughter, who by this time had fallen in love with him.[98]

Tales about forced marriages are gruesome but rare compared to the numerous stories of frustrated passion one may find in Napier's casebooks and elsewhere. Strictly arranged marriage was being eroded by new ideals and by increased geographical mobility. Legal practice and public opinion were firmly against forced marriages in the seventeenth century, and even among the aristocracy, parents were becoming more concerned about their children's happiness. Stuart preachers and pamphleteers labored hard to fashion a new and more liberal notion of the ideal courtship. The old vices of romantic love and premarital sexual attraction were transmuted into the virtue of "first liking" – now deemed essential to the spiritual harmony of the family.[99] No one, however, advocated allowing young people complete freedom to marry for love, and all the handbooks and sermons insisted that parents retained absolute authority to forbid their children to marry unacceptable suitors.[100] Lucy Hutchinson described her husband's behavior as a model of passion and prudence, and her story is an epitome of the new ideal that balanced love and parental authority: "One thing is very observable and worthy of imitation in him," she admonished her children; "although he had a strong and violent affection for her as ever any man had, yet he declared it not to her till he had acquainted first his father." Another match with a wealthier woman had been arranged for Hutchinson, but when he told his father about his feelings for Lucy, the older man readily consented to the new match. "His father was no less indulgent to his son's affection than the son was strict in the observance of his duty," she noted.[101] This new ideal slowly spread up the social scale, and by the end of the seventeenth century aristocrats had relaxed their constraints on the children somewhat.[102] Even the cynical Marquis of Halifax, who emphasized to his daughter that women of her class were not free to make love matches, nevertheless granted that the possibility that daughters might "refuse when their parents recommended."[103]

Although some parents were as attentive toward their children's affections as Colonel Hutchinson's father, young people who fell in love risked terrible anguish if their parents disapproved of their choice. Forty-one of Napier's patients attributed their insanity and gloom to the fact that their parents, "friends," or employers forbade them to marry the people they loved. Three-fourths of these miserable young people were women, and only four of them claimed the honor of a title or appellation of gentility (Table 3.6). Mistress Mary Blundell's case is typical in every way except her somewhat elevated rank (her family, Napier's neighbors, had a purely local claim to be counted among the gentry): "Much grief and sighing touching a young man that promised marriage of his own accord, and after . . . broken off by his father that would not consent."[104] In most cases the children appear to have assumed the initiative in courting, leaving the necessary step of alerting their parents about their intentions aside until they had formed a strong emotional commitment or even agreed to marry in the sanguine expectation that there would be no opposition. Sometimes parents intent on arranging good matches for their children were dismayed to discover that they were already in love. Jane Clarke complained that her daughter rejected a fine marriage because she was in love with Thomas Fletcher: "Her friends would place her well, and she cannot look there, but where she should not, there she would fasten." Jane's indignation is plain in the astrologer's language. She informed him in her interview that she had no intention of forcing the girl to marry against her will, but she was equally determined to prevent her from marrying Fletcher.[105]

Parents typically rejected prospective husbands because they were not rich enough – which at this social level often meant simply that they did not have the means to support a wife. Ann Alworth's parents, for example, made the first objection, that her suitor was "not rich enough," and Dorothy Geary's family argued the second, that her choice "had nothing to maintain her."[106] Re-

Table 3.6. *Courtship stresses by social status (N = 767)*

Nature of complaint	Peer/knight	Mr./Mrs.	No title	Totals
Patients in love	1	9	62	72
Lovers' quarrels	1	5	53	59
Jilted	0	2	21	23
Seduced and betrayed	0	0	4	4
Other premarital sex	0	1	12	13
Marriages broken off				
No culprit/lovers blamed	1	4	14	19
Parents object	0	2	19	21
"Friends" object	0	2	15	17
Master/Mistress objects	0	0	3	3

Note: Because cases sometimes included more than one stress, some of them have been counted more than once.

actions when socially unacceptable marriages were proposed could be spectacular. Master Fettiplace, a twenty-two-year-old Bedfordshire gentleman, sent his mother into a rage when his heart was captivated by a poor servant maid. "Loved one that his mother despised," Napier wrote, "came to me not of his own accord but by the appointment of his . . . mother." He retreated into a willful madness, vowing that "he will have his wench Ann" and growing mopish and furious. Eventually he persuaded the astrologer that if he did not marry the girl he would "continue foolish and idle-headed," and Napier advised the matron to "let him marry where his mind is set."[107] Such victories were exceptional. Jane Longe's father refused to let her marry her lover, a servant in the house, even though she was pregnant, preferring the shame of illegitimacy to the prospect of his daughter marrying such a "poor fellow."[108]

Habits of deference were so strong that anguished children seldom challenged their parents directly when their romantic hopes were shattered. There are few cases of clandestine marriage mentioned in Napier's papers, although some defiant youths doubtless simply ignored their elders and risked the consequences.[109] But parental disapproval was plainly a psychologically devastating experience for many who were forced to follow duty instead of love. A gruesome tale told by another rural healer with a reputation for assuaging emotional disturbances, John Spencer, illustrates the brutal presumption that their elders' wishes should always prevail over children's desires. When her lover's father prevented them from marrying, a young woman "fell into a great discontentment and fell distracted." She sought Spencer's help, and his treatments worked. Soon her father was sent for to fetch her home. But when he arrived she refused to speak to him, "nor do any reverence unto him," no doubt because he had not saved the match. Spencer tried to persuade her to honor her father's authority, and when persuasion failed he seized a pair of tongs and wrenched her mouth open as if he were going to yank out her teeth. He tortured her until she repeated the Fifth Commandment and spoke to her father "in a passion of weeping."[110]

The relaxation of prohibitions against premarital affection exposed young people to more psychologically perilous stress, but it had positive effects as well. It was more appropriate to the social and economic conditions of the late sixteenth and seventeenth century than arranged marriage, and probably merely legitimized already common practices. Many children migrated far from their homes to serve their apprenticeships and work as servants, and direct parental supervision of these youths was impossible. Masters and mistresses sometimes acted in loco parentis, thwarting the illicit love affairs of their servants, but the rapid turnover among servants, who often moved from job to job and village to village, must have inhibited even this check on their covert courting. The migratory habits of young people in service provided opportunities to meet prospective marital partners as well as to find work, and many parents were probably content to let their chidren shop around in the marriage market, reserving to themselves the right to reject undesirable proposals.[111] All that we know about the mobility, sexual habits, and anxieties of young people suggests that children of low and middling status often selected their own mates and that love matches were very common.

When affection and authority went hand in hand, the young accepted their parents' rule as lightly as they doffed their caps and bent their knees to acknowledge their subordination. Traditional ideals, which insisted that good order in the family and the state depended upon children's deference and obedience, were repeated in sermons, homilies, pamphlets, and imaginative literature. Habits of obedience were so strong that the yoke of parental dom-

Table 3.7. *Reported causes of conflict between generations (N = 767)*

Disputes about courtship	
Parents and children	21
"Friends" (elders) and children	17
Total	38
Other disputes and unspecified	
Inheritance	9
Others and unspecified	40
Total	49

ination became insupportable only when the needs and expectations of the child and the aspirations of his parents conflicted over an issue critically important to them both. Because divorce was very difficult to obtain and the family was the center of social, economic, and emotional life, deciding whom children should marry was the greatest single source of conflict between generations among Napier's patients (Table 3.7).

The freedom young people were permitted was tempered by the retention of their parents' right to block unsuitable matches. But their choices were also restricted in more subtle ways. They themselves were encouraged to internalize the social values and economic realities parents had traditionally been concerned about. Many learned their lesson well. An anonymous miller was crushed to find that his beloved preferred a richer man: "Intoxicated with love to one that hath a match of £500 offered her and now upbraideth him that he is but a miller and also hath a strong breath," Napier wrote of him.[112] Contemporaries tempered love with practicality in ways that look callous to modern observers who are able to earn wages sufficient to free them from the need to depend upon their parents to provide the capital for setting up a new household. Young Mistress Stafford observed of one of her suitors: "Content if he had any living, doubteth that he hath not so much money as he boasteth of. Hath proffer of many with fair livings; [yet] loveth him best if he had wherewithall to maintain her."[113] When love, economics, social status, and parental approval all coincided, the result was a marriage that was sustained by the tough, internal bonds of mutual affection as well as by the external constraints of neighborly condemnation and ecclesiastical laws that made the dissolution of miserable unions very difficult.

HUSBANDS AND WIVES

The social and intellectual trends that encouraged individual initiative and emotional attachments between courting couples also transformed the psychological complexion of marriage. During the sixteenth and seventeenth centuries ties of blood and vow with those outside the immediate family weakened. Mobile and compact, the nuclear family made husbands and wives, parents and children dependent chiefly upon each other for emotional satisfaction.[114] Puritan writers encouraged the formation of new ideals for marital conduct, emphasizing the importance of intimacy and emotional intensity between married couples. Husbands were encouraged to be mindful of their wives' spiritual and psychological welfare.[115] The double standard of sexual morality, which had made arranged marriages tolerable (at least for men), was attacked, apparently effectively.[116] The aim of Protestant pamphleteers was to persuade their readers that marriage should be built on a foundation of religious and psychological compatibility. A few who were venturesome drew the logical conclusion that divorce should be allowed when harmony was impossible; but most writers scorned divorce and were content that it remained very difficult to obtain.[117] The ideal of an emotionally autonomous marriage founded on sentiment rather than economic and social advantage resembled the consensual unions of the very poor. Cajoled by Puritan moralists and pressured by changing economic conditions, the middling and upper strata of society gradually reduced the sizes of their households and embraced the emotional intensity small families fostered. Companionate marriage spread gradually up the social ladder. The ascent, however, was very slow.

The principal impediment to the adoption of the Puritan ideal of marriage was patriarchalism. Tudor and Stuart men were cottage despots, and the subordinate position of women was sustained by customs that kept them economically dependent and socially deferential.[118] Childbearing remained the chief social obligation of women during the period, and they had few opportunities to achieve power, wealth, and status independently. Within the family itself, wives were subordinate to their husbands and often were unable to take direct action to remedy troubling situations. Contemporary tracts and imaginative literature declared that wives ought always to be deferential. The conventional aphorisms of the Marquis of Winchester include this advice: "I would counsel women not to presume to command their husbands and admonish husbands not to suffer themselves to be ruled by their wives; for in so doing I account it no otherwise than to eat with the feet and travel with the hands, to go with their fingers and to feed themselves with their toes."[119] Women who bullied their husbands or controlled their businesses turned the natural order topsy-turvy and invited retaliation by their neighbors. After it was rumored in the village that Mary Taylor, one of Napier's clients, had scratched her husband, she became afraid to leave her house for fear of being attacked and remained shut up in the cottage for two months.[120] Her reaction carried prudence to the point of phobia, but it was true that contemporaries thought that feminine violence and insubordination was a grave offense to community mores.

The chief feminine virtues were obedience and chastity. Perhaps the most telling expression of the patriarchalism of the age was enacted by an obscure Northamptonshire clergyman in 1634: He christened his infant daughter "Silence." Although wife-beaters were widely condemned, the weapons of domestic combat were unequally distributed, and the stereotypical bad wife was not a thug but a scold. Wrangling women like Shakespeare's shrewish Kate were frequently presented before church courts and Quarter Sessions.[121] The burden that customary restraints and motherhood placed on women was admitted in the most widely repeated discussion of marriage of the period – the homily on marriage, which was appointed by the crown to be read out regularly in every parish church in England: "Truth it is, that they must specially feel the griefs and pains of matrimony, in that they relinquish the liberty of their own rule, in the pain of their travailing, in the bringing up of their children, in which offices they be in great perils, and be grieved with many afflictions, which they might be without, if they lived out of matrimony."[122]

Marital problems were very common among Napier's disturbed clients, and most of those who complained about turbulent unions were women. He recorded 135 cases in which anxieties were caused by marital strife, and in 114 instances, or 84%, the sufferer was a wife. Their complaints reflect both the limitations that patriarchalism placed upon them and expectations that conformed to the new ideal of companionate marriage. The most detailed stories about bad husbands naturally describe appalling failures to be financially responsible, sexually loyal, sober, and kind. Nineteen wives reported that their husbands failed in their duty to support their families. Some, like Mistress Dorothy Abrahall, were vexed because their husbands were "unthrifts" and squandered their small resources carousing.[123] Stephan Rawlins was one of these. His distraught wife told Napier that he "thinketh little to gad a-drinking. Careth not to return until his wife fetch him home when he fondly spendeth his money amongst ill company." She had also to endure beatings and abuse each time he went on a drinking spree.[124] Elizabeth Easton's husband was joined by his family in mistreating her. She owed her despair to "her husband's friends, as mother and brother, that would rate her and slap [her] as a dog – and a husband ready to beat her. She brought some money and her husband's friends, as father, mother, brother, helped to spend it; now they live poorly."[125]

Unless women were very wealthy, they could not gain legal aid to protect their own inheritances from irresponsible husbands, and the financial dependence of wives made them vulnerable to hardship because of their husbands' economic failings, whether they were caused by malicious stupidity or simple misfortune.[126] Just over half of the 99 cases of mental distress blamed on economic problems involved women, and none of the 50 wives was upset about the failure of her own efforts to make money. Women who took the lead in providing for their families might be subject to abuse by neighbors who were outraged by violations of the normal sexual division of labor. A childless woman named Mary Gilberte complained to Napier about aches and pains in 1602. He remarked that she "taketh much grief because her neighbours envy her welfare. They scarce will look on her and speak to her . . . Grieveth and weepeth. She governeth her husband and he prospereth the better. And some repine at it and bid him knock her down. They start to put debate betwixt her and her husband [and] mock her for a barren woman."[127] Later in the century the diarist Richard Gough described with disapproval the behavior of a man who vexed both his first and second wives with his efforts "to concern himself with all things both within doors and without."[128] It is true that farming husbands and wives labored side by side to support their household; but the sphere of activities appropriate to each was sharply bounded, and even women viewed their economic activities as less important than those of their husbands.[129]

Some wives reported that their husbands were brutal, abusive, and openly adulterous. Mistress Mary Robinson said that "her husband curseth her and is dogged with her and loveth her maidens."[130] Alice Maryot's husband throttled her for going out to milk the cow at night when he had forbade it; and Mistress Podder told the outraged physician that she had been "beaten blue about her eyes. Mightily wronged and beaten by her husband that cannot brook her and calleth her a whore . . . Seven years come Shrovetide her husband through jealously hath wronged her . . . Her husband with his foot trampled on her chest, breast and belly."[131] Adultery was very common during the period, as any set of church court records shows, but almost everyone surpassed the moral standard set by Peter Ladimore, a curate whose wife was beside herself because "he loved another man's wife and kept her in the house . . . He drove away her own husband."[132]

The prevalence of miserable women among the ranks of the mentally disturbed undoubtedly owes much to the fact that wives could do very little to escape a brutal or immoral husband. Financially dependent and encumbered by children, they could not easily run away. Although deserted wives were familiar figures among the urban poor, abandoned husbands were distinctly rare.[133] Napier treated 10 patients whose spouses were runaways; 9 of them were women. Divorce with the right to remarry was very difficult to obtain (although there is evidence of popular "divorce" in defiance of the rules), and even the more accessible remedy of legal separation was offered more readily to men than to women.[134] Entirely male and committed to the ideal of marital stability, the church provided some meager consolation and very little remedy for women trapped in intolerable marriages. Women who did manage to leave their husbands were routinely ordered to resume living with them.[135] In fact, although Napier did not condone men who stole away from their wives, his attitude toward women who wanted to live apart from their husbands was much more severe, and in this he was typical. He thought that wives' urges to escape their marriages were signs of mental imbalance.

He judged Alice Harvey, who was living with her parents, "mopish" (a rather pejorative diagnostic term for sullen depression) because she could not "abide to be at home with her husband."[136]

Naturally, there were limits to the force husbands could use to impose their rule. Wife beating was prosecuted in the church courts and at Quarter Sessions. An Essex official charged William Staine in 1587 with "misusing his wife with stripes contrary to all order and reason"; and our physician repeated the view that violent husbands were not merely wrong but irrational in remarks like "her husband [is] light-headed and beateth his wife."[137] Neighbors played an active part in enforcing conformity with the normal standards of acceptable behavior. A noble foreigner was informed by one countryman in 1602: "In England every citizen is bound by oath to keep a sharp eye at his neighbour's house, as to whether the married people live in harmony."[138] Jeremy Taylor described patriarchal authority as "not a power of coercion but a power of advice"; and he, too, thought that a man who beat his wife was brainsick: "This caution contains a duty in it which none prevaricates, but the meanest of people, fools and bedlams, whose kindness is a curse, whose government is by chance and violence; and their families are herds of talking cattle . . . Marital love is infinitely removed from all possibility of such rudeness."[139] The homily on marriage also equated wife beating and violent lunacy: "How can it not appear then to be a point of extreme madness to intreat her despitefully for whose sake God hath commanded thee to leave thy parents? Yea, who can suffer such despite? Who can worthily express the inconvenience that is, to see weepings and wailings be made in the open streets, when neighbours run together to the house of so unruly an husband, as to a Bedlam man who goeth about to overturn all that he hath at home?"[140]

The grave abuses we have been discussing were not taken for granted but were deplored as deviations from an ideal of marital conduct. Most of the complaints distressed wives made to Napier reveal that they were upset because they expected to be treated fairly and affectionately. Marital problems are not easy to classify precisely, but at least half of the 135 cases Napier recorded involved women who were disturbed simply by their husbands' quarrelsomeness or apparent lack of affection for them. A Mistress Podder, for example, was sent to him for advice about how to cope with "her forward husband, herself being also stubborn"; Frances Spencer was dismayed because her husband was "too hasty with her."[141] Jealousy was not uncommon among his patients, and 5 clients complained that their sexual relations with their partners were rare or unsatisfactory, as in the case of the Earl of Sussex and his second wife, who were troubled with "a frigidity and unableness, having been both able before."[142] Some wives were anxious because their husbands neglected them for their boon companions: Mistress Nueman was "very fond of her husband and taketh grief that he is long ere he come to her, making merry with his good companions."[143] Other women who were concerned about financial catastrophes fretted as much about whether their husbands loved them or how their bond of mutual trust might be affected as they did about the economic problem itself.[144] Napier remarked of one woman that she took "no pleasure or delight in her husband, nor child, nor anything, as others have," and the majority of the cases of psychological stress involving marriage in his notebooks suggest that many women expected the tie between their husbands and them to be a bond of love and not merely of obligation.[145] The sober Puritan William Gouge felt that it was necessary to advise the readers of his compendious treatise about family life to avoid using nicknames and terms of endearment, which implied undignified familiarity. He warned wives not to address their husbands with their Christian names or with tags like "Brother, Cousin, Friend, Man," because such words corroded the patriarchal ideal. He also castigated affectionate nicknames. No more should wives call their husbands "Sweet, Sweeting, Heart, Sweetheart, Love, Joy, Dear, etc," or still worse "Duck, Chick, Pigsnie."[146] It is not easy to imagine the austere men and women depicted by modern historians calling each other Love or Joy, much less Chick or Pigsnie.

Touching accounts of the grief husbands and wives felt when their partners died also testify to the strength and intimacy of the relationships of many couples. Death ended far more marriages prematurely than it does today, and the need to continue the economic and social activities of households prompted survivors to remarry rapidly.[147] And yet almost a third of the episodes of illness, despair, or madness among Napier's bereaved patients were triggered by the death of a spouse. Of these 42 tormented survivors, 33 were women. Granted that the financial peril following a spouse's death was greater for widows than for widowers, these women were nevertheless genuinely grieved. Jone Wells recognized that she ought to remarry and could do so easily, but she remained unhappy because of "grief touching the death of her last husband."[148] Another case described by Napier also shows that there was no necessary connection between quick remarriages and widows' lack of affection for their late husbands, as some historians have inferred: "Hath taken a grief touching the sudden departure of her former husband, dying in a field returning homeward, whom she loved. Is now to have another husband."[149] Bereaved women displayed all the signs of intense mourning that we associate with the deaths of husbands and wives today. To cite but one example, Margaret Lancton: "Took a great discontent and fretting by the death of her husband." Soon she fell to pacing up and down restlessly and even suddenly attempted suicide. Four years later she still recalled her husband's passing unhappily.[150] Nor was it only women who loved their partners and were grieved to lose them. Master John Flesher's wife died in childbirth and soon afterward the child perished, too. Here is how Napier depicted his condition: "Now taketh not that pleasure that he was wont, either in reading or working as heretofore he did . . . Very heavy and apt to weep; and at others times very choleric and cannot endure crossing."[151] Sir James Whitlock was shattered by the death of his wife of twenty-nine years. A second shroud would soon be necessary, the grieving patriarch told his servants, and in little more than a year it was.[152]

Stories like these do not prove that most seventeenth-century marriages were happy. Love matches and workable partnerships existed even among aristocrats, whose marriages were negotiated like corporate mergers, but sentiment undoubtedly flourished best where status and property were least important. Napier's clients were mostly of low and middling rank, and the stresses they endured show that although the families of ordinary villagers remained strongly patriarchal, most wives among his clients desired and expected close and affectionate ties with their husbands. Such expectations were encouraged by influential writers, especially Puritan divines, who called upon their readers to found their marriages on the inward grounds of spiritual harmony rather than on the outward grounds of status and property. The evidence in Napier's practice books and in other contemporary sources suggests

Table 3.8. *Conflicts with peers outside the household*
(N = 767)

Sex of patient	Male	Female	Total
Siblings and other kin	11	22	33
Neighbors	13	22	35

that as the complementary forces of rapid social mobility and intellectual change were felt by families of some substance, their members, too, focused their emotional needs and expectations on their husbands and wives.[153]

THE VILLAGE COMMUNITY

All of the measures we can devise agree: The emotional lives of ordinary men and women were centered primarily within the nuclear family. Despite the relative infrequency with which neighbors precipitated the mental disorders of Napier's clients, fellow villagers were nevertheless important. Strife is one test of emotional propinquity, and disturbed patients were reported to have quarreled with their neighbors about as often as they fought with brothers, sisters, and more distant kin.

None of the figures in Table 3.8 is large, and no patient attributed his emotional disturbance to the death of a friend or neighbor. Lovers, husbands and wives, parents and children accounted for almost all of the unhappiness clients blamed on troubling or severed relationships. Neighbors caused individuals much less stress than members of their households, and yet they played a larger part in the psychological world of contemporaries than other kin or than our neighbors play in our lives.[154]

The good opinion of neighbors mattered very much to seventeenth-century villagers. Children drilled in the catechism were asked to recite the Ten Commandments and tell what they learned from them. The proper response was: "I learn two things: my duty towards God and my duty towards my neighbour."[155] Chief among those duties was the obligation to keep a sharp eye out for illegal or irregular activities. The enforcement of all social regulations still depended greatly upon the willingness of members of local communities to assume personal responsiblity to uphold them.[156] They exercised this responsibility in a variety of ways. Because there was no police force, ordinary rustics were appointed constables, and villagers themselves sprang forth to answer the hue and cry, for apprehending criminals was up to them. Perhaps this helps to explain the alarm Englishmen felt about vagrants. Historians have shown that the criminal underground contemporaries imagined did not exist, although there was an increase in crime during the late sixteenth century, when hard times fostered thievery. The fears experienced by 21 of Napier's clients, who had been threatened with robbery, assault, and rape or had actually been attacked are understandable enough. But apprehensions about crime must also have been a "normal" anxiety, an endemic condition that prompted people to feel personally responsible for law enforcement, even during periods when thieves and rogues were scarce.[157]

Most acts of civic virtue were less exciting than the hot pursuit of thieves and thugs. Neighbors also presumed to enforce customs that regulated intimate kinds of behavior, such as the habits of domination and deference of the couple next door and the sexual behavior of wayward husbands and unmarried servants and apprentices. Even if they did not resort to the rough music of a skimmington, social pressure was usually very effective, and to those accused of misbehavior their neighbors' actions looked oppressive and meddlesome, very disturbing and even dangerous. Cases of slander filled the dockets of church courts, and anxious patients sometimes complained to Napier that they had been its victim. Rural life could be oppressively public. Women who were actually pregnant out of wedlock sometimes fled their homes, like one desperate gentlewoman who sought an abortion from Napier, or even committed suicide.[158] Mercy Mallet was disturbed because her village thought that she was pregnant. She remarked that she had not menstruated since her father's suicide, and the neighbors knew it.[159] Threats of formal legal action worried 13 of Napier's distressed clients. Christopher Skynner was "troubled in mind" because a serving-maid had brought him to the bar, probably for molesting her sexually; but the prospect of becoming involved in a court case was upsetting even for the innocent, such as Alice Lockley, who was grieved to receive a summons to appear in a case as a witness.[160] Witchcraft suspects were often beaten and abused, "scratched" to nullify their demonic powers, and four women came to Napier to try to clear themselves with his help. One of them had been searched in vain for witch's marks by the order of a local justice, and she brought a letter from a neighbor attesting to her innocence. Still she was anxious about the suspicion and wanted the astrologer's testimony of innocence as well.[161]

Witchcraft accusations were part of the arsenal of formal and informal sanctions local communities employed to enforce orderly, conventional behavior. The circumstances that provoked them deserve attention, for they highlight the duties and standards of neighborly conduct. More than 500 of Napier's patients, 264 of whom were mentally ill, thought that they were bewitched. Their allegations confirm the view of Alan Macfarlane and Keith Thomas that witchcraft suspicions normally focused upon people with whom the victim had a personal relationship.[162] In most cases only the suspect's name is known, but there are more details in about one in six cases. They show that three kinds of previous interactions between accuser and accused normally preceded accusations. Either the accuser had neglected to perform a neighborly duty and exorcised his own guilt by accusing the slighted woman of being a witch; or the victim and the suspect had quarreled, and the accusation was touched off by an already charged incident; or, finally, the accuser simply tossed in his lot with others who believed that an irksome or eccentric character had supernatural powers to do mischief. This last kind of accusation was rather uncommon: Just 5.7% of the persons suspected by Napier's mentally disturbed patients or their families were "bad" women, feared also by others.

Thomas and Macfarlane argue persuasively that the neighborly obligation that figured most prominently in witchcraft prosecutions was the duty to provide alms. Charitable attitudes and practices were changing, and spontaneous, personal relief was being replaced by organized institutional aid. Almsgiving became a source of anxiety for contemporaries, in whom the habits of good neighborliness and the new ideal of economic individualism jostled together uncomfortably. Several cases of witchcraft accusations in Napier's notes fit this thesis precisely. John Woddle and his wife told him they suspected "Goody Hall of Crawly that cometh and beggeth and hath it, and departeth to their knowledge, thankful. Yet her husband [Woddle] forbade his wife, [she] should not give her any alms."[163] When he fell ill, Woddle recalled the incident and his guilt found a suspect with a grievance. Parnell Payne, Ann Buckingham, and Elisabeth Clark all told similar tales.[164] Respectable Englishmen feared and loathed beggars and vagabonds, and four other clients had been terrified by mendicant neighbors.[165] A number of suspects were widows, who were probably poor and dependent upon their fellow villagers for aid, and a few others displayed physical peculiarities. One of these "lame and mishappen" suspects was accused (appropriately) by a patient who was himself "a lame fellow."[166]

The allegations Napier's clients made were occasioned by a wider range of social and personal obligations than almsgiving. The most interesting of these concerned the custom of inviting village women to assist at a childbirth. The agony of labor without anesthetic was no less intense for being familiar. Describing the violent madness of one woman, Napier remarked that she was "tormented everywhere, as a women in travail."[167] And because surgical remedies for obstetrical misfortunes were crude and ineffective and infection was incurable, childbirth killed many women. London women died bearing children perhaps as much as a hundred times more often than they do today; and even aristocratic wives were twice as likely to perish than their husbands during the first fifteen years of their marriages.[168] Women who survived were sometimes irreparably mangled.[169] The suffering childbirth caused cannot be estimated accurately, but the fear, stress, and illnesses induced by difficult births contributed to the mental disorders of 81 of Napier's patients, including one man who was so frightened by his wife's awful pain that he went mad.[170]

Nothing could make childbirth safer and easier, so contemporaries attended to reducing the fear it provoked. They depicted it as the natural and necessary culmination of women's lives, and they mocked barren women, many of whom consulted Napier and other physicians to find some remedy for their childlessness.[171] When a birth was at hand, village women were invited to attend. The importance contemporaries attached to these displays of feminine solidarity is plain. The law prevented midwives from delivering babies without other women present; women whose travails had been marred by strife were said to have consequently gone mad. Mary Aussoppe became anxious and utterly depressed after a disgruntled neighbor cursed her during her labor. The woman burst into the house, fell to her knees and "prayed unto God that Mary Aussoppe might never have herself [? i.e., be at peace] . . . The plague of God light upon her, and all the plagues in hell light upon her."[172] Five of Napier's clients thought that women whom they had not invited to their deliveries had bewitched them: Participation in this feminine rite was an essential duty and privilege of village women, and omitted neighbors had reason to be angry.[173]

Seventeenth-century villages bore no relation to the peaceable kingdoms anxious urbanites imagine made up "the world we have lost." Criminal records abound with evidence that hatred, fear, and violence were endemic in rural England before the Industrial Revolution, and many witchcraft accusations were simply extensions of personal hatreds and family feuds.[174] Ten of Napier's clients, for example, who had antagonized suitors by rejecting their proposals accused their spurned lovers of witchcraft when misfortune afterward befell them. Elizabeth Smith told the astrologer: "One that haunteth her and sayeth that he will marry her, and she denieth him of a long time. She feareth that he hath bewitched her."[175] Like several other women, Joan Brytton suspected that her barrenness was caused by invisible malevolence, and she applied to Napier for a magical amulet to protect her, explaining that "an old man that loved her said that she was sure to him and told her in the church where she was to be married that . . . some cross should befall her for denying of it."[176]

Rustic hamlets were relentlessly intimate, and it was impossible to avoid people whom one hated or feared. When Francis Gondone heard his neighbors brawling next door he shared the gossip and made a terrifying enemy: "He found her tugging with her husband and rumoured it and caused the next neighbour to be to the cuckingstool. She threatened to be even with him."[177] A brawl between Jane Clively and a woman of her parish over which of them would have the honor of reading scripture aloud in church provoked the conclusion that she was "haunted with spirits" when she afterward developed gripping pains in her chest and belly: "Was desirous to read a chapter in the church; and a woman took away her book in the pew and turned her to a psalm to read, and she said she would have read a chapter, and so presently took ill and fell sick . . . The woman did it because she scorned she should have the upper place."[178] The intensity of the anxieties that hurt feelings, angry words, and thoughtless actions bred in the intimate world of the village community is plainly set out in this distressed narration that John Welhed related to Napier:

He met a woman of that town as he went into the field, to whom he spake. But she [spake] never a word, whereupon he secretly said to himself that this woman hath never a tongue; and they think she spake not because they had driven out her ducks, out of their yard. This woman is taken for an honest woman and reasonable well to live.[179]

Worried and frightened people like John Welhed were not thought mad or melancholy because they suspected that their neighbors were causing them some supernatural harm. They were articulating the normal anxieties of village life in terms of beliefs that most men and women shared. Witchcraft accusations expressed the hostilities and uncertainties that assailed villagers who were forced to rely upon an ever-shifting group of neighbors and friends to provide them with physical help, credit, protection against thieves and thugs, companionship and support in times of sickness and need.[180] Ellen Bale's plight is emblematic of the anguish men and women who alienated their neighbors felt. After a quarrel with another woman she fell to pacing up and down, wringing her hands and muttering, "What shall I do? . . . Where shall I go?"[181] The only haven in this harsh world was the family, and that fact was also embodied in witchcraft fears. Anxious men and women dared not accuse their families of bewitching them. Napier recorded the names of 428 persons who were suspected witches; only 6 of them, or 0.4%, were related to their accusers, the rest were almost certainly neighbors.[182] The psychological security of seventeenth-century villagers depended far more on maintaining good relations with their neighbors than our peace of mind does, but the focus of their emotional lives was nevertheless the nuclear family, the source at once of their most troubling fears and their greatest consolations.

As numerous as Napier's practice notes are, they cannot show us all the frustrations ordinary people were forced to bear. They contain comparatively little about the problems peculiar to men, save for the anxious fear of want and losses of cash and kind that troubled 99 of his clients. Few men complained of troubles between them and their lords; there are no hints of the anger and resentment that exploded into rebellion in 1607 when men armed themselves to protect the corrosive effects of enclosure in the region.[183] Such tensions were apparently not thought to be plausible explanations for mental disorder, however much they actually contributed to the anxiety of individuals. These notes can only guide us to the problems men and, still more, women believed imperiled their happiness and sanity. Their preoccupation with the difficulties of courtship and marriage emphasizes the necessity for historians to study the emotional dynamics of family life. The complex interplay of love and hate they reveal reminds one again and again of the often profoundly sensitive treatment of youthful love and married life in the poems and drama of the age. Londoners never tired of watching comedies whose plots reconciled the conflicting claims of passion and parental authority; playwrights explored every tragic consequence that violating the divine and natural bonds between husbands and wives, parents and children, could unloose upon an Othello or a Lear.[184] They show us that it is foolish to presume that peasants and artisans did not experience passion and love, for they prove that ordinary villagers thought losing them was sufficient cause for misery or madness.

4

Popular stereotypes of insanity

SYMPTOMS AND TYPES OF MENTAL DISORDER

Midway through his massive compilation of authority and anecdote about melancholy, Robert Burton falls into a pessimistic mood. "The tower of Babel," he declares, "never yielded such confusion of tongues as the chaos of melancholy doth variety of symptoms." Its signs are like the letters of the alphabet, and its manifestations more various than the variety of words the "four-and-twenty letters make . . . in diverse languages." No single sketch can do justice to the profusion of forms that melancholy may take; the character of a melancholy man is more changeable than Proteus. Nor should we expect to find all the tokens of the disease in a single case: "Not that they are all to be found in one man, for that were to paint a monster or a chimera, not a man; but some in one, some in another, and that successively or at several times." Despite such repeated lamentations, Burton denied that the difficulties of composing a single ideal character of melancholy's victims meant that the disease did not exist or could not be discussed at all: "There is in all melancholy *similitudo dissimilis*, like men's faces, a disagreeing likeness still; and as in a river we swim in the same place, though not in the same numerical water . . . so the same disease yields diversity of symptoms."[1]

Burton anatomized a single, comprehensive type of mental disorder and produced a record of the opinions of hundreds of authorities and the experiences of one man, the anatomist himself. Richard Napier encountered every kind of mental affliction his contemporaries knew and produced a massive record of the ideas of one self-taught expert and the experiences of thousands of sufferers. The scholar's encyclopedia and the physician's notebooks are often comparable. Both Burton and Napier were traditionalists: conservative divines who developed a consuming interest in classical medical science and retained confidence in the efficacy of astrology. Neither of them was an innovator; both of them sought to assimilate ancient learning and modern example, arcane studies and popular wisdom. Like Burton, Napier was reluctant to impose patterns on the profusion of psychological symptoms he observed; but the fashions and beliefs of his age nevertheless shaped his perceptions and those of his patients. The modish preoccupation of gentlemen and gentlewomen with melancholy, for example, is reflected in his case notes, and so is the old popular association of suicidal gloom with apostacy and demonianism. *The Anatomy of Melancholy* has often, and rightly, been used as a summation of contemporary commonplaces about mental disorder. Napier's records may be used in a similar manner, for his descriptions of his patients' afflictions provide a remarkable magazine of popular beliefs about the nature and meaning of insanity. Burton's book collects the views of ancient and modern writers and presents them as brief quotations assembled into coherent sequences; Napier's notebooks record the observations of his clients and their relatives and present them in brief summaries organized according to a consistent format. In both instances, the reader can detect many different voices, modulated at the writer's pleasure, not a single voice, expressing only the author's personal opinion. Indeed, it is occasionally difficult to separate the attitudes of Burton and Napier from those of their sources, but it is usually possible to distinguish their idiosyncratic notions from more widely shared beliefs.

Ever since antiquity, insanity has been defined by experts but discovered by laymen. Physicians and lawyers have devised more or less rigorous definitions of mental disorders, but they have been obliged to rely upon laymen's looser conceptions of insanity to enforce them.[2] In seventeenth- and eighteenth-century England, even more than today, laymen identified particular persons as insane and sought medical treatment to cure them and legal action to manage them and their property, for there were no agencies, such as the psychiatric profession and the police, to act on behalf of the community. Popular beliefs about mental disorder were therefore significant in determining who was considered to be insane, and why. All of the principal sources for the study of insanity are conjunctions of official and lay thought: Medical records represent the

physician's thought, but the patients were selected by their relatives; legal documents reveal the lawyer's views, but the defendants were descried by their neighbors. Burton's compilation of
medical authority frequently appeals to common experience, or
more correctly common belief, to validate its assertions. Napier's
case notes reveal popular attitudes about the types and significance
of mental disorders unusually plainly because they are remarkably
free from expert jargon. In many instances he was content merely
to list his patient's complaints and add that he was "troubled in
mind," dispensing with a formal diagnosis altogether. The language with which he epitomized his clients' relations of their
symptoms was closely modeled on their testimony. Sometimes,
despite their brevity, his records convey the authentic voice of
suffering, unimpeded by the physician's own words. Here, for
example, is what Thomas Stiles's father told Napier about his
son's condition:

A strong maddish fellow . . . Was frightened with two fellows that fell
upon him and wounded him in the head . . . Much amiss. Very wild and
will walk all the night and talk with himself with a staff and sayeth that
he would beat him if he could find him. Very fantastical and talketh
much of the Devil and sayeth that he is a fine serving man and that the
Devil doth no man harm . . . He sayeth that he seeth the Devil and that
he is a fine man and doth no man harm.[3]

Taken individually, these notes leave one with the Burtonian impression that the variety of insanity knew no bounds. If, however,
we grasp the force of Burton's remarks about classifying the
symptoms of mental disease, and if we do not expect to find in
each case the typical signs of a single disorder but treat them instead like single letters or words, we can combine them to form
intelligible statements about the thoughts, actions, and emotions
that ordinary men and women considered to be abnormal. Distinct types of psychological disturbance become apparent and the
babel of symptoms can be seen to be coherently related to contemporary social norms and popular beliefs.

Attempting to find coherent social significance in the speech and
behavior of the insane is not an altogether unusual practice. Anthropologists and sociologists have recently produced a congeries
of theoretical and empirical work aimed at showing that the
symptoms of mental disorder are culturally relative and are

viewed as violations of particular social norms.[4] This strategy may reveal attitudes about proper conduct too familiar to contemporaries to be emphasized in legislation or conduct books. This approach is also attractive to historians because it proceeds by trying to make sense of the records left by men and women who actually saw insane or troubled people and by attempting to explain the language and categories they employed. Evidence is interpreted precisely for what it is – the outcome of a social encounter between a mentally disturbed person and another individual who was concerned with assessing the social normality of his thoughts and actions. One may ask, simply, why did this man or woman seem to be psychologically abnormal to his physician, his family, or even to himself? This methodological stance avoids the potential anachronisms that would accompany the use of twentieth-century categories. Its disadvantage is that it sacrifices the capacity to make systematic cross-cultural comparisons and therefore camouflages those facets of psychological disorder that are resistant to the variations of time and space. Although I am aware that many social scientists would disagree, I think that the advantages of the contextual approach for historical research amply compensate for the power of generalization it necessarily lacks.

The simplicity of the methods I have used to analyze the psychiatric symptoms of Napier's clients resembles the famous experiment that is the central device in Wilkie Collins's masterly thriller *The Moonstone*. In that novel a physician's assistant writes down the delirious ravings of his diseased employer in an effort to see if they convey a coherent thought. He leaves spaces between the broken phrases, which he fills in as the patient's repetitions make a connective obvious. "I treated the result thus obtained," he explains, "on something like the principle which one adopts in putting together a child's 'puzzle'. It is all confusion to begin with; but it may be all brought into order and shape, if you can only find the right way."[5] Reading Napier's notes in conjunction with the chief medical treatises and popular literature about insanity of the period, I devised a list of more than one hundred words and phrases that described psychologically abnormal states in seventeenth-century speech. I then tabulated the frequency with which each of these "symptoms" occurred in the 2,483 consultations in Napier's practice books containing one or more of them. Diagnostic categories such as *mopish*, *mad*, *lunatic*, *troubled in mind*, and *melancholy* were then used to produce a second set of calculations. Choosing only those consultations that included one of those afflictions, I counted the number of times each of about fifty other symptoms were found together with the maladies I was studying.[6]

These techniques were not statistically sophisticated, nor were the results necessarily statistically significant. The frequencies and cross tabulations they yielded are valuable because they provide a means of summarizing thousands of shards of information and mapping the locations of their discovery. The advantage of the simple numerical maps presented in the tables is that they permit one to identify typical cases more readily than one could if the data were presented simply as a series of examples. The brevity of Napier's notes, his clumsy, telegraphic style, and the sheer repetition of common ailments make routine consultations seem stupifyingly dull and lend illusory importance to odd or well-presented cases. Moreover, the statistical summaries of the frequencies with which symptoms can be found together are an invaluable aid to reassembling the ideal types that made individual cases of mental disorder meaningful. Just as a classical archeologist might use shattered bits of pottery to reconstruct the vessels from a single site and then by comparing them with pots discovered elsewhere identify the characteristic features of the amphora and psykter, so the historian can use the cross tabulations of symptoms from Napier's notebooks to reassemble the kinds of mental abnormality he recognized and then by comparing them with descriptions found in contemporary sources distinguish the typical signs of madness and melancholy. Thus, although the complete remains of individual vases or cases of insanity are seldom discoverable, it is nevertheless possible to sketch the features of the general classes to which they belong.

Table 4.1 shows the symptoms singled out for special attention, either because preliminary counts showed that they were very numerous or because contemporary literature made it plain that they were important signs of mental disorder. I have grouped some symptoms together because they seemed clearly to describe a single emotion or kind of behavior. In such cases, the variations among the words used to describe the same phenomenon were themselves significant. The vocabulary of mental disorder contained many "complex words" (the phrase is William Empson's),

Table 4.1. *List of symptoms selected for special scrutiny (N = 2,483)*[a]

Symptom	Consultations	%	Symptom	Consultations	%
Troubled in mind	794	32.0	Cannot follow		
Melancholy	493	19.9	business	100	4.0
Mopishness	377	15.2	Despair	97	3.9
Light-headed	372	15.0	Doubts salvation	95	3.8
All sensory symptoms	330	13.3	Mad	91	3.7
Took grief	328	13.2	Raging	91	3.7
Fearful	305	12.3	Too little talk	92	3.7
All religious			Evil thoughts	90	3.6
symptoms	293	11.8	All violence symptoms	89	3.6
All sadness symptoms	271	10.9	Laughs	78	3.1
Moodiness	194	7.8	Stubborn	74	3.0
Simply sad	182	7.3	Too much talk	75	3.0
Idle talk	175	7.0	Screams or cries	74	3.0
Fancies and conceits	174	7.0	Terrible dreams	68	2.7
Took fright	168	6.8	All infanticidal		
Suicidal	158	6.4	symptoms	68	2.7
All harmful symptoms	158	6.4	Furious	62	2.5
All hostility symptoms	143	5.8	Religious		
Mad/lunatic combined	137	5.5	preoccupation	58	2.3
Distracted	134	5.4	Screams	54	2.2
Frantic	131	5.3	Inactive	53	2.1
Tempted[b]	132	5.3	Lunatic	49	2.0
All hallucinations	127	5.1	Curses	46	1.9
Senseless	118	4.8	Solitary	44	1.8
Grieving	107	4.3	Suspicious	45	1.8
Weeping	108	4.3	Wandering	43	1.7

[a] Figures indicate the number of consultations in which the symptom or type of symptom was mentioned. Because the principal aim of the investigation in this chapter was to determine which symptoms were likely to be associated closely, consultations, which record single observations, were thought to be a more appropriate basis for calculations than cases, which lump together all the consultations in a single episode of illness. There were obviously more consultations than cases, and this had the effect of reducing the number of instances in which any two symptoms occur together. The percentages of consultations in which symptoms appear do not sum to 100% because consultations usually record more than one symptom.

[b] When the word *tempted* appeared by itself it probably meant tempted to commit suicide in most instances. But as Napier sometimes had in mind urges to commit other sins when he used "tempted," it has been tabulated separately from suicidal thoughts.

terms that changed their meaning depending on their context. Napier and his contemporaries used the word *despair*, for example, to describe both a sad emotion and a moral and theological state. To preserve the connotations of this word, it was necessary to count it three times, once by itself, once as a description of a feeling, a "sadness symptom," and once as a religious condition, a "religious symptom." This is the only way to assess the significance of despair both as an emotional and as a religious sign of mental abnormality. Because the tables in this chapter preserve the contextual variations of complex words, they are easy to misunderstand. One word may have several meanings, each consultation contains several symptoms, and all of them have been counted; the total obviously far exceeds the number of consultations for mental disorder. Our chief concern is to measure the frequency with which given symptoms appear among the consultations for mental disorder. The percentages given in the tables, therefore, are proportions of the total number of consultations in which particular symptoms may be found. They do *not* sum vertically to 100% because the total of that column would be the sum of all the symptoms in all their connotations. To facilitate comparisons, I have omitted the percentages of consultations in which symptoms, groups of symptoms, and pairs of symptoms (in cross tabulations) do not appear. For example, an entry in Table 4.1 indicating that the symptom "troubled in mind" may be found in 32% of the consultations for mental disorder implies that it is absent from 68% of them.

The symptoms in Table 4.1 are arrayed in order of their frequency in all the visits to Napier by people who suffered from some mental disturbance. Burton, who loved lists, would have delighted in this one. A single creature assembled from the traits in it would be a monster, not an ideal type. It displays some peculiar features. The terms *melancholy, mopish, troubled in mind*, and *light-headed*, which were among the ten most common afflictions, are both symptoms and types of mental disturbance; some patients suffered from one or more of these afflictions at once. The most flamboyant and recognizable kinds of insanity, *madness, lunacy*, and *distraction*, are comparatively scarce. They appear in only about one in every twenty consultations. The distinctive features of the contemporary concept of utter insanity, madness, or lunacy, will thus be found in only a tiny proportion of the total number of psychiatric consultations. Four conclusions emerge from an examination of this table: It includes the symptoms of several kinds of mental disorder; the signs of these maladies are not always neatly confined to separate consultations; disturbances of mood and perception were much more common than extravagant eccentricities of behavior; and the characteristic symptoms of the various types of disorder appear in rather small numbers of consultations.[7]

The frequencies of the symptoms in this list will serve as a crude guide with which to distinguish the principal types of disorder found in Napier's practice. The signs of a particular kind of insanity often may be detected by comparing the distribution of symptoms among all the consultations for mental disturbances with the distribution of symptoms in the consultations for a specific disease or complaint. The tables in this chapter and in the appendixes are provided to facilitate such comparisons. A more statistically sophisticated procedure for isolating the patterns of symptoms characteristic of the major types of mental disorder might have been devised, but my attempts to do so invariably distorted the messy complexity of these very difficult records. Because Napier was not concerned to perfect a general vocabulary of insanity or to organize his material for statistical analysis, he tolerated a great deal of ambiguity in the words he used and often neglected to record information that he thought was self-evident. The consultations with people who were stark mad or who had seen him the day before, for instance, are often cryptic, probably because he did not bother to elaborate the obvious or repeat what he had written down previously. These habits are evident enough to the reader who explores the whole field of Napier's case notes, but they make statistical presentation of them difficult. The simple tabulations recorded here are best understood as measurements of the *tendency* of particular symptoms to be found among the victims of different types of mental disorder. I have tried to be faithful to the complexities and failings of Napier's records. Although it displays some of the fashionable trappings of quantitative history, this study is made largely of old-fashioned historical fustian, woven together from a study of the language of Napier's case notes and the scientific, literary, and theological works of his contemporaries. Burton eloquently described the difficulties of finding patterns in the symptoms of the insane: The signs of melancholy are "irregular, obscure, various, so infinite, Proteus himself is not so diverse; you may as well make the moon a new coat as a true character of a melancholy man; as soon find the motion of a bird in the air as the heart of a man, a melancholy man. They are so confused, I say, diverse, intermixed with other diseases."[8] To make a coat that fits a melancholy or a mad man, the tailor must rely as much on eye and hand as on the numbers on his tape.

Four distinctive varieties of insanity are reflected in the patterns of psychological symptoms Napier recorded and in the descriptions of abnormal thoughts and actions reported by his clients and their guardians. These broad types of mental disorder may also be found in drama and poetry, legal records and medical treatises composed before 1640. The most severe kinds of insanity were identified with two patterns of behavior, one of which resembled criminality, the other sickness. Both of these stereotypes were characterized by terrible energy and mental incoherence, and both of them were called by a variety of names, including, respectively, *madness*, *lunacy* or *distraction* and *mania*, *distraction* or *light-headedness*. The less violent types of mental disorder were also loosely organized into two patterns of thought, mood, and action. These disorders were typified by physical torpor and by emotional disturbances, faulty perceptions, or delusions. One of these stereotypes was the most fashionable malady of the age, melancholy; the other was a much less prestigious affliction, usually referred to by such unflattering terms as mopishness, lethargy, or (in later works) insensibility.

In addition to the symptoms comprehended in these popular stereotypes, there were many emotional and mental abnormalities that were regarded as symptoms of insanity in certain circumstances, but were not assimilated into any specific concept of mental disease. The clients whom Napier diagnosed as *troubled in mind*, for example, suffered from an enormous variety of psychological afflictions, most of which were exaggerations of normal emotions. Thus, although such patients were more anxious and gloomy than mentally sound people, neither these symptoms nor any others identified them with a distinctive type of mental disorder: Melancholy people, for instance, were more typically the victims of anxiety and gloom than the merely troubled in mind. There were also varieties of mental abnormality that were not defined in secular terms. Suicide, for example, was a religious and

civil crime. Churchmen, coroners' juries, and crown officials regarded it to be the embodiment of apostasy and premeditated
murder, not the product of mental disease, and the sufferers of
suicidal gloom agreed that their heinous impulses were frequently
caused by Satanic temptations, rather than by natural disorder.
Popular opinion and the teachings of physicians and theologians
sometimes disagreed about the extent to which secular and supernatural explanations for mental disturbances were or were not
compatible. Many of the ordinary villagers whom Napier treated
thought that demoniacal possession, for instance, might explain
almost any kind of mental affliction, and some writers and
preachers also believed that the Devil could cause natural diseases,
including insanity.[9] Prominent physicians, however, argued that
possession was distinguishable by a narrow range of very unusual
symptoms, which could not be attributed to any natural malady.
The four main types of insanity discussed in this chapter therefore
do not account for all of the tokens of mental disorder recognized
by seventeenth-century people. They were merely the most conspicuous stereotypes of mental illness. In order to understand their
social and intellectual significance, it will, of course, be necessary to consider their relationship to the other important kinds of
mental disturbances contemporaries identified. The justification
for focusing at length on these four stereotypes is that their long
history, wide popular recognition, and medical authority established them as the images most English men and women had in
mind when they spoke about madness.

VIOLENT MADNESS

Renaissance Englishmen were fascinated by fools and madmen.
The Jacobean stage teemed with idiots and lunatics, and popular
writers and ballad makers populated their works with natural
fools, counterfeit madmen, Mad Toms, melancholy gentlemen,
and distempered lovers. It is impossible to think about madness in
early modern England without hearing Lear rage; Webster's
Duchess of Malfi and Fletcher's *The Pilgrim* contain whole troops of
Bedlamites.[10] In the greatest age of English drama, the longest
running show in London was Bedlam itself. Small and squalid, the
asylum housed fewer than thirty inmates during the late sixteenth
and early seventeenth centuries. The offal that shocked inspectors

did not deter the public from coming to gawk at the small company of lunatics. The audience grew so large and mindless of the inmates' interests that Sunday closing had to be ordered in 1657. Fifty years later, in new and larger accommodations, the hospital entertained as many as 96,000 visitors a year.[11] Although Bedlam was the only asylum for the insane in England until the middle of the seventeenth century, it was not the only place where the curious could see actual lunatics. English villages lacked private chambers and specialized institutions that might have served as *oubliettes* for mad relatives. Insane men and women were perforce on public display, a situation that is strikingly illustrated by the well-informed comments of neighbors in legal actions to determine the sanity of putative suicides and lunatics.[12]

The fascination with madness was so strong that it minted new words and proverbs. By the turn of the century Elizabethans had transmuted the name of Bethlem Hospital into "Bedlam," a slang term for utter madness, which was understood everywhere in the kingdom. "Bedlam, Frenzy, Madness, Lunacy, I challenge your moody empire," exclaimed a character in Marston; "Stark Bedlam mad," wrote Napier about one of his patients.[13] Madness was invoked by everyone as a term of abuse or a kernel of wisdom: There were at least twenty-seven proverbs about mad acts, mad folk, madness itself.[14] Abraham men, beggars who pretended to be Bedlamites, and Mad Toms were proverbial figures, traditionally pictured as ragged, dirty, dangerous characters, living like beasts on the highways and in the woods.[15] The popularity of stage lunatics and real madmen and the proliferation of words and phrases describing or invoking insanity are important because these phenomena reflect the diffusion of generally understood stereotypes of insanity. Literary madmen embodied medical and legal ideas about how insane people talked and acted, as well as popular notions of abnormal behavior. Ordinary laymen could test the aptness of these figures of insanity by observing people whom the authorities at Bedlam, the officials of the Court of Wards, or the local magistrates regarded as lunatics. From popular literature and reports of real madmen's behavior, they learned a common vocabulary with which to describe the varieties of insanity. By the early seventeenth century the language of madness had become rich and pervasive; words and phrases about insanity were part of the common coinage of everyday speech and thought, negotiable everywhere in England and not restricted to a small circle of medical and legal experts.

Richard Napier used three plain words to describe men and women who were patently insane: *mad*, *lunatic*, and *distracted*. To these he added a fourth, more ambiguous term, *light-headed*, to describe states of delirium ranging in seriousness from simple giddiness to utter senselessness. Many of the notes he made about patients who suffered from these afflictions were based on the reports of relatives or friends who thought that the patients were too dangerous, ungovernable, or sick to be moved safely.[16] The victims of acute insanity were characteristically described as terrifyingly wild and incomprehensible. Often frantic and raging, they were likely to be hostile, angry, or violent, to laugh strangely, babble or scream incoherently. Within this range of common symptoms one can find two patterns of emphasis, or stereotypes. One kind of madman was violent or menacing, and his behavior was hardly separable from the actions of criminals; others were raving and apparently incoherent, and their behavior was barely distinguishable from the delirium commonly caused by mortal fevers. The influence of these stereotypes can be detected numerically if one examines the symptoms of the patients Napier actually called mad, lunatic, distracted, and light-headed (Table 4.2). The distinctive feature of the behavior of madmen and lunatics was their propensity to rage and threaten violence.[17] People who were distracted were also often violent, but their distinctive action was idle talk – raving, seemingly incomprehensible speech. Those light-headed patients who were plainly insane instead of just giddy were also characterized by a tendency toward idle talk and frantic babble, but they were seldom given to violence.

The kinship of madmen and criminals was not peculiar to Napier's practice. Legal rules that originated in the Middle Ages identified lunatics as a special class of criminal: Together with infants and idiots, they enjoyed immunity from the usual savage penalties for crime. Michael Dalton, in his standard handbook for justices of the peace, emphasized the point in his remarks about murderers: "If one that is *non compos mentis*, or an idiot, kill a man, this is no felony . . . Now there be three sorts of persons accounted *non compos mentis* to this purpose and the like. 1. A fool natural . . . 2. He who was once of good and sound memory and after (by sickness, hurt, or other accident or visitation of God) loseth his

Table 4.2. *Cross tabulations of selected symptoms among acutely insane patients (in percent)*

Symptom	All mental disorders (N = 2,483)	Mad and lunatic (N = 137)	Distracted (N = 134)	Light-headed (N = 372)
Mad and lunatic	5.5	100.0	11.9	4.6
Distracted	5.4	11.7	100.0	4.3
Light-headed	15.0	12.4	11.9	100.0
Frantic	5.3	17.5	9.0	10.2
Raging	3.7	14.6	11.9	3.2
All violence symptoms	3.6	10.2	10.4	3.5
Too much talk	3.0	8.8	11.2	8.1
Idle talk	7.0	6.6	14.2	15.3
Laughs	3.1	8.8	6.0	5.4
All sensory symptoms	13.3	12.4	14.2	17.5
All sadness	10.9	2.2	3.0	7.0
Suicidal	6.4	0.0	.7	5.6

Note: Figures are percentages of consultations in which both symptoms appear.

memory. 3. A lunatic, *qui gaudet lucidis intervallis,* and is sometimes of good understanding and sometimes is *non compos mentis.*"[18] The laymen who composed juries were fully familiar with this principle. Examples of murderers and arsonists whose guilt was excused because of their insanity are not difficult to find, and less heinous infractions by lunatics were also tolerated by lay and ecclesiastical courts.[19] In spite of their leniency toward madmen who had committed crimes, English villagers were terrified of lunatics and often resorted to preventive detention to protect themselves. Petitioners asked Somerset justices to restrain John Day who had "become a lunatic and doth yet so continue, whereby all persons coming near unto him are in danger of their lives." And the inhabitants of the same county were afraid that another lunatic would commit "much mischief and set on many dangerous attempts."[20]

Both the application of the legal rule mitigating the offenses of the insane and the protection of the community by the restraint of dangerous madmen depended upon the capacity of ordinary men and women to recognize a lunatic when they saw one. As jurymen they had also to be able to distinguish between "normal" crime and violations of the law that were irrational. Only the ex-inmates

of Bedlam, a trifling number, may have been officially badged as
lunatics; certification by experts, whether physicians or lay practitioners, was unusual even in disputed cases of insanity.[21] In fact,
some men worried that the gestures of insanity were known too
widely and that the unscrupulous could mimic them precisely
when they wanted to avoid prosecution. Included in the rogues'
galleries published by the scholastics of ruling-class paranoia, John
Awdeley and Thomas Harman, were "Abraham men": malefactors who counterfeited madness in order to beg freely.[22]
Warwickshire justices were informed in 1655 of an Ipsley woman
named Alice Child whose neighbors believed that she was feign-
ing madness, and the case nicely illustrates the importance of community opinion in identifying the insane:

Alice Child . . . pretending herself to be distracted goes peddling up and
down disturbing the peace and is abusive and troublesome to her neighbors . . . Whereupon the advice of the court is desired how to quiet her
and give ease to the people from her abuses which seem to be rather the
actions of one set upon mischief than distracted or lunatic.

The justices appointed one of their number to examine the woman
and determine whether "restraint and correction may do her good
and reduce her into any better order or course of life and be a
means to ease the people of the trouble."[23] No one considered
consulting a specialist to confirm the community view that she
was not actually insane.

Napier's records of the insane conduct of his patients provide
insights into the criteria villagers used to identify acute mental disorders such as madness, distraction, and lunacy. They also show
that those criteria rested upon assumptions about social life and
cosmology that are different from the fundamental beliefs of
Englishmen today. Acutely insane patients, it has already been
said, typically combined three kinds of behavior: They were frantic, talked too much and laughed oddly, and they threatened or
had committed some criminal action. These actions were important because they were evidence pertinent to the two questions
that had to be answered to decide if someone was mad: Did his
behavior violate the rules of good conduct and was the violation
the result of normal thought?

The kinds of crimes perpetrated or threatened were undistinc-
tive: murder, assault, theft, bigamy, bastardy, and begging were

not exotic offenses. But the objects of insane crimes or threats were often unusual. The peculiar nature of much mad crime was that it menaced or destroyed people and property that ought to have been dear to the lunatic. Unreasonable lawbreaking imperiled one's social identity because it attacked the relationships and material objects that situated one in the village community of households and the wider social hierarchy. Such crimes repudiated one's place in the family, destroyed the symbols of social and economic status, and disregarded the conventions of deference and demeanor. The more these acts of social self-destruction were mingled with violence, the more likely they were to be considered signs of the worst forms of mental disorder.

During the seventeenth century the basic garment of social identity was still homespun. The diffusion of individualism had not yet eroded the assumption that every person was before all other considerations the member of a household. To prove that a man was an idiot, one began by showing that he could not name his mother and father. To indicate that a lunatic was insensible, one might note that he did not know his family or "friends." To demonstrate that a melancholy adult's sadness was pathological, one could say that he took no pleasure in his or her spouse or children. Thus the Court of Wards' rules for determining idiocy stipulated that the natural fool should be asked who his parents were.[24] Napier observed that 26 of his clients were so disturbed that they could not recognize their nearest relatives. He wrote of one lunatic, for example, "sayeth that she hath no child nor husband"; and he noted that another frantic woman "knoweth not her own children."[25] Napier also sometimes measured the severity of his patients' gloom by judging their capacity to experience normal enjoyment from their roles as spouses and parents. He reported that one despairing woman "had lost her joy . . . the joy of her marriage, her child and son" and that an unhappy father took "no delight in child or anything."[26]

Because households were hierarchical networks of dominance and submission, another sign of mental abnormality was a patient's failure to acknowledge his superiors. Ellen Hixon was, according to a letter written to Napier, "mopish, apish, foolish, untoward. Will not do anything that her parents bid her, but at her own mind."[27] When William Markes, an Essex man, was charged in an Elizabethan church court for living apart from his wife, he defended himself by answering that she was "a woman many times beside herself and will not be ruled."[28] Napier used the same phrase, "will not be ruled," or near approximations seventy times to describe mentally disturbed behavior. Rose Bateman's decline from melancholy into madness included these symptoms, described to the astrologer by her father: "Was melancholy, now frantic and raging, especially against her father, mother and brother and sisters. Was tempted a year since to do herself harm, but not of late since she was raging. Hath knowledge enough, but will not be ruled by her parents and friends."[29] Rebelliousness was often a token of mental disturbance in the eyes of distressed elders. A young gentleman who raged at his parents, calling them "all to naught," was alleged to suffer from a "strange melancholy."[30] Explaining to Napier that his son's wits had failed him, Philip Hatley's father complained that he "useth outrageous words against mother and father."[31]

The bonds of obedience were tough and enduring. Even if children were adults in their own right and had ample cause to rail against their elders, such defiance might be construed as evidence that they were mentally unbalanced. Ursula Lane (thirty-six years old) was judged light-headed because she would "not pray but curse her husband [and] mother."[32] The symptoms of Thomas Birchmore (twenty-eight) were summarized like this: "Small pox and frenzy. Frantic and unruly about three weeks; cannot abide his mother and his wife."[33] The father of Harry Peach (nineteen) told Napier that his mad son "cryeth out" against his aunt; and Edmund Broughton (twenty-one), who was "distempered in his brains," was reported to "rage against his dearest friends, father and mother."[34] Philip Hatley (thirty-five) and Richard Meadow's son (twenty-one or older) were also believed to be insane because of their hostility toward their parents, even though they had legitimate problems that their parents had caused or refused to alleviate.[35] The customary obligations of deference that children owed their parents did not vanish when they attained their majorities, and women simply exchanged their submission to their parents for obedience to their husbands when they married. Three women Napier treated were called "mad, foolish," "Bedlam mad," and "merry mad" because they treated their husbands with fear, jealousy, and scorn.[36] Although parental authority and patriarchalism were neither absolute nor unchallenged, reverence for the hierarchical bonds between parents and children and husbands and wives was so strong that it shaped popular conceptions of insanity, causing ordinary villagers to identify defiance toward elders and superiors within the family as a sign of madness.

The most heinous crimes in early modern England were violent attacks on kith and kin, and contemporaries were inclined to believe that people who committed them were insane. Women who committed infanticide or child murder seemed mad simply because of the deed's irrational disregard for motherhood, the normal measure of feminine maturity and respectability, unless the victim was illegitimate and hence a talisman of shame.[37] Husbands and wives who attacked their spouses also menaced the relationships that identified them as responsible adults. A Sussex man who axed his wife to death in 1565 was declared insane, "a frantic man," at the assizes. Over a century later Oliver Heywood concluded that a rival clergyman was mad because he "had liked to have killed his wife."[38] Napier and his contemporaries sometimes called men who beat their wives too brutally unreasonable, lightheaded, or brainsick. A Somerset coal miner's wife persuaded the justices to commit her husband to Bridewell because he terrified her with threats and cruelty: "He liveth very idly," the session record reads, "being as she believeth a man distempered in his brain."[39] Alice Maryot's husband told Napier that she had been thrown into Bridewell twice and declared that she was "furious" when she threatened him with a spit; Mary Hanson's husband said that she was "outrageous mad" because she had bit him and ripped his hair out.[40] Violent threats against parents naturally were also likely to be regarded as evidence of insanity. Bitter about his father's continual postponement of his marriage and inheritance, the thirty-year-old George Baker cried out that he would kill him and "master God and do as much as God," behavior that persuaded his mother that he was bewitched and his physician that he was "mad and frantic; mopish, furious and foolish."[41]

Men and women without households and masters were vagrant and pariah; people who attacked members of their households or rebelled against the dominion of their elders therefore repudiated the bonds that fixed them in the social and economic life of the community. The wanton destruction of personal property also often appears as a significant detail in contemporary descriptions of madmen for a similar reason. In addition to meeting specific material needs, possessions articulated one's place in the social hierarchy. Social status in medieval and early modern England was determined at least as much by the prosperity of one's household as it was by ties of blood and marriage.[42] Contemporaries naturally prized material goods, which symbolized high status and wealth. Accounts of the insane destruction caused by madmen call special attention to the demolition of such objects. Breaking windows, for example, was an action frequently mentioned as evidence of insanity during the Great Rebuilding of England between 1570 and 1640. Napier's patients John Collins and Agnes Man were judged mad and lunatic because they broke glasses and windows when they were not restrained.[43] Two accounts of the flagrant insanity of Edmund Francklin emphasized that he had smashed out all the windows in his luxurious house.[44] This apparently odd preoccupation with glass panes is simple to explain: Clear glass was very costly and especially valued during this period as a mark of the prosperity of households climbing up the social ladder.[45]

Nothing signalizes the social rank of a person more plainly than his dress, and Tudor and Stuart observers paid inordinate attention to the clothes – or lack of them – of madmen. Nakedness was included among the symptoms of mania in ancient and medieval times, but early modern Englishmen were uniquely concerned about the expressive possibilities of costume and altered and rehabilitated old ideas about the psychological language of dress.[46] Faced with unprecedented social mobility, sixteenth-century traditionalists reenacted medieval sumptuary laws to regulate the costume of every man and woman so that it conveyed his social rank precisely. These statutes naturally failed to prevent the socially ambitious from masquerading as their betters, and Stuart monarchs gave up the attempt to legislate a hierarchy of dress.[47] The ideal, however, survived; Burton, for example, imagined that in his utopia "the same attire shall be kept and that proper to several callings, by which they shall be distinguished."[48] The Anglican book of homilies and Stubbe's Puritan encyclopedia of contemporary abuses both devoted considerable attention to the neglected decorum of attire.[49] However often it was abused, the social symbolism of dress remained potent, and the Quakers and Ranters provoked violent hatred by refusing to doff their hats and by parading naked in the mid-seventeenth century. Advancements in trade and industry actually heightened awareness of costume in that century by introducing a rich salmagundi of items costly and cheap, foreign and domestic into the English market.[50] Contemporaries devised new conventions that enabled dress to express psychological states as well as rank and occupation. Emblems and portraits, for example, depicted melancholy people in dark and disheveled clothes. "These sad, gloomy people are easily recognised," Roy Strong claims, "for they wander around in black, their clothes untidy and negligent, their arms folded, their hats flopping down over their eyes."[51] Burton accordingly recommended to healers that a depressed client should be neatly dressed, "according to his ability at least . . . for nothing sooner dejects a man than want, squalor, and nastiness, foul or old clothes out of fashion."[52]

Madness stripped men of their reason, the essential accoutrement of humankind, and nakedness was the natural symbol for stark insanity. The image of Lear raging, bare on the heath, has analogues in numerous medieval and early modern descriptions of lunatics.[53] Elizabeth Knot's father told Napier that his daughter tore her dress and "in her mad mood tramped naked on the wet and cold ground."[54] The physician's description of George Katelin repeats the venerable symbolism that equated nakedness and bestiality: "Senseless and beastlike. Senseless since harvest last by fits; and lieth in the straw and will suffer no clothes, but teareth all things and will piss in the chimney corner."[55] The fact that Henry Miller went about bare was evidence worthy to be included with the fear that he was "likely to have killed his father" as proof that he was "Bedlam mad."[56] Many contemporary reports insisted that lunatics disrobed or tore their clothes deliberately and not merely out of anguished negligence. Joan Savage, a mad client of Napier's, "was proud of her clothes and tore them all in pieces." In his wild, mad fits, Christopher Neuman stamped on the ground, talked to himself, saw devils, and, as he grew even worse, "was very outrageous and would tear his clothes."[57] A Lancashire man told justices of the peace in 1661 that his sister "fell distracted and is troubled by a virulent lunacy in which she hath continued pulling herself and her apparel to pieces, to the great danger not only of spoiling herself but to the danger of the neighbours."[58]

Men and women who destroyed their own clothing were irrationally wasteful and socially self-defacing. Apparel was valuable property, which was very expensive to replace, for clothes cost ordinary villagers far more time and trouble than they do today.[59] More important to worried onlookers, madmen who ripped their clothing to shreds repudiated their social pretensions. When John Spencer, an amateur practitioner with a reputation for healing the insane, visited the wealthy lunatic Edmund Francklin, he was dismayed to find the gentleman dressed much below his station: "He was in a slight suit, hardly worth five shillings, like Irish trousers without a band. The hair of his head on both sides being rubbed off . . . and looking so terribly, that he would have terrified a man that was not acquainted with furious objects."[60] Popular writers and playwights costumed Mad Toms and Abraham men in rags; and Napier thought it important to note that 33 of the mentally disturbed patients he treated had reduced their clothes to shreds. The persistent reference to the ruined dress of lunatics, in literary stereotypes and actual descriptions of madmen, seems oddly insignificant unless this detail is understood as a symbolic repetition of essential ideas about insanity. By reducing his apparel to rags, the lunatic repudiated the hierarchical order of his society and declared himself a mental vagrant; by casting away all artificial coverings, he shed all trace of human society. These gestures appeared to normal men and women to be acts of self-destructive violence, a kind of social suicide.

The thread connecting all the kinds of hostility and violence we have been examining is the conviction shared by Napier and his contemporaries that behavior that threatened to destroy the relationships and objects that defined a person's social identity was gravely irrational. The distinction between obviously criminal violence and insane mayhem was that the madman's attacks against people and property were self-destructive: A man alienated from his household and his place in the status hierarchy was socially extinct.

Simpler forms of self-violence were also considered to be evidence of insanity. The jurors who decided that Richard Pudsey was a lunatic in 1652 reported to Chancery that Pudsey recklessly risked his life clambering about on the roof of his house, spoiled his clothes, and cut off his fingers, "saying oftentimes the spirits of the air made him do so."[61] In a similar case, Napier wrote that Ann Smith bit off part of her tongue, "like a Bedlam."[62] Among his mentally disturbed patients generally, 47 had made some self-destructive gesture, 46 had attempted suicide, and 9 had hurt or mutilated themselves. The belief that self-destructive behavior was evidence of insanity, however, paradoxically excluded its most obvious manifestation, suicide. Thus, although Napier treated 158 patients who were tempted to kill themselves, none of them was classified as mad or lunatic and only one was described as distracted (Table 4.2). Suicide was incompatible with severe insanity. A digression to consider this anomaly will illustrate the complex relationship between secular stereotypes of insanity and religious and legal traditions, a theme that will be touched on again later in this chapter.

MADNESS AND SUICIDE

Suicide was a civil and religious crime in Tudor and Stuart England, and custom and criminal law dictated penalties to be exacted from the deceased and his survivors that seem savage to our minds. The seriousness of the act called for condign punishment. Suicides were denied funerals and burial in the churchyard, the rites that marked the transmigration of Christian souls into the afterlife and membership in the community of the dead. Interred hugger-mugger at a crossroads, the body was pinioned through the heart with a wooden stake. The dead man was tried posthumously: A coroner's jury assembled from local men declared him a felon, a murderer, and his movable goods were forfeited to the king's almoner. These penalties expressed a genuine and ancient conviction that suicide was abhorrent. Confiscation of the suicide's goods was encouraged by offering royal officials a portion of the spoils that they secured for the crown, a procedure that was routine in all felony cases. Desperate families were concerned to avoid the stigma that attached to suicide as well as to escape financial hardship, and they sometimes made pathetic attempts to conceal and deny the suicides of their loved ones.[63] The prohibition against the Christian burial of suicides seems to have been widely observed.[64]

The rigors of the penalties for suicide and the occasionally determined efforts to circumvent them show that juries did not return verdicts of *felo-de-se* lightly.[65] The abhorrence of the crime and the machinery of royal confiscation pressured them to certify that ambiguous deaths were suicides; sympathy for the damage done to the reputations and fortunes of the survivors compelled them to find means to avoid such verdicts. Moreover, the stereotype of suicide itself presented them with complexities that were frequently irresolvable. Legal thought and popular belief insisted that suicide was self-murder, a conscious and premeditated act committed by a fully rational criminal. "Homicide," wrote Edmund Wingate in his handbook for local justices of the peace, "may be in a *felo de se* or another . . . He is *felo de se* that doth destroy himself out of premeditated hatred against his own life or out of a humour to destroy himself."[66] Because suicide was a species of murder, the perpetrator was not guilty if he killed himself when he was too young or too mad to be aware that his act was wrong. Dalton's earlier *vade mecum* for magistrates put it this way: "If one that wanteth discretion killeth himself (as an infant or a man *non compos mentis*) he shall not forfeit his goods, etc."[67] Finding out what the state of mind of a criminal was when he broke the law is difficult; reconstructing the thoughts of a dead man is still harder. Few Tudor and Stuart suicides could have left notes, for most of the people who killed themselves were poor and probably illiterate. The scanty occupational evidence and the listings of goods included in the inquests for the suicides from Napier's region suggest that about half of them were propertyless peasants and laborers.[68] Juries were forced to rely on indirect testimony about the character and behavior of putative suicides to establish premeditation.[69]

Traditional religious beliefs reinforced the view that suicides were fully rational criminals. The medieval insistence that suicidal behavior signalized an alienation from God was sustained by clergymen and the vast majority of laymen in the late sixteenth and early seventeenth centuries. Self-murderers are portrayed in a diverse array of sources as people who had turned away from God and yielded to the temptations of the Fiend. This view is implicit in the formal language of coroners' inquisitions, in the depositions and charges presented in Star Chamber suits, in the confessions of spiritual autobiographers, and in the explanations that Napier's patients gave for their suicidal emotions. The Latin formula adhered to in coroners' inquisitions asserted that suicide was committed "at the instigation of the Devil," and although the phrase was standard and was employed in documents about other felonies as well, it was still meaningful in the seventeenth century.[70]

The resolution to kill oneself was routinely equated with the temptation to despair of God's mercy and to abandon all hope of salvation. Napier remarked that fifteen of his patients who were suffering from suicidal compulsions were also tempted to despair of their salvation. Other self-destructive clients actually saw the Tempter. Elisabeth Hayford, for instance, declared that she "cannot be saved, so the Devil tells her. As she sayeth, look where the Devil stands. Will weep much."[71] Robert Toe thought that a "black boy" from whom he bought a knife was actually Satan dissembling; Guiles Southan thought that everything he saw was Satan.[72] Napier believed Robert Lea when the desperate man told him: "It will speak often to him and appear in the likeness of a man, and to kill him, and would draw him away."[73] Sadly noting that Alice Savil had killed herself, the physician recalled: "She said that the Lord had forsaken her and drowned herself." When Joan Kent fell into a self-destructive mood, she warned him with the same literal metaphor, saying that she could not "refuse Satan longer."[74] Such language was not peculiar to Napier's clients. Recording a suicide in 1607, the minister of Terling, Essex, wrote in the parish register: "God grant we may never forsake Christ and fall to the world." Similarly, the curate of Aldgate in London noted in his register that a coroner's jury found in 1590 that "falling from God," one Amy Stokes, "had hanged or murdered herself."[75]

The popular imagination personified evil in the form of Satan, and it attributed the unaccceptable thoughts that accompanied emotional misery to the machinations of the Fiend. Napier's patients appear often to have believed that they embodied both a good spirit, associated with happiness, normality, and piety, and an evil spirit, associated with unhappiness, suicidal despair, and apostasy. Visions of Satan or the urgent conviction that one was haunted by demons were not taken to be sure signs of severe psychosis during the seventeenth century, and we should not dismiss them merely as the delusions of addled minds. Belief in the devil's immanence, his protean craftiness, and his responsibility for the dark, antisocial urges that entered men's minds was general. Conventions everybody accepted gave a shape and name to the despairing temptations of miserable men and women: Their visions embody a universal belief that despair was devilish.[76]

The traditional legal and religious stereotype of suicide provided a precise definition of the act as deliberate self-murder and apostasy and condemned it as a crime and a sin. Contemporaries were nevertheless often confused by the problem of distinguishing between insane acts of despair and self-destruction and true suicide.[77] Such confusion arose because legal ideas about suicide, although logical enough in themselves, did not stipulate how to tell if a person was mad when he killed himself. Juries relied on a mixture of medical psychology and popular wisdom to identify lunatics. But doctors' notions about the connection between the varieties of mental disorder and suicide were inconsistent; and when they were interpreted by laymen, they were further refracted and distorted by common opinion.

Melancholy became a badge of fashion during the late sixteenth and seventeenth centuries, and the fascination with this classical malady fostered the belief that suicidal behavior was a sign of mental illness, rather than a religious crime. Medical writers stressed the connection between melancholy and suicide. Burton, the best and most popular among them, wrote that melancholy men and women often slew themselves: "Hence it proceeds many times that they are weary of their lives, and feral thoughts to offer violence to their own persons come into their minds."[78] Discussing the prognosis of the disease, Burton adds: "Seldom this malady procures death except (which is the greatest, most grievous calamity, and the misery of all miseries) they make themselves away."[79] The link between melancholy and suicide soon became familiar to ordinary laymen. As any reader of Elizabethan and Jacobean drama knows, melancholy characters like Hamlet often pondered, and sometimes committed, suicide.[80] The idea that suicide was an outcome of melancholy illness is reflected in Napier's case notes as well: 5.5% of his melancholy patients were contemplating suicide, as were 7.8% of his clients who suffered from the less specific ailment, "troubled in mind."[81]

These views might have been reconciled with legal and religious ideas about suicide if a rigorous distinction between severe insanity and lesser mental disorders had been maintained. Acute mental disorders shattered the victim's reason and so were incompatible with suicide. Melancholy and anxiety disorders affected the emotions and weakened the sufferer's resistance to suicidal temptations but did not ruin his understanding. Thus the victims of these milder forms of insanity could be said to commit suicide without contradicting the traditional stereotype. Napier did make just this distinction. We have already seen that only one of his 158 suicidal patients was classified as mad, lunatic, or distracted; in contrast, 27 of them were melancholy and 62 were troubled in mind. If one examines the symptoms associated with suicidal thoughts more closely, one finds that they were never linked with violent behavior toward others and that suicidal patients were much less likely to show signs that their sense perceptions and understanding were impaired than typical disturbed clients. The most striking feature of the symptoms consistent with suicide is the frequency with which religious anxiety and despair were added to the other signs of sadness and despondency and the frequency with which self-destructive thoughts were attributed to the Devil or to other evil spirits. Napier therefore succeeded in integrating medical psychology with the traditional stereotype of suicide shared by himself and his patients.[82]

Napier's logical reconciliation of the potential conflict between the medical and religious interpretations of suicide was not generally observed. Medieval medical writings and literary works had presented suicide as one indication of madness or mania.[83] The notion that people who committed suicide or who tried to do so were mad can be found in the comments of seventeenth-century writers as well. Perhaps the best example is John Aubrey's remarks about the death in battle of Lucius Cary, Viscount Falkland. Aubrey thought that Falkland had killed himself with madly dangerous behavior, a suicide motivated by grief because of his mistress's death:

At the fight at Newberry my lord Falkland . . . as the two armies were engaging, rode like a madman (as he was) between them, and he was (as he needs must be) shot. Some . . . would needs have the reason of this mad action of throwing away his life so, to be his discontent for the unfortunate advice given to his master [King Charles] . . . , but I have been well informed by those who best knew him and knew intrigues behind the curtain (as they say) that it was grief of the death of Mistress Moray . . . his mistress, and whom he loved above all creatures was the sure cause of his being so madly guilty of his own death.[84]

Burton himself wrote that when mad or melancholy people kill themselves, they should not be censured as suicides must be: "In some cases those hard censures of such as offer violence to their own persons . . . are mitigated, as in such as mad, besides themselves for the time, or found to have been long melancholy, and that in extremity; they know not what they do, deprived of all reason, judgment, all, as a ship that is void of a pilot must needs impinge upon the next rock or sands, and suffer shipwreck."[85]

The problem faced by juries when they tried to decide whether a self-killer was non compos mentis, and hence an innocent luna-tic, or *felo-de-se*, and hence a guilty sinner, epitomized the difficul-ties faced by laymen in assessing the significance of the behavior of all potential madmen. Until the act of suicide in itself came to be regarded as sufficient evidence of insanity, an eighteenth-century development, jurors had to consider testimony about the victim's state of mind just before his death to decide if his act had been rational. The best evidence we have about how these judgments were made comes from Star Chamber actions disputing the causes of death of putative suicides. The crown, anxious to confiscate the victim's goods, typically argued that he had formed a deliberate plan to kill himself. John Stoner, for example, was alleged to have acted "desperately minded and having as it seemed by the sequel a purpose and full resolution . . to destroy himself and make him-self away."[86] Occasionally the crown itself asserted that the de-ceased was melancholy or troubled in mind prior to his death, but in such cases evidence that he had formed a plan to kill himself was presented and the religious sanctions against suicide were invoked in the language of the bill. Thus a London merchant named Lance-lot Johnson was said to have been "observed to walk in a very sad, deep, melancholy and discontented manner along the river's side, there where he had no other occasion to be, but only to execute his said ungodly resolution" to drown himself in the Thames. Evi-dence that the melancholy Johnson had fully premeditated his "discontented and ungodly purpose" was also presented: He had left behind a note, which his wife destroyed, "containing the rea-sons and causes of his discontentment and purpose to destroy him-self," and he made "desperate speeches" indicating that he was troubled in mind about his business losses and debts.[87]

There were two lines of defense against such charges. Kinsmen could argue either that the death was an accident, countering the crown's circumstantial evidence with claims that the deceased's character was inconsistent with the desperate godlessness of the stereotypical suicide, or they could admit that the death was self-inflicted, answering the crown's case with a claim that the victim was mad at the time of his demise. Ellen Johnson asserted that her husband, Lancelot, was too pious to have committed so ungodly an act as suicide. He had made no "desperate or ungodly speeches" and had attended church regularly. "He lived in good repute and esteem amongst his neighbours and acquaintances and also carried himself in an exceeding honest, upright, godly fashion both abroad and amongst his children and family . . . and never given to any ungodly or unreligious course . . . and hath gone through all the offices in the parish where he lived and died, churchwarden."[88] The other possible defense, that the deceased had been non compos mentis, was more difficult to prove. A defendant in the suit concerning George Copwood relied upon the common knowledge that people with fevers frequently became delirious to make his claims plausible. Copwood, he maintained, "by reason of great want of sleep and other distempers of the body . . . was become non compos mentis and overcome with frenzy or lunacy."[89] In a more complex case, the crown argued that Arthur Peirce, an admitted lunatic, had not been mad at the time of his death. According to testimony, which appears to have come from one or more servants of dubious loyalty, Peirce was wont to walk to the market from time to time to buy necessities and was fussy about his diet. His capacity to buy goods "orderly and carefully for his profit" and his concern about his food were construed to prove that he was capable of acting "as a man of sense and reason" and that he was mindful of his bodily needs, "as a man of sense."[90] His brother answered that Peirce had been capable of speaking "some words which might seem to be sensible" very rarely, but that on the other hand he sometimes had to be bound up because of his "unruly and mad disposition." He admitted that his brother had once gone to town to buy some cloth, but he claimed that this was a unique episode of economic rationality.[91]

PROOFS OF LUNACY

The distinction between rational suicide and insane self-destruction implicit in traditional legal and religious ideas about suicide compelled jurors and survivors to reexamine the victim's words and actions in an attempt to establish his sanity or insanity at the time of his death. Although the act of suicide was the most extreme form of self-destructive behavior possible, it could not be considered insane unless defendants could prove that the man or woman who committed it showed some other sign of mental alienation. A very similar pattern of thought is implicit in descriptions of people who committed other harmful actions. The law and popular opinion demanded that people who threatened or perpetrated crimes – even the kind of pointless and self-destructive crimes characteristic of the insane – must also exhibit some other evidence of madness before they earned the protective cloak of lunacy. It was necessary to prove that the putative lunatic's actions were caused by ungovernable passion. The substantiating proofs of insanity mentioned most often by Napier and his clients were frantic energy, fits of wildly inappropriate laughter or rage, restless wandering or aimless running, and titanic physical strength. To anxious observers, such behavior was an outward manifestation of the chaotic power of a mind in which the rule of reason had been overthrown by the anarchic force of the passions.

Nicholas Culpeper wrote in his medical guide for laymen that the signs of madness or fury were various: "Sometimes laughing, sighing, then sad, fearful, rash, doting, crying out, threatening, skipping, leaping, then serious, etc."[92] Napier's mad, lunatic, and distracted patients displayed all of these symptoms of frantic insanity. Their moods could be changeable as quicksilver and they noisily expressed them in weird laughter, horrible screams, continual babbling, and furious raving. Laughter was the special token of antic madness. The lunatic William Cras did nothing except "laugh, leap and hallow."[93] Eleanor Ashton's case illustrates the distinctive nature of irrational merriment; it was a predicate without a subject, and nobody could tell why afflicted people laughed, not even they themselves: "Will fall into a strange laughing every foot and can give no reason of it."[94] Sometimes these fits of giggling alternated with terror or anger, as Culpeper remarks. Master John Browne, for example, would "laugh and clap his hands upon his face and at other times will be sullen and mopish."[95] Sibyl Fisher's malady was described like this: "By fits will laugh and be merry, and anon after will cry out that she is damned."[96] The "merry mad" William Iremonger oscillated between bouts of laughing and fighting; and Mistress Jane Turney, who whooped with laughter as she tore up everything in sight, showed "no sense, reason, nor understanding at all, but is like a frantic."[97] Even when they were not laughing, madmen made frightening noises. Joan Perkins, who was a lunatic, excelled all normal bounds both in volume and endurance, crying out "Christ Jesus, have mercy on me!" day and night for a whole year.[98] Others among Napier's clients, like Elizabeth Hurrell, cursed and talked incessantly.[99] The lunatic Adam Grave displayed every kind of uncontrolled emotion, save merriment. He had three kinds of fits: "sometimes in quarreling fits, sometimes in mopish fits and most in talking fits."[100]

Fits of rage terrified observers far more than strange laughter and wild moodiness. John Archer remarked that the sort of madness that made men furious and raging was the worst to cure, a statement that sounds more like the genuine distillation of his experience as a healer than his usual platitudes.[101] The Latin tag *Ira furor brevis est* had been transmuted into an English proverb early in the sixteenth century: William Wager paraphrased it as "wrath and madness they say be all one."[102] John Downame, who wrote a whole treatise about the ill effects of anger, agreed and was a more exact Latinist: "Anger is called *Brevis furor*, a short madness, because it differs not but in time. Saving that herein it is far worse: in that he who is possessed with madness is necessarily, will he, nill he, subject to that fury; but this passion is entered into wittingly and willingly."[103] Many of Napier's clients were, like Master Robert Hustwate, maddened or distracted by rage. Here is how the astrologer described Hustwate's case: "From anger grew to a rage. Feared the loss of his senses, finding that by anger he was grown into a raging fit."[104] The proportion of mad patients who were reported to have been raging was higher than the 3.7% that was the symptom's allotment in all the consultations for mental disorder: Mad and lunatic patients raged in 14.6% of their consultations, distracted people in 11.9% (Table 4.2).

The behavior of the insane seemed to observers to be a pantomime of unchecked passion. Lunatics often roamed around like Lear loose on the heath. Three of the clients John Smith claimed to have cured of lunacy early in the seventeenth century were reported to have gone "wandering up and down the country and fields" when they were mad; and another, more ominously, was given to "hunting up and down in the woods."[105] An acutely disturbed patient of Napier's epitomized the wandering passion: "Will wander up and down and did once go into the wood and lived in the wood three days and three nights without any food. Was at the first outrageous. Knoweth everybody, but his sole delight in wandering . . . Six years before did wander, but mended."[106] This portrait of William Akens contains all the images embraced by the theme of wandering in miniature. Directionless as countless allegorical sinners, he roams for three days and nights in a wood. The number and the place are replete with magical associations and identify Akens with the holy wild men of medieval legend, the love-crazed youths in festive comedies such as *As You Like It* and *Midsummer Night's Dream*, and the menacing figures of vagabonds and outlaws who shared with madmen lives outside the normal limits of social convention.[107] Aimless wandering was mentioned in 43 consultations recorded by Napier, 9 of them with patients who were mad, lunatic, or distracted.

Insane people who carried the pantomime of undirected passion further and added chaotic rage to their aimlessness, struggling wildly or striking out at others, were utterly intolerable. Anxious Lancashire authorities in 1668, for example, were concerned about tracking down a woman who, they said, "hath lately pulled out one of her eyes and is wandering about and offers violence to her own children."[108] These were the lunatics whom contemporaries bound up in chains, a measure ordinarily dictated by apprehension rather than cruelty. Terror pervades the descriptions of such people, and men firmly believed that their madness made them extraordinarily strong: "Raging mad and so strong in his fits that none can hold him," Napier wrote of John Baker.[109] Sibyl Fisher's family tied her up hand and foot because, they said, "when she is loose she is so strong that they cannot deal with her."[110] The wife of Thomas Bassington told Napier that he was, "lunatic . . . and rageth and talketh and will strive with three that hold him down."[111] Even restraint did not quell the alarm felt by the neighbors of another Lancashire lunatic: "Hath fallen by God's judgment and visitation into a lunatic frenzy and distraction of his wits and senses – he lying bound in chains and feathers [*sic*] – every-[one] of the neighbours fearful to come near unto him."[112] English villages afforded little privacy and no security. A violent lunatic was a terrifying threat to everyone's safety, and there was seldom a place to lodge a dangerous madman. A seventeenth-century proverb warned: "Take heed of mad folks in a narrow place."[113] The horrors of Bedlam can easily mislead us into believing that contemporaries normally treated the insane sadistically. Chains and fetters were reserved for the most violent and menacing mad-

men, people who terrified their families and neighbors. The man-
acled lunatic was not a sign of the cruelty and stupidity of ordinary
villagers; he was an emblem of their fear.

An image of the popular conception of one of the most severe
types of insanity, the condition Napier labeled madness, lunacy,
and distraction, is reflected in these tales of violence and passion.
English laymen thought that the stark, Bedlam madman was dangerous, inclined to murder and assault, arson and vandalism. Unlike a criminal, however, he could reap no conceivable benefit
from his violence, because he threatened or attacked people and
property that were essential aspects of his own social identity.
Moreover, his behavior and moods suggested that he was helpless
to govern the wild energy of his passions. The chaotic intensity of
his actions set him apart from other people. Sane men and women
were extremely violent by modern standards. They often flogged
their subordinates, especially servants and children. Normal violence, however, was constrained by the conventions of hierarchy
and self-interest, confined to particular social situations, and inflicted upon persons of lesser social rank. Madmen terrified even
the roughest Elizabethans precisely because they were oblivious to
these conventions of family life, social esteem, and deference,
rules that made normal violence predictable and comprehensible.

INSANITY AND DELIRIUM

Seventeenth-century laymen recognized another type of insanity
that ruined its victims' ability to reason and communicate as effectively as madness and lunacy. The distinctive feature of this disorder was verbal pandemonium. Napier called the people who suffered from severe mental alienation and babbled rapidly and
incoherently *distracted* or *light-headed*. Neither of these terms identified this stereotype of insanity precisely. Patients who were classified as distracted were sometimes violent like madmen and lunatics; clients who were said to be light-headed sometimes suffered
from simple vertigo. Nevertheless, distracted and light-headed
patients who talked "idly" were often identified with a coherent
set of symptoms that emphasized the similarity between their sufferings and the delirium that accompanied mortal illnesses.

The friends and relatives of distracted and light-headed people
frequently compared the urgent energy and apparent randomness

of their ravings with delirium. They supposed that like the victims of mortal fevers these insane people were seized by a disease that destroyed their capacity to control or even to understand their own words. Napier made this comparison often, and he remarked that some of his patients were unaware of what they said.[114] Similarly, the clergyman who wrote the preface to Dionys Fitzhue's autobiographical account of her mental disintegration reassured her that the Satanic words and ideas she uttered when she was insane "were no . . . more I think to be accounted yours than the speeches of those that in burning fevers and other such violent diseases speak idly, they know not what."[115]

The men and women who reported the demented ravings of their relatives to Napier sometimes claimed that their speech was nonsense. Thus Mistress Katherine Tyler was said to repeat the same words over and over, no matter what the occasion; Joan Morgan seemed to speak "at random"; Faith Harbart discoursed "without reason"; and Francis Adams and Widow Lovet turned every speech into riddles and rhymes.[116] But Napier's paraphrases and occasional quotations of the actual words that insane people spoke show that there was frequently a coherent message in the sufferers' broken speech. Their language communicated an anguished conviction that the emotional torment of insanity was the same as the agony of mortal illness, and their families responded by treating them as the innocent victims of sickness. They were permitted freely to express normally unacceptable ideas, and they became the center of solicitous attention. This unconscious communication between the insane and their relatives was based upon ideas and conventions that were so familiar that people responded to them without realizing that they had deciphered the mad babble and responded to it.

Perhaps the nature of this exchange will be clarified by an analogy. When we read Lewis Carroll's famous poem "Jabberwocky," it seems at first to be amusing nonsense. If we are prodded into reflecting further on the poem and our reaction to it, we realize that it is funny because it uses familiar conventions in a nonsensical way. Carroll employs language that grafts familiar roots and stems into unfamiliar combinations, and he arranges his jabberwocky into mock heroic meter. The result, a poem that has no literal meaning, is perceived as a parody of heroic verse in the grand manner, and a reader well acquainted with the conventions of English verse will laugh before he is fully aware of the way the poem works. The communication between Napier's insane patients and their relatives happened similarly. The sufferers used language and intonation that invoked a set of symbols and ideas so much a part of the popular mentality that their families repeatedly interpreted their ravings in the same way, although they insisted that what they had heard was "idle talk."

The language of the inner life that most men spoke had a rough and limited vocabulary made up largely of elementary Christian and demonic lore. The allegorical struggle between the figures of good and evil in popular medieval morality plays persisted in the common mind as the conventional representation of emotional turmoil.[117] Several of Napier's patients said that they embodied a good spirit and a bad and indicated their feelings of hopelessness by telling him that their good angel had been vanquished.[118] Mentally disturbed men and women expressed the extremity of their suffering by crying out to God or screaming about the Devil. Alice Harvey "would always call upon God"; and Isabel Hodell fell down in a fright "saying Jesus bless me."[119] They were just 2 of Napier's 23 clients who invoked the Lord's help loudly and insistently. The common thought that these and other insane people had in mind was the terror of impending judgment. Goodwife Rose cried out that "Satan will have her and burns her in hell."[120] Others, such as Joan Simpson and Mistress Jane Kelly, were obsessed by the Fiend's approach.[121] Thomas Richardson's wife, Thomas Stiles, and Alice Godfrey all talked about the Devil incessantly.[122] Stiles's fantastical assertions that the "Devil doth no man harm" might have been interpreted as an effort to reassure himself that he would overcome the forces of death and damnation, as could William Athew's oath that "no ill thing should prevail against him" and Mistress Franklin's distracted claim that she had "beaten down twenty devils and twenty witches,"[123] Recalling his episode of insanity during the Interregnum, George Trosse described his thoughts and feelings like this:

At which desperate madness of mine it seemed to me that all were astonished; and I fancied that every step I stepped afterwards, I was making a progress into the depths of hell . . . Whatever noises I heard as I passed by, my fancy gave them hellish interpretations. For I was now persuaded that I was no longer upon earth, but in the regions of hell. When we came to the town, I thought I was in the midst of hell: every house that we passed by was as it were a mansion in hell; . . . and as we went forward, methought, their torments increased; and I fancied I heard some say, as they stood at their doors with great wonder, and somewhat of pity, "What, must he go yet farther into hell? O fearful! O dreadful!" and the like.

At last, by God's good providence we were brought safely to the physician's house. Methought all about me were devils, and he was Beelzebub. I was taken off my horse, and expected immediately to be cast into intolerable flames and burnings, which seemed to be before mine eyes.[124]

Popular religious beliefs spanned the chasm of incomprehension that lay between the insane and their observers. Although literally incoherent, their thoughts and words conveyed an understandable idea that observers grasped without even being aware of it. That idea was simple: Their anguish was like the pangs of death; the peril of damnation was terrifyingly near.

The fascination ordinary men and women had about acute insanity was stimulated by the fact that it seemed to be a state of mind with only one analogue in common experience, the delirium that attended desperate fevers and usually signaled certain death. Describing how her sister died soon after childbirth, Alice Thornton suggests the extremity of her suffering by pointing out that she lost "part of the use of her understanding" just before she perished.[125] Elias Ashmole noted in his diary a fever that had brought him near to death and made him "raging mad and senseless."[126] As a result of being wounded in the head in a wild brawl in 1580, a Sussex man, according to an assize indictment, "became insane" and then died.[127] In the course of an intricate controversy about the efficacy of the sacraments, Bishop Jewel also repeated the belief that insanity was often a sign of mortal illness. He argued that the authority of the ancient church proved that "if a man, standing excommunicate, had happened to be bereft of his senses, and being in that case had been likely to depart this life, upon proof of his former repentance he should be restored, that he might depart in peace as a member of the church of God."[128] Lunacy was actually listed as a cause of the death in the London Bills of Mortality. John Graunt observed that there were 158 such deaths recorded in the early seventeenth-century bills he studied and commented: "I fear many more than are set down in our Bills, few being entered for such, but those who die at Bedlam, and there all seem to die of their lunacy."[129] Graunt implies that the searchers of the dead did not adequately distinguish between those who died of fevers and other diseases and those who were killed by their madness. He was certainly right to believe that many people found it difficult to tell the difference between the symptoms of mortal illness and true insanity.

Medical thought, which might have been expected to provide some means for helping laymen to make such discriminations, insisted on the contrary that their outward signs were virtually the same. The classical doctrine repeated by popular English treatises asserted that insanity (mania) differed from delirium (frenzy) in only one respect: Maniacs were not feverish. Thus Burton wrote: "Madness is . . . defined to be a vehement dotage, or raving without a fever, far more violent than melancholy . . . Differing only in this from frenzy, that it is without a fever, and their memory is most part better."[130] The influence of such books was enormous, and they nurtured the popular equation of insanity and death. Consider, for example, Oliver Heywood's observations about the sudden demise of three young people in his neighborhood:

I had a sad object, Mistress Elizabeth Rhodes . . . distracted by a fever or frenzy seizing on her. She spoke much, yet in due time the Lord heard prayers for her recovery . . . But her own cousin, Lady Margaret, [began] . . . to be in the like manner yet more raging, and in a fortnight's time died . . . About the same time . . . a godly young man of our society . . . one Joshua Bates, fell into a kind of frenzy . . . [He] was under deliriation. At last it grew to a perfect distraction, that four men had much ado to hold him. He was bound, raved, raged, in a formidable manner, made rhymes, yea (which was sad) Satan used his tongue to swear many dreadful oaths, which he never did in all his life . . . In the morning I went to see him, he was a sad object . . . That evening at ten o'clock he died.[131]

Perplexed laymen often sought the help of physicians and astrologers to find out if the wild ravings of their kinsmen were the harbinger of sudden death or stark madness. James Burser's "friends" consulted Napier because they were "desirous to know whether he will live or no." They had given him up for dead once, and the mourning bell had been rung: "Cryeth out of his former life; talketh of devils; sweareth; idle talk. Distracted and much distempered. Had an ague and hath been since let blood. Talketh wisely until the fit cometh on him."[132] The seriousness of a patient's disease might even be measured by comparison with the symptoms of insanity: "Extreme sick," Napier once wrote of Thomas Page, "like a distracted man. Calleth out on devils, raging, catching and pulling . . . Mind very much troubled; speaketh a little."[133]

Seventeenth-century physicians did not have an accurate means to determine a patient's temperature, and in the absence of any diagnostic techniques that might have allowed them to make sure discriminations, vehement insanity and desperate illness blended together even in medical practice. Ordinary men and women regarded the insane with anxious awe. Already alienated from the everyday world of thought and action, distracted, witless people seemed to be held poised between providential recovery and certain death. A consequence of their ambiguous existence was that they were treated with the tolerance and concern normally reserved for the dangerously ill. Their blasphemies were pitied and excused; anxious families searched out healers in an attempt to find some remedy for their condition. The "myth of mental illness" is not a modern invention, the creation of a "therapeutic state." The idea that insanity is an illness was a natural truth to seventeenth-century laymen, and even the religious language of extreme suffering encouraged them to believe that the insane were sick. That is why physicians were asked to minister to mad and troubled minds.

The preoccupation of Renaissance writers with unreason has caused some modern historians to idealize the concept of madness in early modern society. Lunatics were not treated with superstitious reverence; nor was their privileged legal status the result of a belief that they were goofy sages, ever ready to utter a profundity. Imaginative writers were attracted by the immense satiric and ironic potential of contemporary stereotypes of madness and folly. Lunatics and fools were living tropes, simultaneously man and beast, social creature and natural, "unaccommodated" humanity. Real madmen were terrifying and disgusting, impossible to control and oblivious to the rules of normal violence. Their behavior imperiled the fundamental principles of social life: household and hierarchy. The idle speech of raving lunatics was mystical in a sense, for like the delirious utterances of dying men and women it was spoken by people nearer the unseen world than we, but it held no peculiar authority. Many censorious things may be said about the way lunatics were treated, but if anachronisms are avoided, it appears from contemporary records that the ordinary understanding of insanity resembled Lear's tormented recognition of both Mad Tom's degradation and his humanity: "Thou wert better in a grave than to answer with thy uncovered body this extremity of the skies. Is a man no more than this? Consider him well. Thou ow'st the worm no silk, the beast no hide, the sheep no wool, the cat no perfume . . . Thou art the thing itself, unaccommodated man is no more but such a poor, bare, forked animal as thou art."[134]

DISORDERS OF MOOD AND PERCEPTION

Shakespeare's contemporaries were fascinated by the idea of madness, but when the literary spell was broken by confrontations with real lunatics, they acknowledged that severe insanity was a rare and awesome calamity. During the forty years Napier practiced medicine, fewer than thirty men and women from Bedfordshire, Buckinghamshire, and Northamptonshire were certified as lunatics by the Court of Wards. Although the court undertook the guardianship of some people of middling status and small means, there were certainly more than thirty lunatics in the region.[135] Some wealthy madmen must have been kept privately by their families; more pauper lunatics must have been maintained by their parishes. The disappearance of the quarter sessions records for this period prevents an accurate estimate of the true incidence even of publicly recognized insanity. Nevertheless, it is plain that extravagant mental disorders were comparatively rare. There were at least 200,000 villagers in the three chief counties in Napier's practice.[136] If one adds all the mad, lunatic, and distracted people he treated to the number made royal wards, the total becomes only 6 cases per year for the whole area. Even if the real rate were three or four times that number, one would have to conclude that madness was not a common phenomenon. Moreover, the severely insane were only a small minority among Napier's mentally disturbed clients: Madmen and lunatics together were only 5.5% of the total; those patients and the distracted ones together were just 10.3% of the disturbed, around 8 cases a year. The most familiar forms of mental disorder were afflictions of mood and perception, and these lesser maladies were very common indeed.

Social critics of every persuasion believed that emotional suffering was epidemical by the end of the sixteenth century. The pessimist Godfrey Goodman insisted that everything in nature was decaying and that in corrupt sympathy the minds of modern men were tormented by grief, sorrow, and suicidal gloom. Joseph Hall, the "English Seneca," remarked that everybody knew of men who had committed suicide or been driven out of their minds by grief or disease. "How many millions," he asked hyperbolically, "what for incurable maladies, what for losses, what for defamations, what for accidents to their children, rub out their lives in perpetual discontentment, therefore living, because they cannot yet die, not for that they like to live?"[137] The anatomist of melancholy naturally felt that malady was more common in his age than in any previous period.[138] These worried intellectuals may have been right. We know that almost two out of three of the settlements in Napier's region housed someone who was sufficiently mentally troubled to seek his help, even though there were many other physicians, clergymen, and magicians in the area.

There is, therefore, plenty of evidence that Englishmen were more aware of mental suffering after 1580 than they ever had been before; and only a small amount of the anguish they were discovering was madness. What were the shapes that the other afflictions of the mind assumed? They appeared to be almost as various as the silhouettes that Hamlet's fancy found in clouds. Melancholy, of course, but also mopishness, anxiety and fear, sadness and suicidal gloom, just to mention the most common complaints brought to Napier. Whatever discrete forms were attributed to these maladies, they were all feelings or ideas that were believed to be excessive or evil. They were also detected differently than madness or delirium. Sufferers *themselves* frequently judged that their emotions were abnormal. Lunatics, on the other hand, were unable to scrutinize their own behavior and decide whether or not they were sane.

Most of the lesser mental disorders were emotional disturbances. Contemporaries believed that the feelings experienced by melancholy and troubled people were exaggerations of normal states of mind. The sheer intensity of their moods was abnormal. Summarizing conventional opinion, Burton characterized the emotional signs of melancholy like this: "The symptoms of the mind are superfluous and continual cogitations . . . They [melancholy people] have grievous passions, and immoderate perturbations of the mind, fear, sorrow, etc."[139] Neo-Stoics and faculty psychologists believed that inappropriate or excessive passions were the cause and character of insanity. Hamlet's grief, Othello's jealousy, and Lear's rage dramatized this popular assumption.[140] Many of the 717 patients Napier called troubled in mind suffered from some excessive emotion, which was often an overreaction to an everyday problem. The range of these feelings was so various that clients who were troubled in mind had nothing else in common. They complained most frequently that they were sleepless, fearful (anxious), light-headed, suicidal, or concerned about religion, but the victims of other disorders suffered from all these problems more often. In Napier's lexicon of unhappiness the concept "troubled in mind" illustrates the prevailing view that every person harbored passions that could overthrow the balance of his mind if they were aroused to too high a pitch. On the other hand, contemporaries recognized that there were other types of mental disorder that were distinctively different from normal states of mind because their victims suffered from delusions or false perceptions. Two of them, melancholy and mopishness, were common among Napier's patients.

MELANCHOLY: "THE CREST OF COURTIERS' ARMS"

Melancholy was a la mode in Jacobean England, and the rage for this fashionable affliction popularized medical ideas about emotional distress. Lay interest in melancholy was one consequence of the educated elite's fascination with the literature and learning of the ancient world. Writers all over Western Europe composed vernacular treatises about melancholy in the late sixteenth century, most of them medleys of stories and lore from a few classical texts. Translations of books by the Spaniard Huarte, the Frenchmen du Laurens and Charron, and the Dutchman Lemnius appeared in England. In 1586 Timothy Bright composed an original work in English to console a melancholy friend and reached a multitude of readers: The first edition of the book disappeared within six months and it was reprinted in 1613. Robert Burton wrote the most ambitious treatment of them all and the most popular. Burton enriched the familiar recipe with a myriad of ancient and foreign ingredients and concocted an infusion so suited to native tastes that he became one of the most widely read authors of the age.[141]

Bright and Burton taught educated men and women to speak the language of classical medicine. Literary scholars have anatomized and anthologized their influence on playwrights and poets; and one has only to think of Hamlet and Jaques, any work by Marston, or Jonson's plays about characters in and out of humor to appreciate the popularity of the theme. Melancholy and gentility became boon companions. Noblemen delighted to have themselves painted in the guise of melancholy lovers; and courtly poets scribbled verses that could have been used to caption them. When a lowly barber in Lyly's *Midas* complains that he is "melancholy as a cat" he is chided for his social pretensions: "Melancholy? Marry gup, is melancholy a word for a barber's mouth? Thou shouldst say heavy, dull and doltish: melancholy is the crest of courtiers' arms, and now every base companion, being in his muble fubles, says he is melancholy." John Earle declared that an ordinary country fellow was too stupid to be melancholy: "He has reason enough to do his business and not enough to be idle or melancholy." Burton, who was not as great a social snob as Earle, repeated the idea that melancholy was an affliction of the privileged from the opposite point of view: "And this is the true cause that so many great men, ladies and gentlewomen labour of this disease in country and city; for idleness is an appendix to nobility; they count it as a disgrace to work . . . and thence their bodies become full of gross humours . . . their minds disquieted, dull, heavy, etc.; care, jealousy, fear of some diseases, sullen fits, weeping fits, seize too familiarly upon them."[142]

The influence of these ideas on the way contemporaries thought about their miseries is palpable in Napier's case notes. Melancholy patients were in good company: More than 40% of them were peers, knights and ladies, or masters and mistresses; the ordinary ruck of mentally disturbed people included less than half that measure of gentlefolk. The affinity of melancholy and gentility is especially striking when one compares the social ranks of those who suffered from it with the statuses of clients afflicted with the other most common maladies, the hundreds of people who were called troubled in mind and mopish. These patients were a socially undistinguished lot and included proportionally fewer aristocrats and gentry than mentally disturbed clients in general. If one turns the statistical telescope in the opposite direction and scrutinizes the numbers of peers, knights, and ladies who suffered these various maladies, the social prestige of melancholy is even more sharply

Table 4.3. *Social status of melancholy, mopish, troubled-in-mind patients*

	Melancholy (N = 465)		Mopish (N = 347)		Troubled in mind (N = 717)		All mentally disturbed (N = 2,039)	
	N	%	N	%	N	%	N	%
Peers, knights	40	8.6	4	1.2	11	1.5	62	3.0
Mr. and Mrs.	154	33.1	45	13.0	104	14.5	334	16.4
No title	271	58.3	298	85.8	602	84.0	1643	80.6
Totals	465	100.0	347	100.0	717	100.0	2039	100.0

Note: Figures are computed from cases rather than consultations to maintain consistency with the computations in Chapter 2 and to minimize distortions caused by people (especially rich people) who were treated repeatedly for a single episode of illness.

visible: Almost two-thirds (65%) of the aristocrats complained of melancholy, about one-fifth (18%) were troubled in mind, and only four (6%) were called mopish.

There were two reasons why the literary companionship of melancholy and gentility was realized in Napier's practice. The first is simply that unlike Lyly's barber he was aware of the social properties that governed the naming of woes. The appearance of Burtonian jargon for the first time in his notes in 1624 indicates that the reading of *Anatomy of Melancholy* had rekindled his interest in the technical niceties of humoral medicine.[143] Coincidentally, he was also treating Viscount Purbeck and Lord Compton for emotional disorders during this period, and his growing esteem in courtly circles provided a swelling tide of gloomy gentry whom he could appropriately call melancholy.[144] But the physician's own punctilliousness was not the sole reason why his melancholy patients were often gentlemen and their ladies: Persons of rank and learning frequently judged themselves to be melancholy rather than merely sad, troubled, or fearful. When Master George Spencer became anxious and afraid in 1623 and 1624, for instance, he wrote to Napier: "Desirous to have something to avoid the fumes arising from the spleen," a well-informed response to emotional distress indeed.[145] The husband of Mistress Price was equally precise about her malady when he visited Great Linford: "Deep melancholy fearfulness, almost of every object. Fumes ascending from the stomach, distempering the brain . . . He feareth that it will turn into mania."[146] One surviving letter to the astrologer about a mentally disturbed client shows that Napier's notes about such reports reflect their contents accurately. In 1628 a Londoner named John Evans wrote to him on behalf of an anonymous gentleman. After complaining about his own finances, Evans comes to the point: "That having taken an extreme cold and presently an exceeding grief for the death of his wife . . . [He was] thereby cast down into sickness and melancholy."[147] Melancholy was indeed "the crest of courtiers' arms."[148] No other malady was so strongly linked to social class, and the evidence that gentlefolk were often diagnosing themselves suggests that the figures from Napier's notes are a measure of the diffusion of classical medical ideas among the educated elite.

To find the reasons for the popularity of melancholy one must first ask what the characteristics of this fashionable affliction were. It was, first of all, notoriously like a chameleon: To the eyes of observers, it could fittingly appear wherever the social foliage seemed suitable. Nevertheless, it also had peculiar symptoms that emerge distinctively when one reads many contemporary tracts and huge numbers of actual descriptions of melancholy men and women. These characteristic signs were delusions, fearfulness, and sadness.

Extravagant delusions and hallucinations are today popularly understood to be certain signs of utter madness. Stories about people who think that they are God or Napoleon are familiar embellishments of modern stereotypes of insanity's most severe forms. Tudor and Stuart Englishmen were also fond of such tales. Their favorites, often reprinted, all had long usage by the time they appeared in English late in the sixteenth century. Galen's melancholy men, who thought they were made of ceramic so fine that they would shatter if they were touched, were reincarnated as people who imagined themselves to be made of glass. Two of the most famous yarns were about one man who believed that his nose was as big as a house and another who thought that his bladder was so full that the town would be drowned if he relieved himself. These stories were also first printed by classical physicians to celebrate successful cures. The crafty doctor of the deluded Pinocchio persuaded him by a ruse that he had amputated the offending organ. After putting his patient into a deep swoon, the physician scratched his nose. He then revived his client in front of a bucket of animal guts, which the grateful dupe accepted as surgical debris. The man who was afraid to urinate was cured by a simpler trick. His physician set a fire and made his simple patient believe that the whole town would burn down unless he flooded the fire with the deluge he had been holding back. For delusions such as these, contemporary medical theory offered complex physiological explanations, which identified them as symptoms of melancholy, not lunacy or madness.[149]

None of the famous examples of melancholy delusion was native, and English doctors seem to have encountered very few fabulous fancies in practice. Despite Nashe's claim that "physicians in their circuit every day meet with far more ridiculous experience" than the grand illusions repeated by classical and Renaissance writers, the fancies and conceits Napier encountered seldom defied the common understanding of the physical world.[150] Ordinary credulity concerned everyday matters. Sara Rice, for instance, was "apt to believe any lies and false report."[151] Dorothy Horne suffered from "jealousy proceeding from over-much melancholy," and 21 other clients also were "jealous without any provable cause."[152] The most unusual melancholy delusion Napier recorded was Alice Davys's terror of the century's most ubiquitous substance, dirt:

Extreme melancholy, possessing her for a long time, with fear; and sorely tempted not to touch anything for fear that then she shall be tempted to wash her clothes, even upon her back. Is tortured until that she be forced to wash her clothes, be them never so good and new. Will not suffer her husband, child, nor any of the household to have any new clothes until they wash them for fear the dust of them will fall upon her. Dareth not to go to the church for treading on the ground, fearing lest any dust should fall upon them.[153]

Although this compulsion struck Napier as more bizarre than any other signs of melancholia he encountered, it, too, was an exaggeration of a normal state of mind. Napier treated only a handful of clients whose ideas were exotically incompatible with their identities. One young man proclaimed himself to be God; Jane Travell claimed that she was "a spirit and not herself"; Sir Simon

Norwich was fully persuaded that he had started the Netherlandish revolt; a Cambridge don named William Taylour talked all night of monarchs, emperors, and popes and thought that he was a king or emperor. None of these patients was called mad or lunatic because of his delusions.[154]

The knowledge that exotic fancies were symptoms of melancholy rather than of madness or lunacy was spread beyond the expanding circle of readers familiar with the niceties of psychological medicine by two controversies. Skeptics argued that the confessions of accused witches were melancholy delusion, and the early opponents of religious enthusiasm declared that the inspirations of the enthusiasts were also melancholy fancies. Before the English Revolution, the more influential of these polemics was the attack on witchcraft beliefs by Reginald Scot and his imitators. Scot saw that witchcraft beliefs could not be refuted unless the voluntary confessions of women accused of witchcraft could be discredited. In highly publicized cases, some defendants, who were usually old women, admitted that they had made compacts with the Devil and boasted of their powers and miraculous feats. Borrowing the basis for his argument from Johan Weyer, a Dutch physician, Scot declared that these stories were caused by melancholy, which corrupted the weak imaginations of its elderly victims, and he strongly emphasized the delusive powers of the disease, repeating several of the most famous tales of deluded melancholics. The best publicists for this argument before the late seventeenth century were its opponents, who frequently repeated its medical facts before attacking its conclusions; both the skeptics and their opponents granted that melancholy could cause fabulous delusions. As the opposition to witchcraft beliefs mounted in the century, Scot's view eventually prevailed among the educated elite.[155]

None of Napier's clients thought herself a witch, but some of them were persuaded that they had seen the Devil. Joan Ekins believed that she had given away her soul to Satan; some suicidal patients claimed that they actually saw the Tempter; and several others said that they were possessed. The astrologer did not make a formal diagnosis of Ekins, merely citing her Faustian compact as proof that she was liable to "speak idly" and was "very furious."[156] Although 66 of the 158 clients who were suicidal claimed to have been "tempted by Satan," only one of them was called distracted and none was mad or lunatic. The elaborate fanta-

sies of William Ringe persuaded Napier that he was actually possessed, and although nobody else provided such dramatic evidence
of the Devil's presence, Napier concluded that 17 others were also
possessed by demons.[157] These, then, were the alternatives: Flat
claims that one was in league with the Devil or had been tempted
by him might be evidence that one was suffering from melancholy, suicidal gloom, or (rarely) another mental disorder; or they
might be true. As long as men continued to believe that Satan
could appear to rational people, encounters with him could not be
dismissed simply as symptoms of madness.

Many godly Protestants believed that the Lord might directly
inspire His prophets with visions of the future or doctrinal truths.
When they read in the pages of John Foxe that Protestant martyrs
had supernatural knowledge of the future or in the biographies of
orthodox divines that holy churchmen were routinely prophetic,
most Englishmen assumed the validity of the claims. But when
allegedly inspired prophets were not plausible instruments of
God's purpose, either because they were sectarians or simply unworthy, many thought them insane. The increasing popularity of
secular medical writing about melancholy and the governing
elite's horror of political and religious radicalism converged in the
seventeenth century, and religious enthusiasts were accused of insanity by their Anglican adversaries.[158] Robert Burton cited a
shoal of authorities to the effect that religious enthusiasm was a
kind of melancholy less violent than madness, and Henry More,
Henry Hallywell, and Joseph Glanvill amplified the idea.[159] Napier treated two patients who were reported to have received divine commands. He thought that Mistress May Mydlemore was
"troubled with much sadness and melancholy" and listed among
her symptoms her belief that she had spoken directly with God
who had "promised salvation of fools." Roger Laurenc, a servant
whose master and mother consulted Napier, also held ideas repugnant to orthodox observers. Napier and Laurenc's master
conferred and decided that he was "frantic with a vision that he
should go teach all nations. Talked with a Brownist that said we
had no church nor calling."[160] In each of these cases the patient
was believed to be deluded because his message was theologically
deviant and the person was deemed unworthy to be an inspired
prophet. Mistress Mydlemore was a Catholic, and until his conversion Laurenc had been merely a "witty and choleric" servant.
Napier's casebooks would hardly be the place to look for evidence

that religious inspirations themselves were interpreted as symptoms of insanity; their author conversed with the Archangel Raphael about points of theology, after all. But the fact that his own early biographers, Aubrey and Lilly, displayed his dealings with the Angel as evidence of his piety shows that as long as the possibility for inspiration remained widely accepted, only *individual* prophets could be debunked as madmen. To transmute all such claims into tokens of utter insanity, it was necessary first to persuade people that no rational man, however holy, could speak directly to God.[161]

As the polemical uses of the idea of melancholy suggest, the hallucinations and delusions it was supposed to spawn were so various that the sheer inventiveness of melancholy minds was emphasized both in theory and in practice. Thomas Nashe exclaimed that when melancholy fumes disorder our imaginations, "Sundry times we behold whole armies of men skirmishing in the air: dragons, wild beasts, bloody streamers, blazing comets, fiery streaks, with other apparitions innumerable."[162] Napier remarked upon the helplessly creative imaginations of several of his melancholy clients who had "strange fancies," or "whimsies," or invented "toys."[163] Michael Adams's ruined understanding fooled him into seeing devilish visions: "Mind much troubled with false conceits and illusions. Fearfulness of sin . . . Fearful dreams . . . Supposeth that he seeth many things which he seeth not. A mist in his eyes; a giddiness in his head."[164] Credulous patients whose claims to supernatural portents Napier disbelieved were described as the victims of melancholy, rather than of the more acute disorders, madness or distraction.[165]

Because Elizabethans believed that the world was vibrant with supernatural forces and invisible beings, it was understandable that they were reluctant to presume that fantastic visions and disembodied voices were experienced only by the most insane madmen. But cosmological and religious assumptions alone do not account for the fact that delusions and hallucinations were so often judged to be symptoms of melancholy, whose most common signs were fear and sorrow. There was a logical connection between delusions and pathological emotions. Fear and sorrow were obviously appropriate in some situations, and they were viewed as symptoms of mental disease only when they were aroused without any credible cause or when they far exceeded the intensity of feeling appropriate to the situation. "So I think I may truly conclude," Burton wrote of melancholy people, "they are not always sad and fearful, but usually so: and that without a cause, *timent de non timendis* (Gordonius), *quaeque momenti non sunt.*"[166] Delusion was therefore the mother of all melancholy, for its victims felt grieved and afraid even when they had not actually experienced a significant loss or danger.

Many of the examples of melancholy fear Burton provides are common anxieties that troubled psychologically robust men and women as well. Everybody was afraid occasionally of the perils that many of Napier's melancholy patients complained about: devils, death, illness, accident, disgrace, robbery, and witches, for example. The apprehensions of patients like Clement Horn, Ellen Selbee, Sara Musgrave, Agnes Knit, and Goody Pearson that they would die or be driven mad by disease were tokens of melancholy because they did not seem ill enough to justify such fears.[167] Mary Glover refused to be persuaded that the dog that had bitten her was not rabid after others had concluded that the cur was simply vicious.[168] Ann Wilson thought that the medicine a physician had given her harmed her unborn child. The idea that women should avoid dosing themselves with physic during pregnancy was commonplace; Wilson's fearfulness was melancholy because it persisted even after the child's healthy birth had vindicated the careless physician.[169] Everyone knew that witches sometimes sold people goods that were poisoned or enchanted, but one had to have some grounds for suspecting that the seller was a witch. William Ball's alarmed conviction that he had bought his cow from a "false fellow" was only "his imagination," because his father did not believe it.[170] Similarly, although violent crime was endemic, persons like Ann Kimbell, Anthony Fouke, and Edward Collins, who claimed that some unknown malefactor was going to kill them, turned a legitimate apprehension into a melancholy fear by detaching it from any plausible situation or dangerous enemy.[171]

Englishmen knew that they lived in a perilous environment and that no one could escape fear, no matter how rigid his Stoicism or profound his trust in Providence.[172] They thought that sudden frights could drive men and women mad and even kill them, as we have already seen.[173] They also believed that this ordinary emotion could be provoked by misperception and sustained by delusion, and they called such groundless terror melancholic. Just as no one could escape fear, so all men experienced sorrow and grief. Sorrowful occasions were so common that the causes of such misery and the mood they provoked were both described with a single word, *grief*. The supple phrase *to take a grief* meant more than to have felt some sudden sadness; it also implied that one had been assailed by a sickness or a loss, a *grief*.[174] Like fear, grief and sorrow could be aroused by false apprehensions and amplified by delusion. Baseless sorrow was called melancholic even more readily than groundless fears: Some note of gloom intruded into 20.5% of melancholy patients' consultations with the astrologer.

"Sorrow is that other character, an inseparable companion of melancholy," wrote Burton, and that is the meaning of melancholy that has proved most durable.[175] The black and negligent attire, the bent posture of melancholy portrait sitters and stage players were the visual expressions of dolor.[176] Naturally not every gloomy person suffered from the disease of melancholy. Pathological sadness was unprovoked or far surpassed the normal ratio of "grief" to gloom, of cause to effect. Master Francis Chayne, who knew "no cause of his melancholy," aside from a trifling dispute with a lawyer, fits precisely the traditional stereotype of deluded sorrow.[177] Many instances of sadness had legitimate occasions in the death of loved ones and were revealed to be the sign of melancholy delusion by their unusual intensity and duration. When Agnes Stiff's mother died she could not reconcile her grief and became utterly incapacitated: "Troubled with melancholy, how to live for the death of her mother that died a quarter of a year since. Will weep and cry and wander abroad, she knoweth not whither, to her friends. Can follow no business. Yet can sensibly relate all things touching her infirmity as one that were wonderful well."[178] Excessive grief was a topic that preoccupied contemporary writers. Dramatics, casuists, preachers, and physicians all cautioned against its deleterious effects. The French expert on melancholy La Primaudaye wrote this typical warning in a book popular in England: "Now when grief is in great measure, it bringeth withall a kind of loathing and tediousness, which causeth a man to hate and to be weary of all things, even of the light and of a man's self, so that he shall take pleasure in nothing but his melancholy . . . refusing all joy and consolation. To conclude, some grow so far as to hate themselves."[179] There was plenty of reason to be concerned: After the death of someone they loved, 134 of Napier's clients became mentally disturbed, and many of these men and women were melancholy. Margaret Lancton's plight is typical and closely resembles La Primaudaye's prognosis: "Hath taken much grief touching the death of her husband . . . Full of melancholy and ill thought and cannot rest day nor night. No comfort. Tempted to drown herself. Weepeth all the day long. Craveth God's help and grace."[180]

Whether melancholy crept unprovoked upon the sufferer's affections or stormed into the void created by the death of a child, a spouse or a parent, its effect was to draw him away from normal involvement in the emotional and social world around him. Melancholy men and women lost the capacity to take pleasure from activities they had previously delighted in or to enjoy the social relations that gave happiness to others. Master John Flesher's grief for the deaths of his wife and infant, for instance, was exacerbated by "unnatural melancholy." The evidence for this physiological catastrophe was that Flesher suffered from "melancholy fancies" and "now taketh not that pleasure that he was wont, either in reading or working as he did."[181] Insensible to ordinary delights, Master William Barton found no contentment from being with his family; and Mistress Margaret Gregory, Ann March, and Jane Newell were so heavyhearted that they could "take no joy of anything."[182] The alienation of melancholy men and women from the pleasures of everyday life was symbolized in literature and in descriptions of actual sufferers by their love of solitude. Citing a battery of authorities about melancholy solitude, Burton remarks that "the Egyptians therefore in their hieroglyphics expressed a melancholy man by a hare sitting in her form, as being a most timorous and solitary creature."[183] The aptly named Mistress Experience, a nineteen-year-old gentlewoman, may stand as a single instance of the sad withdrawal of 44 of Napier's clients: "Weepeth often and knoweth not why. Full of fear and melancholy. Loveth solitariness . . ."[184] Melancholy made men and women inner exiles. This is what John Archer had in mind when he wrote that mundane disappointments, if unchecked, could lead eventually to unnatural emotions and acts: Discontent "makes more way for the greatest enemy of nature, *viz.*, sadness or melancholy, it being a true saying, *tristitia omnia mala parit*."[185]

MOPISHNESS: A DISCARDED IMAGE

The lesser mental disorders, it will be recalled, were distinguished from madness, lunacy, and distraction by the relative infrequency

Table 4.4. *Symptoms of melancholy, mopish, and troubled-in-mind patients (in percent)*

	All mental disorders (N = 2,483)	Melancholy (N = 493)	Mopish (N = 377)	Troubled in mind (N = 794)
Melancholy	19.9	100.0	19.9	15.2
Fancies and conceits	7.0	11.6	3.4	8.9
Fearful	12.3	19.7	9.3	12.7
Sadness symptoms	10.9	20.5	10.1	9.7
Suicidal	6.4	5.5	3.7	7.8
Troubled in mind	32.0	24.5	19.1	100.0
Mopish	15.2	15.2	100.0	9.1
Senses disturbed	13.3	11.0	27.9	8.3

Note: Figures are percentages of consultations in which both symptoms occur.

of antic violence and frantic, raging behavior among their victims. The symptoms of melancholy were distinctive enough to show that it was regarded to be a separate type of mental disturbance, although the popularity of the disease encouraged contemporaries to use it to describe virtually any nonviolent emotional disturbance. Napier's usage was comparatively precise. The patients whom he diagnosed as melancholy suffered from deluded fear and sorrow far more often than those who were described simply as troubled in mind (Table 4.4). He also recognized another kind of mental disorder less acute than madness and its companions, whose victims he called mopish. Mopish men and women often suffered from the characteristic symptoms of melancholy, especially gloom and solitude. Mary Kings, for example, was "despairing, heavy-hearted, exceeding sad" and spent her time sobbing and sighing. Another mopish patient, John Askue, was "solitary and will do nothing."[186] Forty-one of Napier's mopish clients were so glum and withdrawn that, like Ann Hector, they sat sunken in "dumpish, sullen silence."[187] Indeed, one connotation of the word *mopish* current during the seventeenth century was a pale kind of melancholy.

Mopishness nevertheless had distinctive social and psychological signs. It was the social antithesis of melancholy. The dumpish moods of idle gentlefolk frequently earned the classical appellation; the sullen inactivity of husbandmen and artisans merited more often the rude and common word *mopish* (Table 4.3). This socially pejorative aura was also reflected in the symptoms Napier associated with mopishness. The idleness of melancholy aristocrats was seldom viewed as a sign of mental illness; it was instead the very mark of gentility, a cause and not a consequence of melancholy. But Napier remarked that his mopish patients were idle and "could not follow [their] business" more than twice as often as his other mentally disturbed patients, with 9.8% of them displaying that symptom compared with 4% of the whole group of disturbed patients.[188]

The truly characteristic psychological evidence of mopishness, however, was a disturbance of the senses. Of the consultations with mopish patients, 105 resulted in notes like "sottish," "foolish," "not well in his wits," "troubled in his senses," or "senseless."[189] Some evidence of impaired sense perceptions is included in 27.9% of the consultations marked mopish, but similar observations occur in only 11.0% of the consultations for melancholy and 8.3% of the consultations in the vague category, troubled in mind. The identification of mopishness with disturbed sense perceptions was not peculiar to Napier. Medical writers seldom used the word *mopish*, but they described an almost identical condition which was called *stupor* or *lethargy* by Galen and his English disciples.[190] A century after Napier's death, William Battie included in his famous treatise on madness a malady called *insensibility*, which he characterized as "a prenatural defect or total loss of sensation."[191] That is precisely the meaning of *mopishness* understood by Napier and his contemporaries. Shakespeare, for instance, used the term to signify a kind of mental disorder that ruined people's capacity to perceive the world and react properly to stimuli without disturbing the passions or provoking irrational frenzy. At the end of *The Tempest*, for instance, Alonso is unable to reconcile the tale of the events Prospero has caused with what he himself has seen and experienced, and he compares the apparent illusions to a kind of mopishness.[192] Hamlet is more specific about the effects of mopishness on the senses when he denounces Gertrude for marrying Claudius:

> Eyes without feeling, feeling without sight,
> Ears without hands or eyes, smelling sans all,
> Or but a sickly part of one true sense
> Could not so mope.[193]

Hamlet would have Gertrude be precisely the opposite of a mopish being, one who in Napier's words, is "not mopish but of good senses and understanding, . . . not mopish but sensible and healthy."[194]

The popular usage of the term *mopish,* which is echoed in Shakespeare's plays and Napier's notebooks, can be precisely interpreted in terms of contemporary psychology. The condition it described was a disturbance of the sensitive faculty, rather than the reason. Mopishness was therefore less severe than the maladies that ruined the reason itself, such as madness and lunacy, because it harmed a lesser faculty and interfered with wit and will merely by depriving reason of normal perceptions, the raw material of thought. As Napier's records show, this was a very useful diagnostic tool, providing a means with which to separate melancholy from the lesser mental disturbances that made their victims remote and insensible but not sad or anxious. The fact that the concept may be found in popular literature suggests that it was commonly recognized as a type of mental disorder. And yet the popularizers of classical medical psychology largely ignored it in their publications and instead encouraged the tendency to broaden the concept of melancholy to include the symptoms of every mental disturbance except outright lunacy.

Despite his lamentations about the elusiveness of melancholy's symptoms, no one did more to stretch and expand the definition of the malady than Burton; and no one did more to persuade laymen of its generality. Burton and Napier may be taken to represent contrasting approaches to the scientific understanding of mental disorder. Burton deferred to the classifications of learned authority, appreciative of nuance and eccentricity. Where his authorities differed, Burton strove to create a structure, an anatomy, that would comprehend every varying symptom they averred into a single disease, melancholy. Napier, on the other hand, preferred narrower empirical categories. When he could not match a patient's symptoms with a distinctive stereotype, he often emphasized the sufferer's principal symptom or simply described him as troubled in mind. Napier did not try to invent a new and more precise psychological vocabulary; he used the concepts and terms that were current in popular medical writing and familiar to his patients. But he did try to employ these popular stereotypes more or less consistently. Writing about contrasting styles of discourse in the Middle Ages, R. W. Southern remarks that "rhetoric is persuasive; logic compulsive."[195] This opposition is analogous to the contrast between the methods followed by Burton and Napier. Burton sought to persuade his readers that the protean disease melancholy could describe the whole fabulous realm of mental disorder that prevailed during the seventeeth century; Napier sought to articulate his patients' maladies into categories that were at once scientifically useful and consistent with popular usage. The physicians encouraged the cult of melancholy. They neglected the empirical distinctions implicit in Napier's methods and popular stereotypes in favor of a vague and confused medical vocabulary. Medical men made few empirically based attempts to improve the nosology of mental disorder before the middle of the eighteenth century. Their preference for the broadest possible application of traditional humoral concepts stemmed in part from the realization that the popularity of melancholy among the educated elite fostered the belief that physicians were the best healers for the maladies of the mind. Doctors were not disinterested taxonomists. They were more concerned to suppress their lay and clerical rivals than to preserve the empirically useful aspects of popular psychology and religious healing.

CULTURE AND MENTAL DISORDER

The major features of the stereotypes of insanity discussed in this chapter were not unique to Tudor and Stuart England. Each of the four main types of mental disorder had roughly equivalent antecedents in classical medical texts. Parallels may also be found in contemporary European literature, and the Renaissance revival of classical medicine made abnormal psychology even more plainly international.[196] English ideas about insanity also had a long domestic history. Many of the individual symptoms of mental disorder recognized in the seventeenth century are evident in fourteenth-century portrayals of madmen in literature.[197] The legal and religious stereotype of suicide, for example, was fully articulated long before the sixteenth century.[198] The cultural similarities among the nations of Northern and Western Europe and the relatively slow pace of social change fostered international and historical continuity in the definition of mental abnormality. Nevertheless, the popular interpretation of the nature and significance of mental disorder was fully integrated into the values and beliefs of early seventeenth-century England. Ideas about insanity were shaped in particular by the high value the English people placed on the nuclear family and by traditional beliefs about the supernatural.

The preservation of the family unit was, as we have seen, promoted by institutional and moral pressures: The ecclesiastical courts prosecuted couples for flagrant marital irregularities; officially sanctioned divorce or separation was very difficult to obtain; penalties of special savagery were stipulated for people who murdered or assaulted their parents or husbands; witchcraft beliefs proscribed accusations between members of the same family. Contemporaries regarded deviations from the norms of family life to be signs of alienation from the fundamental values of their society. The examples of antisocial behavior included in descriptions of the insane very often described actions that menaced the survival or the harmony of the family. Napier's clients thought that people who attacked their families were lunatics or madmen; they believed that children who challenged the authority of their elders were brainsick; they felt that wives who rebelled against their husbands were melancholy and mopish; they presumed that men who beat their wives and neglected their familial responsibilities were irrational; they believed that women who were abused or neglected by their husbands had good cause to become mentally disturbed. None of these attitudes was unique to Napier's patients. Legal documents and literary sources frequently mention violations of the rules of orderly family life as evidence of insanity. I have argued above that an antisocial action by itself, no matter how irrational it seemed, was not proof of lunacy. An early eighteenth-century proverb put the point nicely: "One mad action is not enough to prove a man mad."[199] But when English men and women looked for evidence to show that a person was insane, they examined his relations with his family with an intensity that mirrored the importance of those ties in their own lives.

The social and economic significance of the family in early modern England was even reflected in the sanctions against suicide. The death of an adult member of a household was always disruptive and often disastrous, particularly if it was the husband who died. Existing property arrangements were dissolved and the economic foundation of the family had to be rebuilt if it was to endure. Widows and old people might suddenly lose their livelihoods altogether, and if the surviving spouse remarried, the children of the original marriage might be displaced from their inheritances and the affections of their parent. The death of married adults by disease obviously could not be prevented by social regulation, and until the rise of savings banks and life insurance, little could be done to lessen its consequences. But voluntary self-destruction could be prohibited, and that is what the religious and legal sanctions against suicide attempted to do. Severe economic penalties were placed on the suicide's family, which forfeited all of his chattels, even goods that were necessary for farm work and trade. To the potential economic ruin of the self-murderer's family, traditional religious beliefs added the stigma of association with a demonic apostate and a burden of guilt about failing to prevent the death. Although these punishments were often partially mitigated by official leniency and public sympathy, they nevertheless served as a genuine deterrent to suicide by reminding potential suicides of their responsibilities toward their families. William Fleetwood stressed this function of the traditional penalties when he protested their gradual abandonment in the early eighteenth century:

Who can tell but that a severer sentence passed upon self-murderers would make fewer of them? And the utter ruin of some few fatherless and widows prevent a great many more from being fatherless and widows? The laws of almost all wise nations have had that in their eye in enacting penalties; they have punished wife and children, and undone whole families for the offence of a single person, the head of them, not for want of knowing how innocent they were, but with [the] intention of restraining those heads within the bounds of duty, for fear of hazarding and hurting those who were so innocent, and whom they loved and were obliged to love and secure from want, and shame, and misery, and make as happy as they could.[200]

There is some evidence that penalties for suicide actually worked in the way envisaged by Fleetwood. As he lay dying of a self-inflicted wound in 1672, for instance, a Bradford miller lamented, "I have forfeited my estate to the king, beggared my wife and children."[201] When Nehemiah Wallington was tormented by repeated urges to kill himself early in the seventeenth century, he was at last prevented from doing so by reflections about the disgrace he would bring down upon his father and his family's Puritan co-religionists.[202]

Traditional religious and legal beliefs about suicide influenced the popular conception of severe insanity, as we have seen. The stereotype of raging madness excluded the most obvious form of self-destructive behavior from consideration as a symptom of irrational violence. This example points to another way in which ideas about insanity were shaped by contemporary values and beliefs. Both the specific content and the relative severity of the symptoms of mental disorder were judged by religious as well as secular standards. Popular religious psychology was based on an almost Manichaean dichotomy between good and evil, normal and abnormal. The morality plays of the later Middle Ages dramatized the conventional symbolism of this psychology, depicting the hapless Everyman as the prize in a struggle between God's angels and the Devil. The iconography of the morality play persisted in the imagination of the English people long after the Reformation. Napier's clients sometimes described their emotional conflicts as inner warfare between good and evil spirits. The astrologer recorded that Katherine Percivall "sayeth that she hath the Devil in her, and God also to defend her"; Mary Olive told him that "the evil spirit hath overcome the good"; and mad Harry Peace cried out "against his aunt and the Devil, and sayeth his good spirit is gone and he is haunted."[203] Eminent clergymen shared the popular belief that mental turmoil had a supernatural dimension; Bishop Joseph Hall, for instance, wrote:

There is no man, nor place free from spirits; although they testify their presence by visible effects but in few. Every man is a host to entertain angels, thought not in visible shapes . . . The evil ones do nothing but provoke us to sin and plot mischief against us amongst men, by frighting us with terrors in ourselves, by accusing us to God; on the contrary, the good angels are ever removing our hindrances from good and our occasions of evil, mitigating our temptations, helping us against our enemies, delivering us from dangers, comforting us in sorrows, furthering our good purposes, and at last carrying our souls up to heaven.[204]

Seventeenth-century laymen regarded the drama of the inner life as a moral allegory, and they often elided the ideas of madness and sin, sanity and grace, despair and apostasy, anxiety and spiritual doubt.

Religion provided suffering men and women with a set of common ideas with which they could convey the depth of their an-

guish. When Alice Hearne's father died, she became suicidally unhappy: "Sayeth she cannot serve God, and yet doth sometimes
. . . It is too late to serve God, she sayeth, she should have begun
sooner."[205] It was natural enough after the death of a father to
think that devotion might have averted the loss and to lament that
it was too late to compensate for one's lapses, but Hearne was not
the only patient to express sorrow and anger in terms of her relationship with God. "Her child died about a year since," Napier
remarked about another woman: "Took great grief that she did
not tend it well . . . Weepeth for that she cannot serve God as she
would and is cumbered with idle, sad thoughts and bid to curse
God. Feareth that she cannot be saved."[206] The ethical heritage of
Christianity encouraged believers to conceive of their feelings of
guilt and worthlessness in religious terms. Here is how Alice Darling voiced her profound depression: "Doubteth and in a manner
despaireth for her sins. Sayeth that she is the evil itself, is not worthy of God's creation being a damned creature."[207] Pervasive convictions of hopelessness like Darling's were often not attached to a
particular sin or caused by a specific theological scruple but expressed instead a state of mind. Explaining that William Mercer
was "not sick but vexed in his mind," the astrologer added: "A
heavy heart . . . Cryeth out that he is a grievous sinner. Hath
much minded the word."[208] John Berring fashioned for himself a
Chinese puzzle of apparently pointless self-recrimination: "Took a
grief and is sorry to offend God and yet fear he doth. Cannot settle
his mind."[209] Ann Gregory was simply "troubled with a great
dullness and heaviness" and so grew "doubtful of her salvation."[210]

The most famous preachers of the age fostered the popular belief that spiritual and mental afflictions were identical. They used
the traditional personifications to describe the emotional tribulations of unregenerate sinners,[211] and they wrote elaborate sermons
based on the correspondence between insanity and sin. The most
famous of these was Thomas Adams's *Mystical Bedlam, or the
World of Mad Men*, an eloquent tour de force in which the reader is
conducted through a theological Bedlam, pausing to observe successively the representations of twenty men afflicted with different
types of moral madness.[212] Bishop Hall epitomized the method in
a much briefer compass:

He is a rare man, that hath not some kind of madness reigning in him: one, a dull madness of melancholy; another, a conceited madness of pride; another, a superstitious madness of false devotion; a fourth, of ambition or covetousness; a fifth, the furious madness of anger; a sixth, the laughing madness of extreme mirth; a seventh, a drunken madness; an eighth, of outrageous lust; a ninth, the learned madness of curiosity; a tenth, the worst madness of profaneness and atheism. It is as hard, to reckon up all kinds of madness, as of dispositions . . . Only that man is both good, and wise, and happy, that is free from all kinds of frenzy.[213]

Napier and his pious clients often contrasted godliness with abnormal emotions and actions. "Tempted sorely," he wrote of Agnys Buttres, "mopish and foolish and was godly and religious and well in her wits."[214] Sara Pendred's husband told the physician that his wife's mad rebelliousness was foreign to her pious character: "He came for his wife who is so distracted of her wits and did scratch her husband yesterday, and yet a very godly and religious woman."[215] The inability to pray and perform regular religious duties was a measure of the pathology of some people's emotional problems. Joan Hall's anxieties made it impossible for her to finish her prayers, for instance: "Complaineth of her head and wits, and cannot pray and is troubled in mind . . . If she begins to pray, she cannot end it."[216]

Laymen and clergymen alike assumed that traditional religious psychology and secular concepts of mental disorder were compatible. Writers like Nashe and Burton reconciled religious belief and scientific dogma by asserting that the spirit of evil and the malevolent humors worked together to produce disturbing emotions and ideas: "Melancholy men," Burton observed, "are most subject to diabolical temptations and illusions, and most apt to entertain them."[217] The theory that Satan exploited the weaknesses of people suffering from melancholy even provided an argument with which the most diabolical temptation, the urge to commit suicide, could be explained as both the Devil's own work and a consequence of natural disease.[218] The desire to reconcile the reality of the supernatural forces of good and evil with the stereotypes of mental abnormality shaped contemporary estimates of the seriousness of some forms of insanity. Thus the eschatological language in the ravings of insane people was interpreted to mean that their sufferings were like mortal diseases, the most dreadful and

destructive afflictions. More important, delusions, which are today regarded as the token of the worst kinds of insanity, were
considered to be symptoms of melancholy rather than madness. I
have argued above that as long as perfectly rational people were
believed to receive inspirations from God or to have intercourse
with the Devil few authorities were willing to classify apparent
delusions, the majority of which were religious in content, as
signs of wild irrationality. Some doubt always remained that
strange perceptions might be genuine glimpses of the unseen
world, whose immediate and potent presence was assumed by almost everyone.

   The most compelling evidence for this argument is that when
the educated elite abandoned their beliefs in divine inspiration and
demonology, they also elevated delusion to a prominent place
among the signs of madness. These two changes were closely connected. For more than a century after the English Revolution, the
governing classes assailed the religious enthusiasm of the sects.
Anglican propagandists declared that the visions and inspirations
of radical Dissenters were insane delusions based on false perceptions and diseased imaginings. The earliest opponents of religious
enthusiasm argued that it was caused by melancholy, but during
the eighteenth century orthodox controversialists followed Swift
in claiming that it was a kind of madness. A host of famous
writers and obscure sermonizers trumpeted the belief that "enthusiasm and madness are but the same thing in different words."[219]
The campaign against enthusiasm hastened the spread of rational
religion and skepticism about supernatural phenomena among the
governing classes. Many of the enemies of enthusiasm also attacked popular beliefs in witches and demons. Alarmed by the
favorable reactions to the alleged exorcisms and healing miracles
performed by Quakers and Methodists, they charged that the demoniacs and bewitched people whom the Dissenters were supposed to cure were actually the victims of mental illnesses.[220] By
the middle of the eighteenth century the prevailing view among
the educated elite was that people who claimed to have divine inspirations or devilish afflictions were insane.[221] The incessant repetition of the assertion that religious and demonic delusions were
symptoms of madness fostered a new conception of the symptoms
of severe insanity among the ruling classes. William Battie articulated this new attitude in his famous *Treatise on Madness*, published

in 1758. "All mankind as well as the physician" agreed, Battie maintained, that false perceptions were "a certain sign of madness"; and he concluded that "therefore deluded imagination . . . is not only an indisputable but an essential character of madness."[222]

The campaign against religious enthusiasm also hastened the secularization of attitudes toward suicide among the governing classes. Until the eighteenth century suicide was regarded as a civil and religious crime by almost all Englishmen, and the sanctions against it were widely enforced. The demonianism implicit in the traditional stereotype of suicide was emphasized by Puritan and Nonconformist preachers during the seventeenth century. They taught that suicidal impulses were the familiar torment of the reprobate masses and the chief temptation of the saints. The remedy they proposed was conversion and moral regeneration.[223] The orthodox elite responded to these claims with the charge that religious enthusiasm itself was responsible for fostering despair and suicide. Suicidal emotions were caused by religious melancholy, a natural disease, not by Satan's temptations. These polemical arguments gradually discredited the traditional stereotypes of suicide among the governing classes. As early as 1705 there were complaints that coroners' juries commonly avoided enforcing the sanctions against suicide by classifying self-murderers as lunatics, who were not responsible for their crime. The new term *suicide* was coined early in the eighteenth century to replace the pejorative locutions of earlier ages, "self-murder" and "*felo-de-se*."[224] By 1790 traditionalists such as Charles Moore and John Wesley lamented that the ancient sanctions had been abandoned altogether, and the evidence of coroners' inquests shows that they were right.[225] The idea of the immanent Devil had been cast out of the world view of the ruling elite, and coroners and their juries no longer acted on the old belief that suicide was a Satanic compact.[226]

The consequences of these changes in the governing elite's conceptions of insanity and suicide remain obscure. We do not know, for example, precisely how they were related to the asylum movement, the shift away from relying upon the family to care for the insane toward a large-scale, institutional solution for the problem. There is some evidence that among the lowest orders of society traditional religious psychology and stereotypes of mental abnormality persisted into the early nineteenth century. Beliefs in witchcraft and possession were evidently widespread, and thousands of ordinary men and women rejected the claims that religious enthusiasts were insane and believed the divine and demonic revelations reported by John Wesley, Richard Brothers, and Joanna Southcott.[227] The political pressures that prompted the governing classes to adopt a more secular attitude toward apparently supernatural phenomena were not felt by the poor. The result seems to have been the creation of two, often antagonistic, mental outlooks, each with a different interpretation of insanity. The importance of these developments for the present study is that they show that ideas about the nature and significance of mental disorder were responsive to cultural change. The traditional view of insanity was fully integrated into the prevailing values and beliefs of Elizabethan and Stuart England; the new conception of madness and suicide reflected the secularization of the cosmology of the eighteenth-century elite.

5

Psychological healing

Throughout the seventeenth century most English people continued to believe that mental disorders could be caused by either natural or supernatural forces.[1] A myriad of physical and social catastrophes were invoked in popular literature, sermons, and medical
records to explain insanity: astrological events, psychological
stresses, and physical illnesses. Indeed, the situations that could
provoke mental suffering were so numerous that Burton de-
spaired of listing them all: "In this labyrinth of accidental causes,
the further I wander, the more intricate I find the passage; *multae
ambages* [there are many wanderings], and new causes as so many
by-paths offer themselves to be discussed. To search out all, were
an Herculean work, and fitter for Theseus."[2] Napier's records do
not provide a means to simplify the labyrinth of natural perils, but
they do afford some glimpses of its principal features. Two points
stand out. The astrologer and his clients were seldom content to
list a single factor as the sole cause of a case of mental disorder. For
example, Napier never cited the motions of the planets or the
phases of the moon as the only reason for a patient's insanity. He
seems to have felt that the stars predisposed his clients to suffer
mental disorders peculiar to their particular temperaments, and
that they provided signs with which to detect the immediate
sources of their suffering, but that astronomical movements by
themselves seldom drove men and women mad.[3] There was almost always a more immediate cause as well. The second point
that may be inferred from Napier's records is that disturbing
events affected the physical health and social relationships of their
victims as well as their psychological condition. Like popular

medical writers and philosophers, Napier and his patients assumed a powerful sympathy between mind and body. Emotional stress could cause physical illnesses as well as mental disturbances, and almost any sort of bodily sickness could deprive a person of his reason. The many different events in the natural world that were deemed potential causes of insanity disturbed the entire lives of the people they affected, not merely their mental tranquillity.

The supernatural causes of mental disorder were also diverse, but many popular writers observed that all of them were either divine or diabolical. Thus Burton observed that these "supernatural [causes] are from God and His angels, or by God's permission from the devil and his ministers."[4] A long tradition of popular theology taught that God himself inflicted madness and despair on notorious sinners. Medieval writers interpreted the Biblical fate of Nebuchadnezzar to prove that insanity was one of the wages of sin and the death of Judas to show that suicide was another.[5] This tradition was revitalized in the sixteenth and seventeenth centuries by Protestant controversialists. Following the example of John Foxe, they recounted numerous stories about persecutors of the true church who suddenly fell into stark madness or suicidal desperation because of God's judgment against them. A tale told by the martyrologist's Quaker namesake, George Fox, is characteristic:

Susan Frith was moved to tell him, That if he continued on in this persecuting of the innocent the Lord would execute his plagues upon him. Soon after which, this Justice, whose name was Clark, fell distracted and was bound with ropes; but he gnawed the ropes in pieces and had like to have spoiled his maid; for he fell upon her and bit her; so that they were fain to put an iron instrument in his mouth to wrest his teeth out of her flesh: and afterwards he died distracted.[6]

Although Napier remarked of one of his clients that "pride and covetousness had made her frantic," the practice of attributing insanity to God's wrath was most common among didactic writers and sermonizers.[7] Religious conservatives and common people such as Napier and his patients seldom invoked the doctrine of judgments to explain actual cases of insanity or suicide; they were reluctant to attribute such suffering directly to God.

Ordinary villagers, however, readily blamed the Devil and his minions, demons and witches, for madness and self-murder. Clergymen glossed popular beliefs about demonology and witchcraft by insisting that God ultimately determined the scope of action permitted to evil spirits and witches. They could not harm anyone unless it was consistent with the divine will. All mental suffering therefore ultimately had a religious and moral dimension and might be considered the result of transgressions against God or one's fellow men. But laymen often ignored theological niceties. They attributed great power and independence to the forces of evil. Napier's clients believed that demons could cause almost any mental or physical disease. Malevolent spirits and witches were a constant menace to their happiness and health, and God and his angels represented a source of power and consolation with which to combat devilish wiles. This simple dichotomy between the invisible powers of good and evil was a venerable aspect of popular religion, and it survived among the common people well into the nineteenth century.

The methods of curing the afflictions of the mind were as diverse as the forces that were believed to cause them. There were natural and supernatural remedies, and several kinds of practitioners to dispense them. Medical practice in Tudor and Stuart England presented a rich and varied scene, and psychological healing displayed a similar, crowded tableau.[8] Humanistic physicians, medical astrologers, apothecaries, and folk healers purveyed natural therapies, medicaments, and psychological treatments. Although their potions and methods differed considerably, all of these medical practitioners shared the same aspiration: to heal their patients' bodies and minds by restoring their harmony with the natural order. Astrology was anciently the emblem and the instrument of this aspiration. Its rules and symbols provided a means with which to explore and represent the causes of the sufferer's anguish, and it guided the timing and administration of medication. The medical astrologer could thus manipulate the forces of nature to heal his patients. In the early seventeenth century, practitioners' faith in the principles of astrology and their technical skills varied greatly, but both the highly educated adept and the village herbalist were persuaded that astrology enhanced the effectiveness of their treatments. They also believed that it helped them to detect the influence of malevolent spirits, which possessed the power to exacerbate natural disturbances or to provoke insanity and sickness directly.

Many healers devoted themselves chiefly to overcoming the supernatural causes of suffering. Clergymen, astrologers, and magicians of all kinds treated mental disorders. Religious and magical remedies were not sharply distinguished by laymen, and traditionally the clergy had been the most respected practitioners of healing magic. Protestant reformers, however, effectively eliminated exorcism from the Church of England's liturgy in the late sixteenth century, because they objected to its Popish ceremonies. The church's virtual abandonment of countermagic reduced its ability to satisfy the popular demand for healing magic, and dissenting sects and magicians vigorously exploited their opportunity to win converts and customers by performing exorcisms and supplying charms and amulets. Jesuits and Puritans employed ritual and prayer to cast devils out of possessed people; astrologers and folk magicians fashioned astral talismans and parchment charms to protect their clients against witchcraft. All of these activities were condemned by the church as magic, but most of them were based ultimately on religious beliefs and practices, and to many villagers they seemed consistent with popular piety. However much the authorities lamented the willingness of troubled laymen to seek help from schismatics and heretics, they could do little to prevent them from doing so, and the church itself had, after all, fostered the belief that mental suffering was a spiritual affliction amenable to spiritual remedies.[9]

For centuries the parish clergy had ministered to the psychological maladies of the laity. Preachers taught their flocks to interpret emotional turmoil in religious and moral terms, and priests solaced the mentally disturbed by urging them to repent their sins and seek refuge in God's mercy. The clergy before and after the Reformation acted as mediators between people who were suffering from mental disorders and the normal community; they helped afflicted persons to recognize the abnormality of their thoughts and actions and to repent their sins, thus reconciling themselves with the social norms and moral standards of the wider community. Clergymen also visited the sick and afflicted, and provided much needed consolation and advice in times of acute anxiety. During the reigns of the last Tudor and the early Stuarts, Puritan ministers revitalized the practice of "practical divinity," waging an evangelical campaign to reform the beliefs and manners of the English people. Historians have vigorously debated the psychological impact of Puritanism on contemporaries. Some scholars, led by Max Weber, have argued that the Puritans' zealous propagation of Calvinist theology greatly enhanced the anxieties of ordinary men and women; others have asserted that the Puritans' practice of spiritual counsel and practical divinity strengthened believers' capacity to endure the psychological stress of everyday life in a rapidly changing society.[10] Neither of these views is entirely persuasive, and neither of them can be proved. Measuring the anxiety English people experienced is difficult; showing that high or low levels of misery were caused by Puritanism is impossible. There are individual cases of men and women whose anxieties were increased by Puritan teaching, and there are equally numerous cases of people whose suffering was lessened by their conversion to a godly way of life.[11] The Puritan movement did have, however, important consequences for the treatment of the insane, and these can be studied historically. The Puritan clergy established a tradition of Nonconformist thaumaturgy, which persisted throughout the seventeenth and eighteenth centuries. Partly in reaction to the Dissenters' efforts to heal people who were mad, possessed, bewitched, or tormented by despair, the orthodox elite repudiated all manner of religious therapy for insanity until the early nineteenth century. The indirect result of the controversy over the legitimacy of spiritual healing was that the secular alternative, medical psychology, was established as the only acceptable alternative in the eyes of the orthodox elite.

Richard Napier practiced at a time when it was still possible for learned men to reconcile all of the main types of causal explanations for insanity and to offer all of the remedies appropriate to them. The traditional medieval and Renaissance model of the universe postulated the existence of both natural and supernatural forces at work in a hierarchical order of powers and beings. Man existed at the point of convergence between the natural and the supernatural orders, and he was subject to both kinds of powers.[12] This model permitted contemporaries to explain mental disorder as the consequence of events that occurred on any of the several planes of existence, acting singly or in concert. Most people in early seventeenth-century England saw no theoretical incompatibility among the different kinds of explanation for mental disorders, and many practitioners combined therapies justified by medical, magical, and religious beliefs. Napier was one of these eclectics. Mentally disturbed people and their families followed an eclectic approach to psychological healing as well. Some of them sought the help of several practitioners who specialized in different kinds of treatments; others consulted a single healer who used several kinds of remedies to treat both the natural and supernatural causes of their maladies.[13] Professional rivalries, religious conflicts, and scientific discoveries eventually discredited therapeutic eclecticism, but it still prevailed during Napier's lifetime. The decline of the traditional pluralistic system of psychological healing was largely the consequence of political and social change rather than the advance of medicine and psychology. Some of the magical and religious treatments practiced by Napier and his contemporaries were widely recognized to be more effective than the medical remedies that dominated the treatment of the insane in the eighteenth century. To see why that was so, it will be necessary to discuss each of the principal methods of psychological healing in the light of the conditions that determined its popularity and prestige.

MEDICAL PSYCHOLOGY AND THE NATURAL ORDER

Elizabethan psychology was a synthesis of classical science and medieval cosmology.[14] Its conception of the design and operations of the mind was derived largely from the faculty psychology of Aristotle and the physiology of Hippocrates and Galen. Medieval theologians and scientists had identified the mind with the soul and elaborated connections between the classical scheme and the Christian picture of the universe. According to Robert Burton's lucid and influential presentation, the soul is divided into three parts, each with a distinctive set of functions. "The common division of the soul," he explains, "is into three principal faculties – vegetal, sensitive, and rational, which make three distinct kinds of living creatures: vegetal plants, sensible beasts, rational men."[15] The human mind thus encompasses the essential functions of the three levels of life, the plants, the animals, and the intelligent beings, men and angels. The vegetal soul shares with the plants the powers of nutrition, growth, and generation. The sensitive soul shares with the beasts the powers of perception and motivation. The rational soul shares with the angels the power of understanding and will. The sensitive and rational souls include the lesser faculties within them, and the human soul is therefore a hierarchically divided unity, like the universe itself. Hence, as Timothy Bright remarked conventionally, the possession of even an imperfect rational soul makes man "a creature of middle nature betwixt angels and beasts."[16]

To Tudor and Stuart Englishmen, the analogies between the levels of the human mind and the hierarchy of living creatures proved that men actually embody in miniature the cosmos itself. Celebrating the nature of man before the Fall, Burton invoked this fundamental belief, shared by all his contemporaries: Man, he writes, is "*Microcosmus*, a little world, a model of the world, sovereign lord of the earth, viceroy of the world, sole commander and governor of all the creatures in it; . . . far surpassing all the rest, not in body only, but in soul; *Imaginis imago*, created to God's own image, to that immortal and incorporeal substance, with all the faculties and powers belonging unto it."[17] The powers of the human mind were mutilated by the Fall. Man retained his central position between the angels and the brutes, but he became subject to disease and death, like the lesser creatures.[18] Mental illnesses, which destroyed the relics of his weakened reason, reduced their victims to the level of dumb beasts. The proverbial comparison of madmen and wild animals expressed a literal truth that was redolent with scientific, religious, and moral implications.[19]

Mental diseases were believed to impair either the sensitive or the rational soul, and some brief discussion of the functions of these faculties is necessary to understand how contemporary physicians accounted for the symptoms of insanity and tried to remedy its causes. Returning once more to Burton's description of the soul, we find that the anatomist explains that the sensible soul comprises the five outward and three inward senses that perceive the external world, recognize and remember impressions, create new images, stir the emotions, and move the body.[20] The five external senses are the ones we commonly recognize today; they apprehend the sensible world and present perceptions to the inward senses, common sense, memory, and imagination. The faculty of common sense merely recognizes the impressions presented to it and transmits them to the memory or imagination. Many of Napier's mopish patients were apparently unable to perceive or react to the stimuli that were presented to them and hence were said to have been troubled in their senses or senseless, as we have seen.[21]

Burton and his contemporaries thought that the imagination causes many of the other symptoms of insanity. A powerful and protean faculty, the imagination is an inner sense that acts as the theater of the mind.[22] Characters summoned directly from the common sense, recalled from memory, or newly invented for the purposes of the spectacle are presented on its stage. The appetites and the spirits are imagination's audience, and through their reactions to the images it presents, the passions are aroused and the body stirred to action. Fancy, as the imagination was also called, is the highest faculty in animals, and it is sufficient to cause all of the mental and physical motions that can be performed by man and beast alike. Reason possesses the power of judgment, which permits it to understand universals, grasp innate ideas, and reflect upon one's own thoughts and actions. "Bees indeed make neat and curious works," Burton remarked in this context, "and many other creatures besides; but when they have done, they cannot judge of them."[23] Reason also possesses the power of will, which allows it to command the senses so that the potent drama of imagination conforms to judgment's script and thus to control human passion and behavior.[24]

The imagination imperils sanity when its illusory powers are not plotted and directed by reason. This was believed to be an imminent danger because the effects of the Fall weakened reason's control over fancy, and its fragile sway is easily overthrown by a multitude of inward and outward provocations. Napier accounted for Robert Madison's psychiatric symptoms by observing: "Imagination is strong when the judgment is weak, and an ill affected spleen is able to arm fancy, to exclude reason."[25] The fabulous visions and false ideas conceived by the insane are the consequences of unrestrained imagination. Thus Burton declared: "That melancholy men and sick men conceive to many phantastical visions, apparitions to themselves, and have such absurd suppositions, as that they are kings, lords, cocks, bears, apes, owls; that they are heavy, light, transparent, great and little, senseless and dead . . . can be imputed to naught else but a corrupt, false and violent imagination."[26] The imagination also plays a part in causing the emotional symptoms of insanity. The afflictions that

were attributed to it included: "Disquietness of mind and alienation of right wits, absurd cogitations, troublesome dreams . . . a
mind sorrowful, comfortless, perplexed, pensive and fearful."[27]
Undirected fancy provokes harmful passions without reasonable
cause, counterfeiting the images of reality or amplifying ordinary
emotions until they become pathological. The anatomist of melancholy explains that the imagination performs a crucial mediat-
ing role between the passions and the mind and body: "This imagination is the *medium deferens* [instrument] of passions, by whose
means they work and produce many times prodigious effects: and
as the phantasy is more or less intended or remitted, and their
humours disposed, so do perturbations move, more or less, and
take deeper impression."[28] The imagination was the amplifying
power that transformed the griefs and fears of many of Napier's
patients into destructive passions that sickened their minds and
bodies.

Christian dogma held that the soul was immortal and incorrupt-
ible; Pauline and Platonic traditions emphasized the dichotomy
between body and soul. And yet, as Herschel Baker notes, the
psychologists of Napier's age accepted the Aristotelian-Galenic
predicate that there was a close organic relationship between
them, in spite of the logical incompatibility of these traditions:
"Virtually no one, not even the professed Neoplatonic mystics,
consistently held to the Platonic notion of the soul as a separate
eidos, apart from and unaffected by the body."[29] Elizabethan psychologists accepted the identification of mind and soul and yet
maintained that the diseases of the mind can sicken the body and
vice versa.[30] Thus when the emotions are amplified by a disordered imagination, they endanger people's health as well as their
sanity. Any excessive passion may be harmful, even love and joy,
but the most dangerous passions are fear and sorrow. "Many have
lost their lives with sadness and despair," Thomas Wright observed, "but few with love and hope."[31] The French expert, popular in England, La Primaudaye warned that "present death followeth a great and sudden fear," and Burton emphasized the
devastating effects of "those panic fears which often drive men out
of their wits . . . some for a time, some for their whole lives, they
never recover it."[32]

The idea that heightened passion causes disease and even death
was common wisdom. We have already seen that many of Na-

pier's patients became ill after they experienced grief or fright. They blamed a wide range of physical ailments on their emotional distress, including, for example, consumption, rheumatism, lameness, bloated faces, swollen limbs, amenorrhea, green sickness, and all manner of fevers.[33] A few people were even said to have died of broken hearts or sudden terror. Two women told Napier about maidens who perished from despair after their lovers had jilted them.[34] Joan Haddell, according to the astrologer, "died of a consumption taken by grief of her husband's debts."[35] The Bills of Mortality summarized by John Graunt show that during the early seventeenth century London officials attributed the deaths of about fourteen people to grief and one to fright each year.[36]

A corollary of the belief that mental disturbances endangered physical health was the conviction that disturbed imaginations could actually transmit mental and physical illnesses from one person to another. Napier's rival, the Northampton physician, John Cotta, made famous the cases of two women who were afflicted with sciatica and cramps after their doctor mistakenly suggested that they had those maladies.[37] Stephen Bradwell asserted that people who were terrified by the plague were more vulnerable to the disease.[38] Many of Napier's clients became insane, anxious, or suicidal after they encountered or merely heard about others with similar afflictions: The astrologer noted that suggestion played a part in causing 20 cases of suicidal gloom and 212 cases of other kinds of mental disturbances. The appropriately named Joan Neighbor, for example, "hearing of one that killed herself, and being melancholy, grew ill"; and "frightened by a raving woman," Mary Wooden herself succumbed to mental illness.[39]

The effects of mental turmoil were easier to observe than to explain. Medical texts generally held that tempests in the mind are transmitted to the heart, where they arouse the passions. The disturbance in the emotional climate of the body alters its inner temperature and causes in turn dangerous mutations in the balance and composition of the humors, whose essential qualities of heat and cold, dryness and moisture, make them sensitive to such changes.[40] The anatomists postulated the existence of spirits that acted as mediators between the actions of the mind and body, but they placed perfunctory emphasis on these dubious entities and stressed instead the sympathetic nature of the connection. Thus

Burton wrote that the mind affected the bodily organs "by an admirable league of nature, and by mediation of the spirit."[41] Sir John Davies exclaimed in verse: "The mutual love, the kind intelligence/Twixt heart and brain, this sympathy doth bring."[42] The idea that there is a natural sympathy between the faculties of the soul and the parts of the body was more interesting than the precise physiological mechanism that connected them, because that relationship could be paralleled with the same kind of relationship on the other planes of existence. Thomas Wilson, for example, conceded that there was little agreement among physicians about the manner in which the passions affect the body, but he hastened to point out: "Yet they consent that it may proceed from a certain sympathy of nature, a subordination of one part to another, and that the spirits and the humours wait upon the passions as their lords and masters."[43] This emphasis on the power of sympathy and on correspondence between events on different planes in the cosmological hierarchy enhanced the popular appeal of medical psychology. Astrological connections could be established between the motions of the patient's mind and the movements of the heavens themselves; persuasive analogies could be constructed between mental disturbances and disruptions in the natural and social orders.[44] Moreover, the concepts of sympathy and correspondence permitted people to organize popular ideas about the fragility of body and mind into a coherent system by providing them with an explanation of how events on apparently separate levels of existence – physical, social, and moral – could cause sickness and insanity.

The tyranny of the distracted mind over the regions of the body was equaled in destructive power by the revolt of the provinces against the metropolis of the mind. The physical disorders that were most perilous to mental health were extreme fevers and mortal illnesses. Madness was the familiar prelude to death, a fact that was widely recognized by contemporaries. Describing King John's death, for example, Shakespeare wrote:

> Death having played upon the outward parts
> Leaves them invisible, and his siege is now
> Against the mind, which he pricks and wounds
> With many legions of strange fantasies,
> Which in their throng and press to that last hold
> Confound themselves.[45]

An Elizabethan Jesuit admonished his readers not to postpone repentance until their final hour, for common experience showed that dying people are "scarce able to behave themselves like reasonable creatures," because "their senses are astounded, their minds distracted, their understanding confused, and both their body and mind racked and tormented with throbs of mortal sickness."[46] There was ample evidence, visible to all, that insanity was often the companion of hectic fever and the herald of death. Among Napier's clients alone, 43 victims of mental disorder suffered from fevers and another 56 were "hot." Many others were probably afflicted with acute infections, particularly the 82 women whose insanity followed hard upon difficult deliveries. The majority of people in early modern England died of fevers and infections; villagers visiting the sick and dying had many opportunities to witness the delirium that mortal illnesses could cause.[47]

Physical diseases could provoke any of the symptoms of mental disease. Nevertheless, physicians and philosophers paid greatest attention to the frantic symptoms that signalized grave sickness, emphasizing that they were the terrible spasms of a poisoned imagination. They thought that fevers' heat cooked and burned the humors, turning them into a toxic substance called "melancholy adust," whose fumes roiled up from the crucible of the spleen to pollute the mind. The best description of this fabulous physiology is by Thomas Nashe:

And even as slime and dirt in a standing puddle engender toads and frogs and many other unsightly creatures, so this slimy melancholy humour, still thickening as it stands still, engendreth many misshapen objects in our imaginations . . . So from the fuming melancholy of our spleen mounteth that hot matter into the higher region of the brain, whereof many fearful visions are framed. Our reason even like drunken fumes it displaceth and intoxicates, and yields up our intellective apprehension to be mocked and trodden under foot by every false object or counterfeit noise that comes near it . . . Lightly this extremity of melancholy never cometh, but before some notable sickness; it faring with our brains as with bees, who, as they exceedingly toil and turmoil before a storm or change of the weather, so do they beat and toil and are infinitely confused before sickness.[48]

The doctors' interest in the wild imaginings, raving, and raging of their acutely ill patients was stimulated both by medical tradition and by their clients' anxieties. As we have already seen, classical physicians made a distinction between madness and frenzy, the physiology of which was neatly explained by Thomas Adams:

Physicians have put a difference betwixt frenzy and madness, imagining madness to be only an infection and perturbation of the foremost cell of the head, whereby imagination is hurt; but frenzy to extend further, even to offend the reason and the memory, and is never without fever. Galen calls it an inflammation of the brains, or films thereof, mixed with a sharp fever.[49]

But because the symptoms of these two maladies were identical, save for the presence or absence of a fever, it was in practice very difficult to tell them apart. Napier appears to have found the classical distinction quite unhelpful. He left only one detailed note attempting to divide frenzy from madness in an actual case, and he seldom used "frenzy" or "mania" as diagnostic terms.[50] Like many of his contemporaries, he hoped that astrology would provide a more exact tool for identifying which mental disorders were caused by disease and which were not.[51] He pressured his teacher, Simon Forman, for more information on the matter, provoking that curmudgeon into complaints about his pupil's doltishness. Forman did, however, provide at least one bit of advice that may have influenced his pupil's practice: He insisted that in such cases Napier should take special care to obtain "their particular questions by their own consent."[52] A long tale in Forman's textbook of astrological physic, which Napier owned and read, shows that the practical adept relied upon his knowledge of his clients' symptoms and character as well as upon his horoscopes to unriddle the sources of perplexing maladies.[53] Not surprisingly, neither Napier nor his clients consistently maintained the classical division between the types of insanity, and they preferred to employ remedies that would cure the afflictions of both the mind and the body.[54]

The violent sympathy of mortal illness and stark madness was the most dramatic and alarming manifestation of the intimate connection between physical and mental health, but milder fluctuations in the workings of the body and the mind could also be psychologically significant. The strain of prolonged study, for example, was frequently blamed for the insanity of clergymen, university dons, and intellectually ambitious laymen.[55] Burton's famous digression about the miseries of scholars elaborates the dangers of mental work and physical idleness, which alter the humors and cause either extreme melancholy or Bedlam madness.[56] The passionate tone of Burton's complaints about the travails of impoverished dons and rusticated clergymen betrays his special interest in scholars' melancholy, but the burden of his remarks was accepted by other writers and practitioners. Napier treated 27 men and women who had allegedly grown unhappy or insane because of too much study. The majority were teachers and ministers who, like the schoolmaster Francis Gadstone, were simply supposed to have worked too long without permitting their minds to rest and return to their normal temperature.[57] Several of his clients, however, were laymen perplexed by hard points of sacred doctrine and women devoted to reading and study. Religious and sexual prejudices, which abhorred heterodoxy and denigrated the intellectual powers of women, probably contributed to the conviction, shared by the physician and his patients' families, that the sufferers had caused their own insanity by overmuch study.[58] The bodily maladies that accompanied the mental disturbances of students and unlettered clients alike were usually mild, chronic, and ambiguous. It is seldom possible to tell in retrospect whether they were thought to be the source of their patient's emotional problems or the consequence of them. The most common complaints were about insomnia, breathlessness, trembling, upset stomach, vertigo, headache, ringing ears, and "rising" sensations, all conditions that modern doctors would suspect to be physical manifestations of emotional disorders.[59]

The flux of the humors was believed to affect mental tranquillity in another way. According to the popularizers of classical medicine, each of the four humors has a particular affinity with certain of the passions that share its distinctive qualities of moisture and temperature. Even among healthy people the balance of the humors is seldom if ever exact, and most individuals therefore display the psychological characteristics associated with their dominant humor.[60] There are four main personality types: choleric, phlegmatic, sanguine, and melancholy. The complexions, or temperaments as they were also called, are not in themselves abnormalities. A melancholy complexion, for instance, proceeds from an abundance of the "natural" form of that humor, rather than its corrupted "adust" state, and produces a character that is sober, contemplative, and timorous. But these normal variations in temperament can contribute to mental disorders. They predispose men and women to suffer dangerous excesses of the passions characteristic of their complexions. Medical psychologists used this scheme to explain the commonly observed fact that some people are more vulnerable to psychological distress than others. "According to the disposition of the heart, humours and body," Thomas Wright remarked, "diverse sorts of persons be subject to diverse sorts of passions, and the same passion affected diverse persons in diverse manners."[61] Napier, who was careless about noting his patients' complexions, nevertheless noted that 37 of his disturbed clients were "subject to melancholy," 9 were chronically fearful, and many more were "apt to grief."[62]

Because they believed so strongly that there was a sympathy between body and soul, Tudor and Stuart doctors employed physical remedies to heal mental diseases. The regimen of treatment for mad and troubled people differed little from the measures used to cure other patients. Regardless of their symptoms, almost every one of Napier's mentally disturbed patients was purged with emetics and laxatives and bled with leeches or by cupping. The clients of other classically trained doctors endured the same treatments.[63] The drugs that Napier and his fellow physicians used to purge their patients were a medley of native and exotic plants, traditional recipes, and new inorganic compounds. Many of these substances had their origins in ancient and Arabic medicine. For example, the electuary that Napier preferred above all others to purge melancholy was a classical invention extolled by Ptolemy for that purpose. It was called *hiera logadii*, and it contained, among other ingredients, aloes, colocynth, and black hellebore, all potent laxatives.[64] Another compound Napier often used to treat the troubled in mind was an Arabic concoction known as *confectio hamech*. It also worked a strong purging action on patients' bowels, for it contained myrobalans, rhubarb, and senna.[65] The exotic plants in these preparations were obtained from the East and West Indies. The expansion of trade to the Levant and the New World during the seventeenth century introduced a profusion of organic medicines into English practice.[66] Tobacco, Raleigh's rank gift to England from America, was especially popular as a vomit; Napier prescribed it frequently, and Burton trumpeted both its medicinal virtues and its potential

perils to health and sanity when overused.[67] Apothecaries proliferated to take advantage of the public demand for such new medicines, and remedies compounded from tropical plants became
widely available. Napier was able to purchase quantities of purging concoctions and soothing infusions already prepared by a London apothecary.[68]

Pharmacology was controversial. The apothecaries organized
and challenged the College of Physicians for a greater role in
health care in the lucrative London market.[69] Public interest was
excited both by the importation of exotic flora and by the appearance of new inorganic compounds. These chemical medicines
were made of metals and minerals, and they were associated with
Paracelsus and his followers. Paracelsus espoused a physiological
theory that was antagonistic to the Galenic system of the four humors. He taught that diseases were manifestations of chemical
malfunctions in the body's organs; he devised inorganic medicaments to combat the chemical causes of illness and employed
chemical techniques to prepare organic substances for use as medicines.[70] His advocacy of the superiority of his philosophy and the
remedies he invented was so strident that he became one of the
most notorious iconoclasts of the age. Pamphlet battles between
the Galenists and Paracelsians preoccupied the physicians of late
sixteenth-century Europe.[71]

Many English practitioners nevertheless incorporated drugs
from both systems into their healing regimens. Even the official
pharmacopoeia of the College of Physicians contained chemical
preparations, and several of its most distinguished members in the
early seventeenth century were Paracelsians. Charles Webster has
shown that a thriving domestic tradition of medical chemistry
prepared a congenial reception of the fruits of Paracelsian chemistry and created interest in its medical philosophy. The medical
establishment was not converted to Paracelsianism, but prior to
the Civil War many physicians minimized the differences between
the rival systems and expropriated the medicines devised by the
Paracelsians without accepting their theories.[72] An unabashed defense of such pharmaceutical eclecticism was written by William
Clowes, who declared that the strife between the Galenists and the
Paracelsians was incomprehensible and irrelevant to medical practice: "If I find (either by reason or experience) anything that may
be to the good of the patients . . . be it either in Galen or Para-

celsus, yea, Turk, Jew, or any other infidel, I will not refuse it, but be thankful to God for the same."[73]

Clowes's declaration precisely describes Richard Napier's practice. Napier supplemented his arsenal of traditional organic medicaments with metallic compounds and distillations; he even collected bizarre folk remedies and occasionally resorted to them.[74] Not content merely to rely upon the recipes available in the *Pharmacopoeia Londinensis*, he became an avid medical alchemist, preparing his own chemical medicines with the assistance of the adepts Thomas Robson and Theodore Gravius. He collected and read books and manuscripts in the medieval alchemical tradition, works by such men as Raymond Lull and Roger Bacon. He was familiar with Paracelsus and owned at least some of his many writings.[75] He bought Simon Forman's huge alchemical library after his mentor's death, and he knew many of the leading alchemists of his time, including John Dee.[76]

Although Napier was fascinated by the mystical aspirations of medieval alchemy and probably knew something about the substance of Paracelsus's medical thought, he nevertheless remained chiefly interested in the practical side of alchemy and regarded chemical medicines as a novel and effective complement to traditional therapies. Writing to a flattering correspondent in the 1620s, he protested that "the skill I have . . . is more in the preparation of chemical medicines of the sick than any whit for the philosopher's work."[77] He warned another enthusiast not to persist in his alchemical studies, because the subject was "so changeable and so uncertain."[78] His attitude toward Paracelsianism must be reassembled from scattered shards of evidence. He annotated recipes for medicines in Paracelsus's works and probably followed his directions for preparing compounds containing antimony and mercury; he employed several other medicines, including lapis lazuli and laudanum, which were associated with Paracelsus.[79] But he appears to have ignored Paracelsus's theory of disease entirely. Nothing in his notes indicated that he explained any illness in Paracelsian terms. During a decade in which he was keenly interested in medical alchemy, the 1620s, he also developed a new fondness for humoral jargon, partly as a consequence of reading Burton's *Anatomy of Melancholy*.[80] He employed Paracelsian preparations, such as compounds of antimony, as substitutes for organic remedies that acted as vomits and purges, and he often combined modern chemical medicines with traditional substances. The notes he made about the best treatments for the mentally disturbed illustrate his eclecticism: A prescription for "all melancholy and mopish people," for example, recommends *hiera logadii*, lapis lazuli, hellebore, cloves, licorice powder, *diambra,* and *pulvis sancti,* all of which were to be infused in a solution of white wine and borage. This olio of plants and chemicals would act as a violent purge.[81] Napier collected many other recipes for medicines to cure melancholy, the majority of which were steadfastly traditional.[82] Burton himself recommended a similar melange of Galenic and chemical medicaments, and Napier's eclectic habits mirror the pragmatism of English physicians, such as Clowes and Burton, who were chiefly concerned to discover effective medical treatments regardless of their sources.[83]

Although Napier provided his patients with the best medicaments that were available, his practice provides chilling illustrations of the hazards and inadequacies of contemporary medicine. The new pharmaceuticals provided patients with relief for the symptoms of a few diseases, notably syphilis, but they were both extolled and attacked chiefly for their violent action. The only medicines that eased the torments of mental disorder were opiates. Administered as opium grains, unguents, and laudanum (a tincture invented by Paracelsus), they were recommended as soporifics and analgesics and were widely recognized to be an effective sedative.[84] Both Galenists and Paracelsians sang their praises, and they were probably used more freely in the seventeenth century than ever before in England.[85] Napier employed them in his treatment of the insane to ease the torment of insomnia and calm the raging of stark madness. Although the statistics are disfigured by his failure to record his prescriptions in every case, his notes provide a numerical indication of this practice. Opiates are mentioned in only 8.2% of his consultations with melancholy patients, but they are included in notes about 16.1% of his sessions with madmen and lunatics, in 21.6% of his meetings with distracted people, and in 18.4% of his consultations with light-headed patients. A similar pattern of prescription may be found in the practice books of other seventeenth-century physicians.[86] Opium is unquestionably effective, and it must certainly have brought relief to many of the frantic men and women who turned to doctors for help.

No other drug used by the physicians of the age can be said in retrospect to have provided a pharmacologically effective remedy for specific symptoms of insanity. Although drugs were praised for their powers to cure particular diseases, the purges and emetics that were the mainstay of medical practice were intended to expel humors that caused a wide range of disorders and symptoms. The way in which Napier used them contrasts with his tendency to prescribe opium to relieve a limited range of ailments. He developed enthusiasms for various medicines, favoring them over other laxatives and vomits for a time and then replacing them with other staple preparations. In the middle of his career, for example, he discarded *confectio hamech* and embraced antimonial compounds; the new favorites, like the old, worked as vomits and purges.[87] Individual variations in the drugs Napier prescribed were influenced more by the size of the patient's purse than the precise nature of his complaints. Like other physicians, he provided the rich with medicines that were pleasanter, more numerous, exotic, and expensive than the nostrums handed out to poorer clients. These concoctions complemented ordinary treatments in Napier's practice, and they ranged from diet drinks made out of spices and wine to a controversial infusion of liquid gold.[88]

Whether one was rich or poor, the medical cure for mental disorder characteristically included orders for a variety of purges and vomits and often phlebotomy as well – all of which were meant to expel noxious humors from the body and restore the balance of the four essential fluids. The amount of blood to be drawn from patients' veins and the placement of the leeches or lesions were included in the physician's orders to surgeons, who performed the actual bloodletting. The afflictions of the mind were generally treated either by extracting blood directly from the patient's forehead or by tapping the cephalic, saphenous, or hemorrhoidal veins to draw the corrupted humors down, away from the sickened brain.[89] Although his records are incomplete, they seem to show that Napier was rather restrained in his use of phlebotomy and that he was adjusting his treatments to suit their constitutions rather than their maladies. It was a maxim of good medical practice that the Galenic physician should take care to prescribe remedies that would not overtax his sick clients. It was for this reason, and not to improve diagnostic precision, that doctors needed carefully to consider their patients' age, sex, and bodily condition, according to Thomas Brian.[90] Bleeding could easily endanger the lives of diseased women and children.

The classical regimen of purges and bleeding often worked terrible effects, even when the physician was mindful of his patients' strength and his medicines were prepared by artful alchemists or apothecaries. The traditional drugs were strong and unpredictable; the Paracelsian substitutes were even stronger. Although Viscount Purbeck received the best treatment Napier and his assistants could devise, his richly documented case includes several descriptions of pharmaceutical disasters. "Took a gentle purge," Napier recorded in one place; "it wrought twenty times, and he said he would never take any more."[91] Another time, after Purbeck drank his purge, he "cast it up and was very sick until all was up, and then had nineteen stools and went to bed."[92] Small wonder that he occasionally refused to take his medicine until Napier himself had swallowed part of the potion.[93] The new chemical medicines devised by medical alchemists and Paracelsians were notoriously violent and dangerous. André Du Laurens condemned the use of antimony to treat cases of melancholy because it was too toxic to be safely employed as a vomit.[94] Napier himself recorded a case in which mercury treatments, probably for syphilis, poisoned a man and made him stark mad.[95] Sir John Hayward echoed the cries of many of his contemporaries when he declared: "Hereupon diverse others also have settled their opinions, that it is the best physic to take no physic at all."[96]

Laymen were thus painfully aware of the perils and discomforts of seventeenth-century medicine, and many of them were persuaded that nature or magic were surer cures than any physician's lore. Nevertheless, the public craving for purging potions and chemical remedies grew, and there were bitter complaints about the cost and social exclusiveness of classical medicine.[97] The huge number of patients treated by Napier alone testifies to the popular faith in physic, for even though he also employed magical and religious treatments, classical medical remedies formed the basis of his therapeutic practice. Some people even welcomed the surgeon's blade because they believed that bloodletting would cure them. Purbeck himself once asked Napier to have him bled.[98] A friend or neighbor of Joan Martyne's reported to him that phlebotomy had cured Martyne a year before: "Easter Monday last was twelvemonth, was troubled in mind. And now well, God be thanked, with letting of blood."[99] Many of the patients Napier treated were probably similarly referred by clients who had apparently found relief because of the classical regimen of purges, vomits, and bleeding.

Because it is perfectly apparent that the noxious potions physicians prescribed and the painful phlebotomy surgeons performed rarely in themselves cured anybody of a mental or physical affliction, how are we to account for the evidence of popular faith in their powers?[100] Part of the answer to this problem is that they sometimes seemed to work. Patients whose recoveries fortuitously followed the administration of medical treatment were likely to attribute their recoveries to the active measures taken by their physicians. But medical nostrums did not merely win gratitude owed more properly to God and nature. They also produced psychological effects that assisted the healing of many maladies, particularly afflictions that were caused by mental distress. Because seventeenth-century doctors lacked modern diagnostic techniques, neither they nor their clients could distinguish between illnesses that were psychosomatic and those that were not. Contemporaries therefore placed even greater emphasis on the curative powers of the imagination than we do today. When Burton sought to explain the evident effectiveness of the magical remedies that he and his colleagues regarded to be ineffective, for example, he attributed their successes to the charlatan's capacity to work upon sufferers' imaginations. The "spells, words, characters and charms" of quacks and mountebanks create "a strong conceit and opinion . . . which takes away the cause of the malady from the parts affected."[101] Although he could hardly be expected to admit that medical treatments worked in the same manner, he did remark that faith in the healing virtues of orthodox physicians was also necessary; no melancholy person can expect to be relieved unless he has "sure hope that his physician can help him."[102] The belief in fancy's curing powers was the reciprocal of the belief in its pathological capacity. Modern sudies show that beguiling scientists dispensing brightly colored placebos can actually produce recovery rates in mentally and physically ill patients higher than those among people who are simply neglected. Such reports suggest that a certain number of seventeenth-century sufferers were undoubtedly cured by their faith in the remedies their physicians prescribed.[103] Their recoveries would be impossible to distinguish from evidence of the actual effectiveness of the medicines they took.

The "placebo effect" cannot take place unless patients are persuaded that the medical system that the curer represents is valid, and it would beg the larger questions of contemporary faith in an ineffective medicine to say simply that medical science was plausible because it sometimes appeared to work. The appeal of medical psychology lay ultimately in the elaborately simple aspiration it espoused: to restore the harmony between the patient's mind and the operations of the natural order. Medical science was holistic. Its theoretical framework postulated that insanity could be caused by events on several planes of existence, within the victim's body or without, and that a distinctive disturbance on one plane would be answered by a disturbance on another. Physicians therefore attempted to correct their clients' disorders on at least three levels simultaneously – the corporeal, the cosmological, and the social.

Astrology was the instrument that permitted physicians to determine the relationship between their patients' health and the order of the universe. The configuration of the stars revealed the sources of the sufferer's dissonance and helped the healer to orchestrate his use of natural remedies to restore his client's sanity. The herbs he selected and the metals he compounded possessed qualities that linked them with things that shared those attributes – diseases, passions, humors, and even the stars and constellations. Ideally, the medicines physicians prescribed were collected or prepared at astrologically propitious moments, so that the relationship between the patient's health and the structure and rhythms of the cosmos could be restored through the power of sympathy. The realities of the pharmaceutical trade probably made this degree of scrupulousness unusual. Some astrological physicians, including Napier, supplied their patients with astral sigils bearing the symbol of an appropriate astrological entity with which they were to stamp their medicines before taking them.[104] Many more doctors probably shared Napier's habit of carefully instructing clients to dose themselves with medicaments and secure phlebotomy at astrologically selected times.[105]

The rituals and calculations that were a necessary part of medical treatment before the decay of astrology served to remind the patient that his sufferings were as much a part of the natural order as a tempest and to make him feel that his anguish was a crisis that had ramifications throughout the universe. The healer's art lay in manipulating the sick person's relationship with the forces of nature, the sources of life and power. Men could see and feel the tangible elements of this artistry – the fluids they identified as humors exist, the passions can be recognized and classified, diseases have distinctive qualities of heat and moisture, the motions of the tide-pulling moon and the planets can be charted. The cosmological framework that ordered all these parts was as evident to the Elizabethans as the Einsteinian structure of space and time is to us (or more so). It was supremely plausible that achieving physical and mental health consisted of restoring the original harmony between the microcosm and the macrocosm.

Medicines and phlebotomy were only two means to that end. To restore the balance of the humors and the tranquillity of the mind, physicians also regulated their patients' physical environment and social actions directly. This was achieved largely by controlling the "six non-natural things" that can affect health – diet, retention and evacuation, air, exercise, sleeping and waking, and the passions.[106] There were lengthy recommendations about how to manipulate these factors in popular medical texts; Burton's remarks about regulating them to cure melancholy occupy an entire volume and range from advice to avoid too much drink and indolence to instructions for using music to create an emotionally soothing atmosphere.[107]

The passions are most frequently aroused by personal relationships and social activities, and contemporary writers devised programs to calm the mentally disordered by rectifying their disturbing relationships and ill habits. The most famous regimen of this kind required melancholy people to seek merry company, play at honest amusements, dress gaily, and haunt light and lovely places and to avoid solitude, banish gloomy contemplations, put away dark and disheveled garb, and eschew black and moldering settings.[108] Young people afflicted with lovers' melancholy were traditionally advised to exchange passion for austerity, to discard the abnormal attachment to their lovers and resume their normal regard for their parents.[109] Napier and his fellow Anglican clergymen often recommended regular church attendance as a form of therapy for the troubled in mind, because in their view acting like a sane and dutiful Christian would inevitably promote sanity and social normality.[110] An unusual example of a therapy designed to force a mentally disturbed person to behave normally is a Skinnerian terror devised by John Spencer to cure Sir Robert Carr's brother of a sottish melancholy. Spencer ordered that Carr be forced to enact a martial exercise that pantomimed the military duties a normal aristocrat performed:

If you find him inclining to a sottish humour, put an armour upon him and beat a drum before him. And let one attire himself like a captain, and put on his gorget and a plume of feathers in his hat and a truncheon in his hand and make him march and exercise his arms, or else set him upon a bounding horse and trot the ring and run a career. And in these martial exercises let the captain command him as a soldier and if he finds him peevish and forward, give him a good knock upon his helmet, and if he finds him willing and tractable, then to [*sic*] commend him and praise him.[111]

The course of blows and compliments worked wonderfully to restore Carr to his former sanity, a result that could be explained as the forced resumption of reason's sway.

The notorious practice of flogging madmen was also a form of social therapy. A Bedlam lunatic comported himself like a beast or a wild child, oblivious to the normal rules of social conduct. The justification for whipping lunatics was the same as the justification for birching backward schoolboys: It taught them to behave well by punishing them for their lapses. The great physician Thomas Willis explained the necessity to flog madmen in his famous *De anima brutorum*, published in 1672:

The first indication, *viz.* curatory, requires threatenings, bonds, or strokes, as well as physic. For the madman . . . must be so handled both by the physician, and also by the servants that are prudent, that he may be in some manner kept in, either by warnings, chiding, or punishments inflicted on him, to his duty, or his behaviour, or manners.[112]

Men who whipped lunatics to bring them to their senses were exempted from legal punishment for assault, because they were no more guilty of a crime than parents who corrected their children.[113] Evidence that village authorities ordered the insane to be whipped can be found, but flogging was certainly not the principal mode of therapy for madness during the seventeenth century.[114] Most mentally disturbed men and women do not appear to have been physically abused, except in asylums and Bridewells.

Napier treated only 20 clients who had been either chained or beaten. Burton does not mention the rod as a remedy for melancholy, no matter how sullenly intractable the patient was.[115] To judge by the lurid descriptions of conditions in Hanoverian madhouses, the practice of beating the insane became much more common during the eighteenth century, when the asylum system spread throughout the nation.[116]

The Tudor and Stuart physician was more than a mere specialist in humoral mechanics. He was a healer who ideally addressed himself to all aspects of his patients' lives and invoked all levels of the natural order in his therapies. From this perspective, it is easier to see why even noxious remedies could be desirable. In practice, however, physicians paid less and less attention to the holistic facets of their craft. They concentrated instead on prescribing drugs and ordering phlebotomy. The decline of astrology in the late seventeenth century removed the most conspicuous emblem of their cosmological aspirations. The sharp controversy over Paracelsian remedies, which erupted during the Interregnum, and the new anatomical discoveries of the century broke the theoretical bond between physiology and cosmology and demolished the intellectual basis for traditional therapies. The psychology of Hobbes and Locke repudiated the classical theory of mind and the medieval identification of mind and soul.[117] These developments deprived medicine of much of its traditional intellectual appeal. Physicians tried to maintain their scientific respectability by accepting some modern ideas and marrying them to ancient remedies, a match that was more attractive politically than philosophically.[118] Restoration medicine was less comprehensive and less consistent than Renaissance medicine. Medical psychology nevertheless displaced its rivals as the dominant mode of treating the insane in the eighteenth century. The increasing prestige of scientific medicine was the result of political strife and religious controversy and not the advancement of psychological theory and medical therapy. The mad and melancholy people of eighteenth-century England suffered the ancient treatments without even the consolation of traditional cosmology. Their anguish was robbed of transcendent significance; their discomforts were stripped of cosmological justification. Properly, we should not speak of the rise of medical science, we should talk instead of the decline of therapeutic eclecticism. To understand the traditional system fully, we must turn now to medicine's siblings and rivals and examine magical and religious modes of psychological healing.

DEMONS, WITCHES, AND MADMEN

In a terrific diatribe aimed in part at Napier himself, the Northampton physician John Cotta lamented that the superstitions of ordinary rustics enhanced the popularity of the physicians' rivals, the astrologers, clerical doctors, and cunning people: "The general madness of this age," he complained, "ascribeth unto witchcraft whatsoever falleth out unknown or strange unto a vulgar sense."[119] Villages and cities were full of men and women who were ready to use magical means to relieve mental and physical suffering, and when ordinary people were afflicted by illness, anxiety, or insanity they often resorted first to such healers. "'Tis a common practice of some men to go first to a witch," Burton wrote, "and then to a physician, if the one cannot the other shall."[120] The physicians sought to change popular attitudes about the causes of diseases, particularly mental illnesses, arguing that even the strangest symptoms were most likely the consequence of some natural disorder. Convinced that the common people were "apt to make everything a supernatural work which they do not understand," Edmund Jorden wrote a famous pamphlet purporting to show that many afflictions that were thought to be caused by witches or the Devil were actually symptoms of a disease he called "suffocation of the mother," which modern psychiatric historians have identified with hysteria.[121] Cotta was more comprehensive and explained that epilepsy could also account for apparently supernatural symptoms and that often very strange behavior was caused by several diseases playing simultaneously upon the same tormented frame. He appealed to his readers to believe that unusual maladies were not more mysterious than jugglers' tricks and that medical men would eventually find the hidden but natural causes of them.[122] Cotta and his fellow physicians did not actually deny the existence of witchcraft and demoniacal possession, but they maintained that patients harmed by these means were very rare and would display some "power, act or deed" obviously above the natural capacity of man: "Hence the sick oft speak strange languages unto themselves unknown, and prophesy things to come above human capacity."[123] In addition to linguistic and prophetic feats, the truly bewitched or possessed might become incredibly strong or perform acts of convulsive acrobatics. Their afflictions would always be impervious to the natural remedies of the most skilled physician.

It is easy to see why arguments that banished Satan and witches from the chambers of the sick in all but the most baffling cases appealed to classical physicians. Most of the "ignorant practisers" Cotta attacked were technicians of the sacred who employed occult means to detect the causes of mental and physical illnesses and remedy them. The skeptical approach to the powers of the unseen world also provided a useful excuse for physicians when their science proved ineffective, and there is plenty of evidence that doctors who were forced to confess ignorance and failure were as ready as the most credulous bumpkin to descry the Devil and his minions.[124] Most men and women had not invested as heavily in natural science as the university-trained physicians, and they retained a much wider notion of the harmful actions of the supernatural. Napier treated hundreds of people of every social rank, who feared that they were haunted or bewitched. At least 513 of his clients suspected that they or their sick relatives had been harmed by witchcraft; 264 of these men and women were mentally disturbed. Another 148 patients who suffered psychological symptoms were believed to be haunted or possessed. The most exalted victims of witchcraft that Napier treated were the Earl and Lady of Sussex, the Earl of Sunderland, and Viscount Purbeck. A randy pair of adulterers before they were married to each other, the Earl of Sussex and his wife complained that the zest had gone out of their copulation since their spouses had died and their union was legalized; they attributed a "certain frigidness" they experienced to the evil work of sorcerers hired by their former mates.[125] Sunderland blamed a lingering, mortal, but unremarkable illness on witches' work and even named a possible suspect to Napier.[126] Purbeck and his wife hurled accusations of witchcraft at each other in their notorious and sordid struggle to escape a wretched marriage. Laud and Buckingham took these charges seriously, but Napier did not – perhaps because the circumstances themselves amply explained Purbeck's lunacy.[127] Hundreds of obscure rustics who repeated their fears to Napier attributed a similar medley of ordinary problems and illnesses to witchcraft and possession.

Popular indifference to the physicians' restrictive definition of the symptoms of supernatural affliction is obvious in the pattern of complaints reported by the alleged demoniacs treated by Napier. These tormented men and women, and their physician, apparently thought that the Devil could harm the mind more readily than the body, because almost all of them complained of some form of mental disturbance. Few of the people who feared that they were possessed or haunted, however, suffered from severe insanity or displayed spectacular symptoms. Most of them complained of lesser disorders: anxiety and worry, religious perplexity of fears, or evil thoughts. About one-third of them were suicidal or "tempted," probably to self-destruction or religious apostasy. As a group, these clients were distinctive because over one-fourth of them related incidents in which they saw or felt the presence of supernatural beings. Most of these experiences would be classified as hallucinations or delusions today, and I have described them in the tables as "hallucinations." Although Napier dismissed some of these tales as "strange fancies" or "conceits," he was more reluctant than we are to dismiss them as fabulous inventions. In the early seventeenth century perceptions of the invisible world were taken very seriously. Encounters with spirits and angels were rare, but they were not by themselves signs of mental abnormality. Napier regarded the unusual sights and sounds reported by these patients as evidence that their fears about demons might be correct; most of his contemporaries would have done the same (Table 5.1).

Keith Thomas has remarked that many of the famous cases of demonic possession occurred in family atmospheres that were oppressively pious. Protected by a cloak of devilish license, Satan's victims screamed spectacular curses and shocking blasphemies.[128] Religious rebellion and apostasy were common themes in published cases of possession, particularly after the appearance of Nathaniel Bacon's popular narrative of Francis Spira's dramatic struggle with the Devil early in the seventeenth century.[129] Several of Napier's clients were tempted by Satan to commit apostasy. Ann March, for example, told the astrologer that "the Devil would have her . . . make as much of him as of God."[130] Twenty-eight of Napier's patients thought that Satan or his minions, appearing to them visibly or as disembodied voices, had urged them to commit suicide, the embodiment of apostasy in popular reli-

Table 5.1. *Patients fearing demons or reportedly possessed (in percent)*

	All mentally disturbed (N = 2,483)	Demoniacs (N = 164)
Mad, lunatic, distracted	10.3	4.8
Light-headed	15.0	9.8
Melancholy	19.9	11.0
Troubled in mind	32.0	41.5
Suicidal	6.4	17.1
Tempted	5.3	18.3
Evil thoughts	3.6	8.5
Religious anxiety	11.8	28.0
Hallucinations	5.1	26.8
Mopish	15.2	11.6

Note: Figures are percentages of consultations in which these symptoms appear. Demons were mentioned in 148 cases.

gious tradition.[131] The spiritual agony of William Ringe rivaled the religious dramatics of notorious cases like Spira's. Tormented by guilt because he had committed adultery, Ringe first became persuaded that Satan himself was leading him to despair, controlling his thoughts to "suggesteth so his sins as that he would persuade him that he is damned for it."[132] Four months later he was possessed by four spirits, whom he named to Napier, as Legon, Simon, Argell (or Arragon), and Ammelee, the tempter.[133] Then, at the climax of this torment, the tempter struggled with Ringe's good angel for the possession of his soul. The spirits spoke with Ringe's lips, and the ready scribe of the archangels recorded their words faithfully:

First the tempter said unto Will Ringe: "Leave tempting
    of me and I will my soul freely unto thee."

Then his good angel bid him say: "Christ shall have
    my body and soul."

Then he tempted him again to say that: "Then thou must
    take it out of God's hand."

And his good angel bid him say: "God shall have it from
    thee."[134]

The religious background of Ringe's family, like that of Napier's other possessed and haunted patients, is unknown, and it is impossible to tell how many of them may have been rebelling against the tyranny of domestic theocracy. Many of these obscure victims of Satan were, like Ringe himself, tormented by guilt, and their psychological motivations seem to have been much simpler and more commonplace than those of the famous demoniacs.

Medieval and early modern villagers normally personified their unacceptable feelings and actions by ascribing them to the instigation of the Devil. Napier's clients were typical in attributing a wide range of evil thoughts and forbidden urges to the temptations of Satan, and for them, as for the majority of their compatriots, these personifications possessed palpable reality.[135] The Fiend appeared to some of them to tell them that they would be his creatures in hell, condemned to suffer for their sins. "Thinketh that she hath an ill spirit within her," Napier wrote of Joan Brawbrook; "the spirit telleth her that he will burn her and damn her and seemeth to speak within her."[136] Joan Perkins "said that she had heard a voice . . . that said he would have her to give her body and soul."[137] The inner voice of William Dudley accused him of killing his wife and persuaded him that he would soon die for his imaginary crime.[138] Patients sometimes told the astrologer that demons urged them to commit heinous sins. Supernatural beings tempted six men and women, for example, to slaughter their children, their parents, or their spouses.[139] Thomas Langly was driven out of his senses by spirits who enticed him to "uncleanness" and blasphemy; he spoke of a witch at Dodford and complained that he was "troubled with whirlwinds."[140] Napier practiced during the height of English anxieties about witchcraft, and his patients blamed witches as well as demons for their forbidden urges. One example will stand for many of the astrologer's clients. Edward Cleaver was "surely tempted with profane and ungodly thoughts, and sometimes with an inward smiling and laughing in his heart." One day after thanking the Lord for his supper, "an ill motion came into his mind, saying 'Kiss my arse.' "[141] Demonology and witch beliefs provided ordinary men and women with a means to express their unconscious yearning to violate moral imperatives and a way to mitigate their guilt by attributing their sins to supernatural beings.

Because the Devil and his ethereal attendants were essential aspects of popular psychology, it is not surprising that some people thought they had detected visible proof of the presence of the unseen world. When men and women were anxious and upset they readily believed that a supernatural agent had brought their trouble down upon them. Even the language with which the sick described the sensations of their diseases blurred the distinction between metaphor and reality. Here is a spectrum of Napier's reports of his clients' descriptions of their symptoms, arranged to show how easily such speech could move from trope to true conviction that evil spirits worked within:

Feeleth a thing at her heart as if it were alive.[142]

Miserably troubled in her stomach as if rats should gnaw.[143]

Supposeth that thing which leapeth within him . . . [so] that he cannot go nor do anything is some ill spirit.[144]

She is haunted, as she thinketh, with an ill spirit, and feeleth some living thing roll up and down in her, and it will pluck her and gather all together then down in the bottom of her belly and then up to her heart and side.[145]

Feeleth something as it were to creep into his cheeks, lips, nose and his eyes . . . Feareth something to haunt him because he is so ill handled.[146]

Much troubled in his brain and supposeth that he is haunted. A thing cometh from without like a breath fiddling about his legs and goeth into his mouth and goeth into his body and then turneth up to his head and troubleth his brain [so] that he thinketh he seeth strange things.[147]

He told his mother he saw a winged thing flew in the air, and then was like to a bird and did fly into his mouth and ever since he will not be ruled.[148]

A thing running about like a mouse. Suspecteth ill things. She thinketh that she seeth a mouse running about her head.[149]

As the frightening physical sensations of anxiety or illness became more urgently real, they revealed themselves as familiar creatures. The visible spirits that haunted Napier's troubled clients looked like dogs, cats, rats, mice, birds, bees, a weasel, and a colt.[150] These were the same kind of animals that were mentioned as the servant spirits of witches in witchcraft trials, and the common name for such demons, "familiars," suggests a simple psychological explanation for the shapes they assumed.[151] Afraid of madness or death, miserable men and women such as the people Napier treated personified their feelings in the form of routine pests, the kind of banal vexations that surrounded every villager and seldom caused grave injury, an association that probably provided some reassurance that their maladies were not entirely mysterious.

The imagined enemies of ordinary people were much more mundane than the evil spirits and hallucinations artists and writers attributed to demoniacs and melancholy souls. Even Satan himself was described by sufferers who feared possession in disappointingly ordinary guises. Everybody knew that the Devil could dissimulate a serpent, a cloud, a chimera, a talking bush, a thousand horrid monsters, or an angel of light.[152] But to Sara Chalice he appeared simply "in the likeness of a man"; to Guiles Southan he was all too protean and looked like "everything he seeth."[153] The enemy was as commonplace as his minions: Satan appeared as a man or even a woman or as a disembodied voice or as a presence with an identity but without a shape remarkable enough to mention to the physician.[154] Men and women who were overwhelmed by anxiety sometimes personified the threat to their lives and everlasting souls simply as flashes of light or fire, a metonym of obvious significance. Agnes Holder, for example, was "troubled by a shaking fear, fearing lest she be carried away; she thinketh that she seeth flashes of fire."[155]

Worldly wise intellectuals found it easy to mock the pedestrian iconography of popular demonology and ridicule the credulity of bumpkins. Thomas Nashe employed his quill in this sport:

There be them that think every spark in a flame is a spirit, and that the worms which at sea eat through ships are also; which may well be, for have not you seen one spark of fire burn a whole town and a man with a spark of lightning made blind or killed outright? . . . Now for worms: what makes a dog run mad but a worm in its tongue? And what should that worm be but a spirit? Is there any reason such small vermin as they are should devour such a vast thing as a ship, or have the teeth to gnaw through iron and wood? No, no, they are spirits, or else it were impossible.[156]

The rich were certainly less preoccupied by vermin than the poor, but they suffered the same anxieties when they fell mad or sick, and there is no obvious material reason why they should have repudiated the solace of common superstitions. Nor did contemporary science offer any better means to cope with guilt and fear than demonology and exorcism. The famous published cases of possession, which many educated people repeated, were actually more fabulous than the fears Napier's clients voiced. Notable demoniacs babbled learned languages, vomited pins and nails, toads, and other creatures; they spoke Satan's words in his own timbre and leaped and jerked like puppets. Often they were adolescents with a grudge against the crew of stern adults who enjoyed so much power to frustrate their wishes and flog them for their misdeeds.[157] Still, they were frequently believed, and when they turned their hostility on elderly scapegoats they became the focus for savage witch-hunts. The notorious trials of groups of witches in Essex and Lancashire had their local analogues in Napier's region. Such a panic in nearby Northampton claimed at least four lives in 1612 and left many others tainted with suspicion.[158] Napier encountered several cases of demonic children whose actions closely mimicked the behavior described in famous cases. Here is his account of the behavior of two of them, a brother and a sister, who were not older than fourteen or fifteen when the incident occurred: "They would leap out of their beds and feel things rising. They had ten spirits haunted them, and would form faces and make strange signs and cried out of a woman called Bing's wife, who was ducked and did swim."[159] When the Countess of Bridgwater's children began to act strangely, as if they were tormented by demons, she turned to Sir Richard Napier to help her discover whether they were truly possessed. The young astrologer wrote to his uncle, reporting that although the countess feared the worst, the cause of the children's affliction was unclear.[160]

Although physicians like Cotta and satirists like Nashe ridiculed the propensity of rustic villagers to descry the Devil or witches in every illness or misfortune, some learned and famous men remained convinced that supernatural evil was an omnipresent peril. Burton, who was one of the most widely read authors of the age, was outraged by the suggestion that evil spirits did not cause insanity and revealed themselves only to the overly credulous minds of superstitious bumpkins and madmen: "Many will not believe they [spirits] can be seen, and if a man shall say, swear, and stiffly maintain, though he be discreet and wise, judicious and learned, that he hath seen them, they account him a timorous fool, a melancholy dizzard, a weak fellow, a dreamer, a sick or a mad man, they contemn him, laugh him to scorn."[161] Throughout the seventeenth century traditionalists published defenses of old demonological lore, but the educated elite's faith in the active powers of the Devil gradually deteriorated, in part because of religious controversy. The physicians' assault on popular credulity was obviously colored by their rivalry with astrologers and village wizards whose countermagic was very·appealing to people terrified by spirits and witches.[162] It is unlikely that this parochial campaign would have had a wide influence on the educated classes had it not become part of the larger and more profound turmoil of religious politics. The Protestant repudiation of the "supernatural" rituals of the medieval church stripped the orthodox clergy of most of their magical powers. The English people, however, continued to believe in the Devil's power to possesss them, and during Elizabeth's reign the Jesuits exploited the church's reticence about the ritual expulsion of evil spirits by touting their own traditional power of exorcism as proof of their superior spiritual authority. The Anglican hierarchy apparently did little to counter this propaganda tactic until the turn of the century, when the Puritan wing of the church began to take advantage of the same weakness. Developing a method of casting out devils by group prayer and fasting, which did not offend precisionist distaste for ritual, the Puritan clergy found a highly effective publicist for their cause, the famous exorcist John Darrell. Alarmed by Darrell's spectacular and well-dramatized activities, the bishops launched a campaign to discredit him. The official pamphleteers, Samuel Harsnet, John Deacon, and John Walker, labored to prove that the victims Darrell claimed to have dispossessed were impostors. The threat that other clergymen would follow his example was countered by a canon enacted in 1604, which forbade ministers to attempt to exorcise the afflicted by prayer and fasting "under pain of imputation of imposture or cosenage and deposition from the ministry."[163]

Paradoxically, the Church of England became the champion of secular interpretations of mental disorder. Harsnet, Deacon, and Walker could neither deny the scriptural basis of demonology nor show that every modern demoniac was dissembling. If their arguments were to be effective against exorcists who were more ingenuous than Darrell and his clients, some of whom had been carefully coached, they had to deny that it was possible for the Devil to possess the minds and bodies of men. All exorcism was a mummer's play, they claimed, because the age of miracles had passed and modern attempts to cast out demons were false and unnecessary.[164] They embraced the physician's argument that strange mental symptoms were caused by illnesses of the mind and body, and they went still further than Cotta, asserting that even the signs of supernatural malevolence he allowed were naturally caused. Lycanthropy, for example, was declared to be a species of melancholy, but "some unskillful physicians do rashly ascribe this humourous disease to the operation of the Devil, and that the ignorant people do absurdly imagine the party thus affected to be undoubtedly possessed of devils."[165] The pamphleteers rejected the possibility that even the wildest feats of mental and physical action might be caused by spirits. Such maladies arise instead

from disordered melancholy, from mania, from the epilepsy, from lunacy, from lycanthropy, from convulsions, from the mother, from the menstrual obstructions, and sundry other outrageous infirmities. For the animal parts being marvellously affected with some disordered fantasies . . . and the mind being mightily troubled by means of noisome fumes, black and gross, vapouring up to the brain like the foot of a chimney, they imagine themselves to be vexed eftsoons of some hurtful spirits, and do strongly persuade themselves, that the devil assaileth their minds.[166]

The official spokesmen of the church were, as Burton complained, not merely denying that people could be possessed by devils; they were accusing the men and women who thought they were haunted of being crazy. Anglican propaganda, like medical self-promotion, regarded demonism and medical thought to be mutually exclusive systems of belief, and it encouraged the public to believe that apparent demoniacs were sick in mind, not merely deluded or mistaken. Precisely the same argument had been used by Reginald Scot in his famous attack on witch beliefs, *The Discoverie of Witchcraft*, to explain away the tales of old women who confessed that they were witches.[167]

It must have been astonishing to hear Arminian churchmen, polemical physicians, and radical materialists singing hymns in praise of the natural scientific explanation of mental disorders. But few educated men and women could entirely ignore the facts that the arguments involved were feeble and the voices were singularly ill-matched. The churchmen and physicians persuaded the educated elite to moderate their views of the Devil's powers and so widened the gap between orthodox religion and popular belief, but complete skepticism remained rare throughout the seventeenth century. Richard Bernard, in his influential *Guide to Grand-Iury Men*, adopted a compromise of the kind that became commonplace. Stressing at length that many strange diseases were caused naturally and emphasizing that putative demoniacs might be counterfeiting or deluded by melancholy, he nevertheless insisted that maladies of the kind Cotta declared to be devilish were actual instances of possession. He remarked that signs of extreme lunacy, such as extraordinary strength, attempted suicide, flight to solitary places, refusal to be "tamed," convulsions and cries, were sometimes caused by Satan, and he commended the Puritan method of curing such sufferers by prayer and fasting.[168] During the Revolution the sects, particularly the Quakers, reinvigorated congregational exorcism, and it was only in the aftermath of the bitter struggles of the Interregnum that demonology began rapidly to lose its respectability among lay conformists.[169]

The fact that the Anglican hierarchy's repudiation of demonology was only partially accepted by the educated classes during the earlier seventeenth century may be explained as the result of both intellectual and social factors. Theologians and learned laymen were quick to see that materialist arguments denying the powers of demons and witches could easily be extended to question the potency of God and his angels.[170] Furthermore, popular credulity about witchcraft provided the governing elite with a means to reshape public attitudes toward poor and marginal members of the village community, and gentlemen were slow to abandon their faith in the existence of witches.[171] Because demonology and witchcraft were so closely allied, the vitality of witch beliefs retarded the spread of skepticism about possession.

Most people continued to believe that witches could make men sick or mad, kill their cattle and children, and spoil their crops and provisions. The carefully circumscribed set of symptoms designated by Cotta as the tokens of witchcraft was vastly distended by popular fear. Napier's clients reported an enormous variety of mental and physical ills that they blamed on witches; indeed, the symptoms of mentally disturbed patients who were alleged to be bewitched are statistically indistinguishable from the pattern of complaints among the whole group of insane and troubled clients.[172] Occasionally Napier remarked that the symptoms of a sick patient were like the torment experienced by a person who was haunted or bewitched. Most of the clients he described with this comparison suffered from plucking sensations or convulsions that made them look as if they were manipulated by invisible creatures. Mistress Paul, for example, was noted to be "fearfully handled as one that were bewitched"; she was "tormented with a strange disease and pain that taketh her by fits . . . in such violent sort that you would think she would presently be plucked in pieces."[173] Of Gillian Woodrosse, Napier wrote, "will start as if she were beworded."[174] The notion that convulsive symptoms were especially likely to have been caused by witches is plainly an extension of the popular urge to personify illnesses as the actions of invisible creatures. Thus another patient who feared supernatural malevolence, Ann Turvey, was "vexed with a live, stirring humour."[175]

Jerking helplessly like a marionette controlled by a careless puppeteer was to the popular mind a strong reason to suspect witchcraft, but such symptoms do not appear very frequently in actual descriptions of bewitched people. It was somewhat more common to mention that their illnesses were lingering or strange. George Gifford, an acute contemporary student of witchcraft, thought that lingering diseases were most likely to have been caused by witches, and Alan Macfarlane has shown that Essex villagers shared that belief.[176] It is reflected in Napier's case notes as well. He remarked, for instance, that Thomas King, who was suffering from an ordinary ague, suspected "some evil tongues because it hath continued so long."[177] The diseases of other purportedly bewitched or haunted people are called "strange," both in the witchcraft accusations by Essex villagers and in Napier's records.[178] Sometimes the ailments described as strange were genuinely odd. Mary Morgan was "strangely taken out of her bed and thrice cast down to the ground"; Robert Enfild had "strange fits" during which he would "sit naked and crieth that 'now they come.' "[179] But in seventeenth-century parlance "strange" often connoted rare intensity and not eccentricity. Thus the illness of Bodley's librarian, Dr. James, was epitomized, "strangely taken with a palsy on the left side of the face and leg."[180] Christian Maunfild similarly reported that he suffered from a pain in the right leg, which "shooteth strangely."[181] In sum, one can say that most of the sick men and women who told Napier that they feared witchcraft were the victims of ordinary physical and mental afflictions, although their diseases sometimes lasted longer and hurt more than such illnesses ordinarily did. In spite of the contemporary readiness to believe that convulsive diseases were caused by supernatural powers, there was no single malady or cluster of symptoms that was popularly considered to be typical of witchcraft.

The belief that one was bewitched served, like the conviction that one was haunted by demons, to relieve the fears of anxious sufferers and their relatives by attributing their illnesses and insanity to familiar agents and comprehensible forces. Witchcraft beliefs were especially attractive in this respect because the malefactor might be identified and punished, removing the cause of misfortune and satisfying simultaneously both the desire for ways to combat long and baffling diseases and the craving for revenge against one's enemies.[182] Many of Napier's patients named people whom they suspected had bewitched them; the mentally disturbed patients alone reported 222 suspects.

Napier's attitude toward his clients' suspicions confounds modern distinctions between superstition and rationalism. He employed divination to confirm or deny the allegations of his patients. Sometimes he conjured the Archangel Raphael and beseeched him to reveal whether or not his clients were bewitched and whether they would be cured. He believed that his necromancy succeeded occasionally. For instance, a rare transcript survives that includes questions and responses that passed between the magician and the Angel during a seance in 1619. It records Raphael's opinion that five of Napier's patients were bewitched and predictions that two of them would recover.[183] Angelic magic was difficult to perform and spiritually perilous, and Napier seems more often to have used astrology to detect witchcraft. When he received his nephew's letter describing the tormented behavior of the Countess of Bridgwater's children, for example, he immediately erected a figure that testified to the truth of her fears that they were bewitched.[184] Scattered throughout his practice books are lists of queries to be answered astrologically, and they often contain entries asking if individual patients are bewitched or haunted.

Nevertheless, in spite of his faith that magic and astrology could discover supernatural evil, Napier was often critical of the information he got by divination and skeptical about his client's allegations. At some time after the 1619 seance, for example, Napier corrected the Archangel's predictions. The spirit had foretold that Mistress Panton would survive the dangers of witchcraft and live to marry; "not so," the astrologer wrote beside this entry, "she died of consumption."[185] The stars were even more difficult to interpret correctly than the communications of the archangel. As we have already seen, Napier very frequently revised his figures in light of the outcome of his patients' illnesses, and he seems to have been reticent to declare that his clients were bewitched or possessed solely on the basis of astrology. He confirmed the fears of only 9 of his disturbed clients who suspected that they had been bewitched and of only 18 who claimed that they were possessed or haunted. More important, he was openly skeptical about the tales that some of his clients told him, and he placed great weight on the public support they gained for their accusations. L'Estrange Ewen, the pioneering historian of witchcraft in England, placed Napier among the pantheon of early rationalists because of his testimony in the notable case of Lady Jennings's daughter, Elizabeth. Alone among the prominent figures involved in the incident, Napier declared that the charges that the girl was bewitched were "all false," and he ascribed her symptoms to the "suffocation of the mother," a disease that mimicked supernatural effects according to Jorden's famous pamphlet.[186] Napier's use of the scientific arguments of the skeptics in this case was not a unique episode of incredulity. When an old woman approached him in 1619 complaining that "something hurteth her and inwardly possesseth her," he concluded, as Cotta might have, that she simply suffered from "epileptic fits of the mother in most pitiful manner."[187] A Hanslope man, who came to Great Linford lamenting "his losses and fearing witches," received rougher treatment: "I would not talk to him," the physician noted later, "but chided him for making such idle questions to me."[188]

Napier placed great weight on his patients' characters and on the public support they won for their accusations when he evaluated witchcraft accusations. Fussbudgets like the man and woman just mentioned did not command his confidence, even if other people believed them.[189] When his client was not given to anxious fantasies, however, Napier was greatly influenced by the confessions and convictions of putative malefactors. Mistress Mary Robinson's chronic fits of distress and fainting worsened in 1628, and she claimed that she felt something "striking within her, as if it were quick." Napier was convinced that her malady was caused by witchcraft when Isaac Richardson, whom she suspected, confessed his "witchery."[190] Sometimes Napier changed his evaluation of a patient's afflictions when a jury confirmed the sufferer's accusations. He originally diagnosed Mistress Elizabeth Belcher's illness as melancholy, but he revised his opinion later when the people she suspected were brought to the bar for their crime.[191]

Napier's attitudes toward witchcraft thus were complex. He thought that it was very difficult to detect supernatural diseases, and he used every means available to him, angelic magic, witchcraft, and even folk rituals, to find out if his patients were bewitched.[192] At the same time his judgment in individual cases was shaped by the circumstances of his client's illness and suspicions. The patient's personality, the credibility of his accusations, and the public response to the case all influenced his decision. Unfortunately, Napier's notes are too laconic to permit us to discover all of the psychological and social factors that distinguished convincing witchcraft accusations from frivolous ones. The inadequacy of characterizing Napier, or any of his contemporaries, simply as a superstitious traditionalist or a progressive rationalist is nevertheless evident from his records. He accepted both traditional beliefs in witchcraft and magic and new arguments against their indiscriminate application. He regarded magic and science as alternative methods of evaluating individual cases, and did not view them as antagonistic belief systems. Depending upon the circumstances of a particular case, he emphasized either the natural or the supernatural causes of his client's symptoms. The methods of divination he used no doubt strengthened his confidence in the judgments he made, but they do not seem to have determined them. Napier's world abounded with natural and supernatural perils that struck down men and women invisibly and indiscriminately, and nothing was more obscure than the etiology of mental disorders. The magical and scientific beliefs of his age complemented one another and facilitated a broad range of responses to illness and misfortune. Witchcraft beliefs assuaged the anxieties of unfortunate people by enabling them to relieve their guilt and punish their enemies; scientific theories enabled physicians and magistrates to discredit the baseless accusations of malicious hysterics. Although religious controversies and professional rivalries sharpened the contrast between magical beliefs and medical theories in the early seventeenth century, many educated people assumed like Napier that old magic and new science could be reconciled.

Seventeenth-century villagers believed whatever cunning made their misery, pain, and squalor easier to bear. They sought relief from folk healers, astrologers, physicians, and clergymen without scrupling to consider the legitimacy of philosophical compatibility of the treatments these groups of practitioners purveyed, a cause for considerable dismay to ambitious doctors and zealous preachers. Learned men could also reconcile the conflicting claims of natural magic and religion, and there were many practitioners who combined the methods of several kinds of healing. Napier was remarkable because of the breadth of his eclecticism but not automatically a medical or clerical apostate because of it. He treated mentally disturbed people who thought that they were possessed or bewitched with folk magic, astrology, humoral medicine, and earnest prayer. Many of the devices and prayers he used were meant specifically to be effective against both mental illnesses and the malevolence of demons and witches. He recognized that these alternatives were considered incompatible by some physicians and divines, but he did not accept the point of their arguments – that only one system was legitimate. Here, for example, is a general memorandum he once wrote about how to cure "anyone that is mopish and distempered in brain or else [harmed by] any witchery, sorcery or inchantment": "First let them blood . . . then say, 'Lord, I beseech Thee, let the corruption of Satan come out of this man or woman or child that doth so trouble or vex her or him that he or she cannot serve Thee as it may please Thee to call them . . . into Thy heavenly kingdom.' "[193] In such cases he often used astrological amulets, which were "good against all spirits, fairies, witcheries, sorceries . . . That [*sic*] be lunatic . . . or out of their wits" or "good for many infirmities . . . against all evil spirits, fairies, witcheries, possessed, frantic, lunatic."[194]

Simon Forman taught Napier how to make astral talismans in 1611, and he quickly incorporated them into his treatment of maladies that might have had supernatural causes. Sigils, as they were called, were metal emblems with astrological designs on them. They were made of metal, usually brass or tin, sometimes silver or gold, and cast at a propitious time, the moment the planet corresponding to the metal used was ascendant in the heavenly house that influenced diseases. Ribboned with taffeta or silk, they were hung around the patient's neck at another astrologically significant time. Sometimes they were used to stamp the celestial design on the patient's medicines before he took them.[195] Napier believed that sigils were ineffective unless prayers were repeated when they were prescribed and when they were put on. The tin sigil "that hath the planet Jupiter and his characters," for example, was potent against all manners of maladies if it was used "with good prayer."[196] Sir Thomas Myddleton, the younger, was anxious that the sigil he had engraved according to Napier's instructions be effective, and he wrote to the astrologer assuring him that he would put it on, "God permitting upon Sunday morning, preparing myself aforehand to be gracious in His eyes that must give it a blessing, humbly desiring the assistance of your prayers which I know will make it prosper the better . . . desiring that this ambitious desire of mine may not be offensive to His Majesty, but that my will may freely submit to His will and pleasure."[197] Napier used these amulets to protect his clients against further mystical infection, and he dispensed them most freely among his mentally disturbed patients to men and women who were tempted to commit suicide or apostasy or who feared they were haunted by demons or bewitched.[198]

Sometimes Napier followed the example of folk curers and wrote down prayers and charms to supplement the power of the amulet. These devotions were almost all traditional scraps of Latin liturgy that had been used time out of mind by cunning men to treat the sick. A memorandum about how to make paper charms to protect against evil spirits, frustrate the malevolence of witches, and soothe troubled minds includes a pseudo-scriptural prayer and the names of God and the archangels; these were to be set down "in a little paper close written and tied with taffeta with a leaf of mugwort or St. John's wort" and worn around the patient's neck.[199] The objections of Puritan clergymen to his use of these ancient techniques of natural magic was understandable enough; more unexpected was the opposition Napier met from the Catholic dowager Lady Dormer, who stripped her servant of the amulet and charms he had given her: "My old Lady Dormer would take from her both sigil upon her neck and her prayer." She may have been offended by the magical use of Catholic liturgy by a Protestant wizard.[200]

Napier also exorcised his possessed clients. To expel malevolent spirits he either used Catholic formulas or composed his own texts to remove their Popish connotations; he also adjusted the prayers to the sufferer's own sensibilities and fears. Thus he addressed the spirits possessing the Bedford gentleman Edmund Francklin with a long and pious peroration followed by this command:

Behold, I God's most unworthy minister and servant, I do charge and command thee, thou cruel beast, with all thy associates and all other malignant spirits in case that any of you have your being in the body of this creature, Mr. E. Fr[ancklin], and have distempered his brain with melancholy and have also deprived his body and limbs of their natural use, I charge and command you speedily to depart from this creature and servant of God, Mr. E. F[rancklin], regenerated by the laver of the holy baptism and redeemed by the precious blood of our Lord Jesus Christ, I charge you to depart from him and every part of his body, really, personally.[201]

This kind of healing was plainly at odds with the Anglican hierarchy's intentions, and it is well to recall that Napier had orthodox partners in his reluctance to discard exorcism. Nevertheless, in his efforts to relieve the suffering of his clients he was unusually ready to set aside scruples about the legitimacy of natural magic and ritual exorcism, a flexibility that was perhaps justified by success.

Many men and women believed that amulets and exorcisms were effective remedies for mental torment. Gentlemen and their ladies wrote to Napier asking him to engrave sigils for them when they were melancholy or anxious.[202] The victims of vaguely defined illnesses and chronic fearfulness sometimes felt better when they were given an amulet for protection, and they attributed their improvement to the talisman. Margaret Franklin, for example, was marvelously well when she wore her sigil, but as soon as she lost it she once more experienced ghostly pains and fretted that she was harmed by an "ill tongue."[203] Michael Musgrave also suffered relapse of his chronic distress when he misplaced his amulet.[204] Maryon Norman's emotional turmoil abated as soon as she put on a necklace fashioned out of a ribbon and a piece of paper with a passage of scripture written on it.[205] The testimonials of these grateful patients may be vastly amplified by numerous stories of satisfied customers treated by cunning people employing amulets and charms.[206]

Exorcism was also widely believed to be effective. The exorcisms performed by Puritans and Jesuits often produced spectacular successes that they publicized energetically.[207] Such propaganda served not only to strengthen dissident religious groups' claims to divine legitimacy, they also sustained popular beliefs in possession and exorcism. The popular faith in exorcism was so intense that the rituals sometimes worked even when they were not performed by a clergyman. Mistress Sara Wheelowes was successfully exorcised by her father. The sight of the corpse of a woman who had been buried alive had caused her to be "strangely taken with strange fits." Napier wrote that her father bravely confronted the Devil and cast him out of the tormented girl: "Her father commanding Satan to leave her, she is rid of her fits."[208] Half a century later John Blagrave recorded a similar example of the popular faith in exorcism. Called in to treat a young woman who had been paralyzed for a year, Blagrave asked her father to help restrain her as the astrologer cast out the spirits who deadened her limbs. Although he was terrified by the supernatural danger, the father courageously swore that "whatever came of it he was resolved to live and die with his child, rather than fail." The exorcism was successful.[209] Like the rituals of obtaining and donning amulets, exorcism worked because it simultaneously invoked the unseen powers in which the patient had faith and prompted displays of concern and affection by the sufferer's physician, family, and friends.

Magical beliefs were strong and enduring. People continued to believe in demonology and witchcraft and in countermagic during the seventeenth century in part because these ideas and practices were socially functional. They helped vulnerable men and women to cope with the terrifying mysterious forces that threatened their health and sanity. They enabled families and villages to unite in support of suffering people and against vexatious members of the community. But magical beliefs also survived because they were an essential aspect of the mental world of ordinary people. Indeed, the distinctions between magic, religion, and science, which were increasingly important to the educated elite, had little meaning for the majority of English villagers. They believed that the supernatural beings and forces in the universe were divided into two kinds, good and evil. Angelic spirits and holy rites protected them against evil spirits and witchcraft; magic was the dark side of religion. This simple dichotomy between dark and light, good and evil, extended beyond popular conceptions of the supernatural. Humble men and women like Napier's clients organized their understanding of emotional states, social actions, and physical events by associating them with good and evil spirits. They attributed the dark and troubling motions of the mind to Satan, and they sought recovery from anxiety and guilt by invoking the assistance of God and his benificent creation, the angels and the heavens. They stigmatized antisocial urgings and immoral behavior by making the Devil their prime mover, and they valued altruism and proper conduct by identifying them as signs of godliness. They viewed misfortunes such as illnesses and insanity as the work of witches or demons, and they often regarded escape from death and madness as a miracle, the work of God. Thus their faith that the Devil could possess a person's mind and that a witch could drive a man mad was an extension of the fundamental conceptual dichotomy in popular thought. It created a chain of associations that linked insanity with all the other kinds of evil and misfortune in the world, and conversely it tied sanity together with all the types of good and well-being they knew. Because people are naturally more mindful of those things that threaten their happiness than they are of those that sustain it, villagers made the association of misfortune with black magic more often than they recalled the dependence of good fortune on religious faith. At least that was the view of the pious elite, who in the seventeenth century endeavored to transform the beliefs and behavior of the masses by persuading them to accept a more rigorous variety of Protestantism. They failed to convert the largest part of the English nation, the men and women without property, because the abandonment of the old, semimagical view of the world was impossible without a vast transformation in the material lives and educational standards of the whole society.

SPIRITUAL PHYSIC

The Puritan clergy spearheaded the attempt to reform the beliefs and conduct of the English people. Emphasizing the anxiety and despair that were the fruits of an unregenerate life, they sought to convert ordinary men and women to Calvinist theology and godly behavior by convincing them of the urgent necessity for reformation in their own lives. In their sermons and writings they developed a rhetorical strategy that appropriated the dualistic imagery of popular religious psychology and transformed its meaning by placing it in a new theological context. They used traditional symbols and plain speech to convey a simple lesson: The root of all wretchedness is sin; the only cure for sin is repentance and conversion. The intensity with which the Puritans preached the need for a reformation of manners was new, but their evangelical techniques were based on a conventional belief that the clergy were the physicians of the soul. All of the churchmen of the earlier seventeenth century, whether or not they were Puritans, agreed that one of the principal duties of the ministry was to administer spiritual physic to the diseased souls of the laity. Dissension arose within the Church of England at first over the strength of the medicines that Puritans prescribed rather than their practice of ministering to troubled minds. The conforming clergy grew alarmed that strong doses of Calvinist doctrine would sicken diseased laymen still further and eventually poison the body of the whole commonwealth. The political struggles of the mid-century intensified this conflict and linked it with the rivalry between the physicians and their competitors, the folk magicians and faith healers.

The Puritan evangelists used language and ideas very similar to those voiced by Napier's troubled clients.[210] They depicted the human condition as a terrible struggle to sustain happiness and sanity in a world abounding with natural misfortunes and supernatural evils. The outward occasions of mental turmoil they enumerated were the familiar catastrophes of everyday life, physical illnesses, children's deaths, marital discord, and economic disasters.[211] These afflictions were sometimes enough to bring people to deep sorrow by themselves, but they were particularly dangerous because they made men and women vulnerable to Satan's temptations. The Devil stood always ready to introject evil thoughts into the minds of the unwary, habitual sinners, and people distracted by griefs and cares. He was especially adept at intensifying the suffering of melancholy men and women. Robert Bolton, for example, warned that these people were in grave spiritual danger, because "Satan, God suffering him, . . . hath great advantage to raise and represent to the fancy many fearful things, terrible objects, grisly thoughts, hideous injunctions, and temptations to despair, self-destruction, etc."[212] Even more than the other clergymen of their time, the Puritan writers liked to organize their discussions of the psychological tribulations of the reprobate with the traditional metaphor of spiritual warfare. William Haller commented years ago: "For them the ancient Christian images of spiritual struggle were the thing wherewith to catch the conscience of the common man."[213] Satan appears in their writings as he does in *Paradise Lost*; he is man's great adversary, his tempter, and the author of his torment. The Fiend is woven skillfully and often into John Bunyan's famous story of his protracted battle to overcome religious anxiety and doubt: "Thus," he wrote in a characteristic passage, "by strange and unusual assaults of the tempter was my soul, like a broken vessel, driven as with the winds and tossed sometimes headlong into despair."[214] The vivid heightening of popular religious symbolism in Puritan and, later, in Nonconformist literature encouraged believers to interpret their own emotional disturbances as manifestations of battles between grace and sin, the clash of antithetical forces represented by God and the Devil. Spiritual autobiographers described their duels with Satan, bouts of anxiety and despair that frequently were the prelude to their conversion to the godly way of life.[215]

The task of the physicians of the soul was to purge the sinner's complacency and show him how to govern his mind and body so that he was better able to withstand the infection of sin.[216] Striving was the key to the Puritan solution to the problem of curing anxiety and despair. Preachers and casuists taught their audiences to submit themselves to rigorous self-examination. To attain spiritual health and maintain it, believers had to practice "the often and careful viewing of ourselves in the looking glass of the law, beholding there our most sinful and most woeful estate, and labouring ourselves to have knowledge and some feeling experience of it."[217] Laymen were cautioned to be especially vigilant during periods of emotional turmoil, for passion weakened their self-control and made them vulnerable to the temptations of Satan.[218] The Puritans' emphasis on introspection and self-discipline caused them to reinterpret the Devil's role in religious psychology. Although they repeated the popular beliefs that Satan introjected evil thoughts into people's minds and tempted them to despair and suicide, they insisted that pious men and women were nevertheless chiefly responsible for their own thoughts and actions.

The Fiend cultivated the seeds of sin that grew into choking weeds of guilt and despair, but he did not have to plant them in men's hearts. Writing for a moment as the Devil's advocate, Richard Capel complained, "I think that the Devil hath a great wrong done him when men to excuse themselves, derive their sins upon him."[219] There were no shortcuts to spiritual peace. Ritual exorcism and healing magic were in vain because they did not remove the ultimate cause of all human misery, sin. Sufferers could not even hope to escape grief and affliction: The saints themselves were tested by doubts and feelings of hopelessness.[220] The psychological reward of conversion and regeneration was an enhanced capacity to endure misfortune rather than an anesthetized indifference to it. "There is an art or skill in bearing troubles, . . . ," observed Richard Sibbes, "without overmuch troubling of ourselves, as in bearing of a burden there is a way so to poise it that it weigheth not over heavy."[221]

Napier's art of spiritual physic contrasted sharply with the Puritan's astringent prescriptions. He pursued his ministry to troubled minds in the same spirit as George Herbert's ideal parson: "The country parson when any of his cure is sick or afflicted with loss of friend, estate, or any ways distressed, fails not to afford his best comforts."[222] Many anguished people repaired to Napier to seek consolation for their earthly afflictions and advice about their spiritual maladies. Almost 300 of his disturbed clients suffered from some kind of religious anxiety or spiritual problem. Their complaints ranged from simple religious lassitude to desperate fears that they would not be saved; 91 patients, 19 men and 72 women, told Napier that they were "doubtful of salvation" or that they were "tempted to despair of salvation."[223] The theological grounds of these people's fears are unknown. Napier recorded that 43 of his clients were tortured by guilt about the sins they had committed, and often they had become convinced that they were damned because of them, but he never wrote down their beliefs about the nature of sin and redemption. Indeed, it is unlikely that he explored their doubts in depth or engaged in theological dispute with them. Napier was deeply hostile toward Puritan Nonconformity, and he had scant sympathy for people whose sufferings seemed to be the result of overly zealous questioning of the tenets of the faith. Elizabeth Whitter's gloom and anxiety were to his mind the consequence of her untutored enthusiasm for Biblical study: "Zealous and religious . . . Busieth herself with reading the scriptures, and not well understanding the meaning, all fearful of her salvation."[224] In an almost identical case, he wrote that Archbishop Abbot's niece, "always praying and studying," had become melancholy; her faith was weakened and she was persuaded that she had sinned against God.[225] He coldly described Robert Kays as a rich man "puritanically affected by over-much studying of the scripture"; Kays was actually desperately ill, and he died a few days later.[226] Thomas Astill, who "followeth preaching up and down," seemed to Napier to be surfeited with godliness: "He hath no joy or comfort in this wicked world."[227] The poetic anguish of Goody Bonner left him unmoved, for she, too, followed sermons, a Puritan habit forbidden by the conservatives in the church: "For her sins despaireth much . . . A follower of sermons, threatened by the minister for leaving his sermons and going to others. Will rise at the crying of birds, saying that they cry out against her for her sins."[228] When he was confronted by a real Separatist, the Brownist Roger Laurenc, he concluded that the young man was "frantic."[229]

Napier believed that the antidotes to religious worry were relatively simple. His views resembled those of Burton, another orthodox divine who abhorred Nonconformity: "Faith, hope, repentance, are the sovereign cures and remedies, the sole comforts in this case"; explained Burton, "confess, humble thyself, repent, it is sufficient."[230] He certainly did not encourage his distressed clients to intensify their introspection and gain "some feeling experience" of their sins, as the Puritan divine Thomas Wilson advised.[231] His religious counsel seems instead to have consisted chiefly of "comforting speeches" intended to fortify his patients' faith and remind them of God's mercy. Napier unfortunately did not write down the substance of his counseling. A typical memorandum notes that Goody Hill was "tempted of the enemy" and sought his advice: "Often tempted in my presence, but by our prayers, the Lord be thanked, greatly comforted."[232] His papers do show that he favored formal prayer to searching self-examination as a means to restore his patients' confidence in God's mercy. He often prayed together with his troubled clients, and he sometimes composed prayers for them to repeat by themselves. When

Jane Ringe, for example, was troubled by the "affliction of Satan," he wrote out a prayer to say with her: "Lord Jesus comfort and strengthen her faith and mightily defend her against ghostly enemies."[233] He urged his patients to pray and perform regular religious exercises, for he felt that they would foster piety and happiness. He wrote hopefully of one woman that she "prayeth often to put out all evil thoughts," and he scribbled anxiously of another, "always praying and calling in God, yet can feel no joy nor inward comfort."[234] Napier's preference for a style of religious counsel that emphasized ministerial guidance, set prayers, and participation in the rituals and sacraments of the church was a consequence of his theological conservatism. He preferred to stress the traditional authority of the church and the value of formal piety rather than to expound upon the mysteries of the scriptures and the threat of damnation. Not surprisingly, his attitudes are consistent with the views that Sears McGee has characterized as the Anglican approach to conversion and redemption. The divines whom McGee has identified as Anglicans commended the imitation of Christ as a means to achieve regeneration and viewed genuine felicity as one of the fruits of a pious life lived in obedience to the guidance of the established religious and civil authorities.[235]

In addition to comforting speeches, formal prayer, and regular religious exercises, Napier often prescribed magical and medical remedies for his patients troubled by religious problems. When he suspected that demons or witches might be involved in his clients' sufferings, he sometimes gave them a sigil to protect them against those perils. He regarded astrological amulets as a means to bolster the religious faith of his patients, not as an alternative to orthodox devotions. Thus when Cicely Stonell became deeply melancholy and anxious about her salvation after her daughter's death, Napier gave her a sigil to wear and was disturbed when it failed to work. "Fearful of her salvation," he wrote, "fearful judgments dreamed . . . Hath S ♃ [a sigil] yet faithless."[236] Few orthodox clergymen were likely to have shared his confidence that such talismans were compatible with legitimate religious practice, but most of them would have agreed that medical treatments were a good and useful supplement to pious counsel and religious exercises. Ministers of all shades of Protestant opinion frequently undertook to heal the bodies as well as the minds of parishioners. Medical practice was, in fact, a natural extension of the pastor's duty to console his flock in time of sickness.

Napier, like the other educated men of his day, believed that physical maladies and spiritual afflictions were often conjoined. The sympathy between natural and supernatural maladies was explained in two ways. Writers as diverse in their religious opinions as Burton and Sibbes agreed that melancholy was "Satan's bath." The Devil exploited the weakened reason and overpowerful imaginations of people sickened by melancholy and tempted them to despair of their salvation.[237] Even, however, when the patient's spiritual distress was not preceded by a humoral disorder, his mental turmoil was often sufficient to disorder his body. Richard Baxter, who advocated both spiritual and medical remedies for "overmuch sorrow," observed that "physic, even purging, often cureth it, though the patient say that physic cannot cure souls, for the soul and body are wonderful copartners in their diseases and cure."[238] Napier acted on these commonplace assumptions by prescribing the same medicaments for his patients troubled by religious anxiety and sorrow as he dispensed to his other mentally ill patients. He recorded orders for purges, vomits, and other pharmacological preparations in over half his consultations with his spiritually distressed clients, roughly the same pattern of prescription found in his notes about patients suffering from other mental disorders. Napier's methods of psychological healing were therefore based on a traditional view of the causes of mental disorder in which natural and supernatural forces were seen as complementary sources of emotional affliction and therapeutic power. He was distinctly hostile toward the Puritans' effort to transform the minister's duty to provide spiritual consolation into an obligation to convert suffering men and women to a more rigorous and saintly way of life.

As the century progressed, Napier's anxieties about the perils of excessive religious zeal came to be shared by more and more clergymen in the established church. Even before the Arminian capture of the church government in the 1630s, Burton had laid the groundwork for the Anglican attack on the Dissenting clergy's methods of psychological healing. Alarmed by the threat he perceived to ecclesiastical and civil harmony posed by the Puritans, Burton declared they suffered from a mental disease, which he named "religious melancholy," and that they spread this malady to the populace through their fiery preaching. He argued that the deluded imaginations of the Puritan ministry prompted their resistance to the rituals and authorities of the established church:

We have a mad giddy company of precisians, schismatics, and some heretics, even in our own bosoms . . . that out of too much zeal in opposition to Antichrist, human traditions, those Romish rites and superstitions, will quite demolish all, they will admit of no ceremonies at all, . . . no interpretations of Scriptures, no comments of Fathers, no councils, but such as their own phantastical spirits dictate, or *recta ratio*, as Socinians; by which spirit misled, . . . they broach as prodigious paradoxes as papists themselves.[239]

Burton charged that the rustic prophets who appeared from time to time, claiming direct inspirations from God, were even more demented than the clerical Nonconformists: "Great precisians of mean conditions and very illiterate, [for the] most part by a preposterous zeal, fasting, meditation, melancholy, are brought into those gross errors and inconveniences . . . . They are certainly far gone with melancholy, if not quite mad, and have more need of physic than many a man that keeps his bed, more need of hellebore than those that are in Bedlam."[240] Religious madmen were dangerous because they persuaded other people to follow their deluded teachings. The Puritan clergy was especially culpable because their preaching stressed the perils of damnation and the rigors of salvation. Instead of strengthening the people against the psychological miseries of the sinful life, they shattered the mental composure of their audiences:

The greatest harm of all proceeds from those thundering ministers, a most frequent cause they are of this malady . . . Our indiscreet pastors, many of them . . . in their ordinary sermons . . . speak so much of election, predestination, reprobation . . . by what signs and tokens they shall discern and try themselves whether they be God's true children elect . . . still aggravate sin, thunder out God's judgments without respect . . . they so rent, tear and wound men's consciences, that they are almost mad, and at their wits' end.[241]

The Puritan ministry reacted strongly to the suggestion that their religious teachings and the sufferings of their proselytes were caused by natural disease rather than spiritual insight. Sibbes was emphatic that godly behavior could not be attributed to melancholy: "The world's objection is that of all kind of men in the world, those that profess religion are the most melancholy . . . But if that be so, it is because they are not religious enough . . . The true character of a Christian is to be cheerful and none else can be truly cheerful and joyous.[242] Bolton denied that pious study and religious contemplations made men mad, even when they were predisposed to be melancholy: "Religion . . . and religious courses and conformities do not make melancholic men mad, as the great Bedlams of this world would bear us in hand."[243] Robert Yarrow responded bluntly to the charge that the spiritual griefs of godly laymen were symptoms of mental disorder: "The causes of these griefs some inconsiderably have referred unto melancholy, whereas it is nothing but sin."[244] Thus in the two decades before the English Revolution the contrast between the Puritan approach to psychological healing and the traditionally eclectic methods favored by conservatives like Napier became a matter of political controversy within the church. The opposition to Puritanism had momentous effects on the treatment of mental disorder.

The attack on religious enthusiasm intensified during the Interregnum and continued for over a century after the Restoration. Horrified by the proliferation of radical sects with socially subversive political aspirations, the ruling elite developed a powerful and lasting aversion to religious groups who claimed special powers of holiness and revelation. Following Henry More's influential *Enthusiasmus Triumphatus*, published in 1656, Anglican pamphleteers transformed Burton's argument that religious Nonconformists were victims and the carriers of mental disease into a ruling-class shibboleth. The hostility of every shade of Anglican opinion toward the practices associated with sectarianism was deepened and sustained by the church's repeated efforts to discredit radical religious movements during the late seventeenth and eighteenth centuries. The Quakers, the French Prophets, and especially the Methodists provoked fusillades of tracts and sermons aimed at proving that the sects were based on mad delusion and fostered religious melancholy or outright lunacy among the common people.[245] The charge that religious enthusiasm was a kind of madness remained an effective polemical weapon because it contained a kernel of truth. The Protestant sects emphasized the spiritual significance of mental turmoil, and during the Interregnum they actively ministered to the spiritual afflictions of ordinary men and

women. After the Restoration, all types of Dissenting congregations practiced spiritual physic. The Anglican clergy, on the other
hand, redoubled their opposition to exorcism by prayer and fasting and grew increasingly reluctant to provide the kind of spiritual
counsel that had been a popular aspect of pre-Civil War divinity.[246] The church's antipathy to religious therapy encouraged the
orthodox elite to regard mental disorders from a secular perspective. Scientific theories were the only kind of explanation for mental disturbance entirely free from controversial religious associations; medical treatments were the only methods of healing
insanity that did not meet with the disapprobation of the established clergy.

The demand for religious remedies for mental disorders nevertheless persisted long after the Restoration. Their popularity
among the common people was sustained in part because of the
glaring inadequacies of medical science. Although the physicians'
commitment to science was ancient, the flourishing of lay interest
in natural science won the doctors as many critics as admirers.
Bacon himself remarked that medicine had made very little progress since the Greeks: "Medicine is a science which hath been . . .
more professed than laboured, and yet more laboured than advanced; the labour having been, in my judgment, rather in circle
than in progression."[247] Bacon's opinion was echoed both by radical critics hostile to the pretensions of the new science and by the
champions of innovations in anatomy and chemistry.[248] The physicians were particularly vulnerable to attack because they failed to
make any advances at all in their therapeutic methods while new
discoveries demolished the theoretical foundations on which they
were based. The College of Physicians scrambled to associate itself
with scientific progress, but it was forced to defend its traditional
therapies with the lame assertion that time had proven them to be
effective, an argument that implied experimental science was, after all, irrelevant to medical practice.[249] A climate of lay cynicism
about the doctors' treatments was created by published attacks on
the college and by numerous vernacular medical works, which
revealed the traditional secrets of the guild and printed new, alternative directions for preparing medicines. Criticism of the medical
profession was especially intense during the Interregnum, but it
continued at a high pitch after the Restoration. A popular quip
attributed to Pope Adrian declared that doctors covered up their

mistakes with earth, and Flecknoe's character of a physician added sarcastically that "another reason why never physician yet held up his hand at the bar for killing patient [*sic*] is because coroners' quest [*sic*] have found it self-murder in those who take physic of them; certainly they do more harm than good."[250] The author of *Poor Robin*, an astrological almanac, predicted brutally that in 1688 the physicians "would all be busy 'killing sick people.' "[251] Marchmont Needham's important *Medela Medicinae*, published in 1665, argued that because medical remedies were discovered by experiment upon hapless patients, the soundest doctors were the empirics, who were guided solely by vast experience. Needham was especially critical of the physicians' traditional technique of curing mental disorders because experience proved that they did not work:

The like may be said concerning people of a sorrowful frame of heart, or those that are broken in their fortunes, who are usually sick in mind rather than body, and the mind disorders the body. Be their disease what it will I never saw them prosper with bleeding, or the other evacuations, upward or downward, if violent or frequent.[252]

Many people believed that experience showed that religious remedies cured the maladies of the mind more effectively than medicine alone, and the Dissenters took advantage of this widespread opinion to win admirers and adherents to their creeds. Nonconformist clergymen and sectarian congregations continued to practice three kinds of psychological therapies after the Restoration, spiritual counsel, group prayer and fasting, and charismatic healing. Prominent divines preserved the Puritan tradition of practical divinity, pastoral counsel, and consolation. They visited the homes of people suffering from mental and physical illnesses to help them, and they taught younger clergymen to be sensitive to the personal problems and emotional condition of their followers. Richard Baxter taught this lesson forcefully: "Another part of our work is to comfort the disconsolate, and settle the peace of our people's souls, and that on sure and lasting grounds. To which end, the quality of the complaints, and the course of their lives, had need to be known, for all people must not have the like consolations that have the like complaints."[253] A second way to comfort the disconsolate was prayer and fasting. Every kind of Nonconformst group seems to have organized meetings to pray and fast with insane and unhappy men and women. The practice evidently began as a method for helping people who were possessed by the Devil, and the meetings retained a strong element of psychomachy, the allegorical contest for man's soul, which heightened the emotional force and effectiveness of these displays of community concern and solidarity. For example, the author of a detailed account of a Baptist congregation's successful struggle to restore a madman to sanity employed demonological language to describe the stages of his recovery. Each time they met in the sufferer's house to pray and fast for him, he made another step toward regaining his self-possession and resuming his normal activities; the report concludes that the Lord cast "as it were, three spirits visible, to be seen, out of him."[254] Such personification forged links between Nonconformist thaumaturgy and the ecclesiastical magic of the medieval past and must have enhanced its appeal to villagers indifferent to the orthodox elite's preference for rational religion.

Finally, some of the leaders of Dissenting sects possessed special powers of persuasion and healing. George Fox in particular enjoyed an extraordinary gift for calming raging lunatics and people who were thought to be possessed or bewitched. He believed that his miraculous cures were an extension of his mission to teach troubled souls God's truth, and he repudiated the use of force to restrain or treat violent madmen. The key to healing the insane, in Fox's view, lay in his ability to communicate his conviction that the inner light resided in everyone. The remarkable narratives of his dealings with mad people show that he could, through gentle persuasion, somehow establish a bond between himself and men and women whose capacity to understand was apparently ruined.[255] Although Fox rejected violent medical treatments of insanity, neither he nor the other Nonconformist healers condemned medicine altogether. All three of the principal methods of religious therapy were sometimes supplemented by medical remedies, and it appears that the Dissenters preserved in practice the traditional belief that mental and physical afflictions were closely allied and should be healed by treatments that succored both the minds and the bodies of suffering people.[256] Religious therapy was a potent political weapon in the Dissenters' battle to capture the hearts of the English people. The Anglican clergy angrily decried its use and tried to blunt its effectiveness. They charged that prayer and fasting for the insane violated the canons of the church and that the practice was a clandestine method of organizing conventicles. Bishop Stillingfleet refused William Bates's invitation to participate in a meeting to pray for his own kinswoman because he thought that it was contrary to church law:

When the Lady Barnard was deeply melancholy and troubled in mind, Dr. Bates made a motion to Dr. Stillingfleet, who was her kinsman by marriage, that they might fast and pray, that they might seek the comfort of the Comforter. Dr. Stillingfleet said that it was against the canon. Then, said Dr. Bates, the canon is no canon . . . because the canon reduceth all fasts to Lents and Ember week.[257]

Oliver Heywood gloated like a victorious campaigner when his successful fast for a melancholy girl left the local Anglican vicar raging at his parishioners. The minister, who had himself refused to organize a meeting to pray for the girl, denounced his flock for attending a conventicle, but the villagers were completely won over to the Presbyterians' side in this case. After teasing his neighbor for permitting his house to be used for the "conventicle," one man remarked to his friend: "Thou didst well. That's the best means, fasting and prayer is good. I should have taken that course myself."[258] Spokesmen for the church claimed that the Dissenters were staging bogus attempts to imitate the miracles of Christ and the apostles. Orthodox hostility to religious therapy deepened during the eighteenth century, when John Wesley and George Whitefield enhanced the popular following of the Methodists by curing mad people and the putative victims of diabolical possession and witchcraft.[259]

Over a century of official denunciation of Nonconformist thaumaturgy failed to reduce the common people's faith in supernatural maladies and spiritual therapies, but it did persuade the upper classes that physicians were the proper healers of the mind, whatever the inadequacies of contemporary medicine. Medical psychology became the sole basis for the treatments of insanity sanctioned by the ruling elite. There was no alternative. Religious therapies were politically dangerous and magical remedies were slowly being discredited by a combination of factors: their association with political radicalism during the Interregnum, the advance of natural science, and the growth in the size and respectability of the medical profession.[260] The expansion of the medical profession was, in part, another indirect consequence of the governing elite's reaction against religious zeal. The eighteenth-century church provided neither intellectual vitality nor financial security for parish clergymen, and the sons of gentlemen looked to medicine and law for more rewarding careers.[261] Skepticism about traditional supernatural explanations for mental disorder gradually prevailed among the educated elite. Parliament repealed the witchcraft statute in 1736 and collegiate physicians refused to diagnose cases of demonic possession, a matter for dismay to John Wesley and for satisfaction to his opponents.[262] Sustained religious controversy discredited the eclectic approach to psychological healing practiced by Napier and many of his contemporaries, and it discouraged the physicians from borrowing therapeutic strategies from religious healers and empirics.

The governing elite in eighteenth-century England treated insanity as a medical and social problem. Asylums proliferated all over the country in the century after the English Revolution. This phenomenon was the consequence of a new consensus among the governing classes about how pauper lunatics should be treated, for the asylum movement was begun and sustained largely by private entrepreneurs with very little direction from the government.[263] The dominance of medical therapies over the other kinds of psychological healing was embodied in the regimens of private and public madhouses, and as their numbers grew, more and more mad people were subjected to physical restraint and confinement, purges, vomits, and bleeding. Because of their religious connotations, supportive and nonviolent methods of curing insanity remained suspect until the end of the eighteenth century, when the "moral therapy movement" succeeded in curbing the abuses of the worst English asylums. These reforms were pioneered by the Quaker asylum, the York Retreat, and they closely resembled the healing methods employed by George Fox and his fellow Dissenters.[264]

The rise of psychological medicine has often been represented as a saga of scientific progress. It was not. It was instead a tale of religious hatred, political conflict, social antagonism, and, at last, intellectual advancement. The eighteenth century was a disaster for the insane. Confined to madhouses and asylums, or even to workhouses and prisons, they waited for more than a hundred years before medical men significantly improved their methods of curing mental disorders, methods that had been criticized as ineffective in the seventeenth century. Many of the successful practices employed by Napier and his contemporaries were discarded because they were associated with religious radicalism and popular superstition. The traditional fusion of natural and supernatural beliefs about disease and misfortune was discredited; the eclectic methods of psychological healing that had been grounded upon it were stigmatized as base ignorance and quackery. The formation of an elite culture compounded of rational religion, neoclassicism, and natural philosophy created an atmosphere in which Richard Napier's fame could not long survive. His reputation as a healer and a magus continued to be brightly visible for a generation after the Restoration and then vanished. His patients died; his arts declined; in time, he was forgot.

APPENDIX A

Age and sex of Napier's mentally disturbed patients

The age counted for each patient is the figure reported to Napier at the time of the patient's first consultation for each episode of illness. If a gap of more than twelve months separated visits to Napier, any subsequent consultation is treated as a new episode of illness. In a very few instances, clients continued to consult him without a break for more than one year. Table A.1. and Figures A.1 and A.2 include the cases of five patients, aged 18, 22, 26, 35, and 60, whose sex could not be determined; not included are 203 people, 90 males and 113 females, whose ages were not recorded.

Table A.1. *Age and sex of disturbed patients*

Age	Male		Female		Totals	
	N	%	N	%	N	%
0–4	2	0.3	1	0.1	3	0.2
5–9	6	0.9	4	0.3	10	0.5
10–14	14	2.1	14	1.2	28	1.5
15–19	43	6.5	75	6.4	119	6.5
20–24	106	16.1	177	15.1	284	15.5
25–29	107	16.3	217	18.4	325	17.7
30–34	110	16.7	174	14.8	284	15.5
35–39	59	9.0	109	9.3	169	9.2
40–44	68	10.3	137	11.7	205	11.2
45–49	39	5.9	67	5.7	106	5.8
50–54	44	6.7	77	6.6	121	6.6
55–59	14	2.1	38	3.2	52	2.8
60–64	27	4.1	35	3.0	63	3.4
65–69	7	1.1	22	1.9	29	1.6
70–74	5	0.8	16	1.4	21	1.1
75+	7	1.1	10	0.9	17	0.9
Totals	658	100.0	1173	100.0	1836	100.0

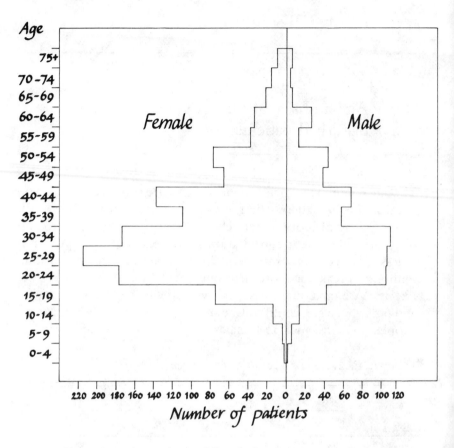

Figure A.1   Age and sex of disturbed patients

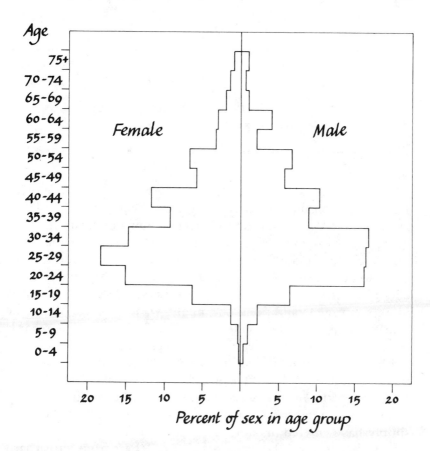

Figure A.2   Age and sex of disturbed patients (percentages)

APPENDIX B

Yearly incidence of mental disorder in Napier's practice

The dates tabulated in Table B.1 and Figure B.1 are those given for the first consultation in every episode of mental illness Napier treated. Thirty-six cases for 1610 were eliminated from this table and graph. Most of these records simply noted that the patient was "melancholy," and except for that survey year, I considered such notes to be insufficient evidence that the client was actually mentally disturbed. The pattern of lost records is so complex that it vitiates any generalizations one might want to make about the yearly variations in the incidence of mental disorder. The records for 1614 and 1626 are especially defective, but cases are also missing from many other years. Because Napier sometimes kept more than one notebook simultaneously, it is impossible to be certain that gaps in the records written on physically continuous manuscripts represent periods in which he did not practice. He may simply have entered his notes elsewhere, in books that have not survived. The handful of cases dated 1635–41 are from Sir Richard Napier's continuation of his uncle's practice.

Table B.1. *Yearly incidence of mental disorder*

Year	Cases	Year	Cases
1597	7	1619	76
1598	23	1620	71
1599	13	1621	52
1600	29	1622	93
1601	38	1623	64
1602	28	1624	78
1603	40	1625	67
1604	24	1626	35
1605	41	1627	90
1606	44	1628	102
1607	47	1629	65
1608	57	1630	84
1609	35	1631	66
1610	43	1632	96
1611	39	1633	88
1612	43	1634	13
1613	25	1635	6
1614	36	1636	2
1615	52	1637	1
1616	54	1640	3
1617	74	1641	1
1618	55		

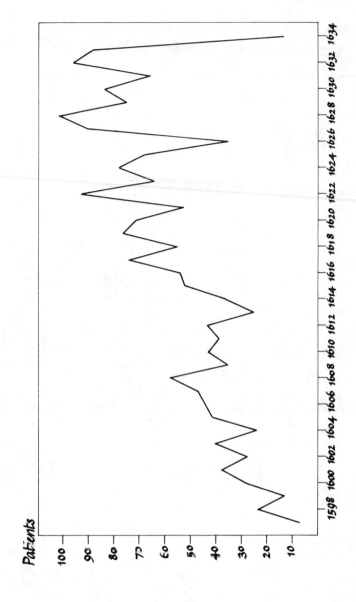

Figure B.1   Cases of mental disorder per year

Stresses reported by Napier's disturbed patients

Table C.1 records every stress reported by Napier's disturbed patients. Many clients complained about more than one problem, and the total number of stresses counted therefore exceeds 767, the number of patients whose predicaments are described in Napier's notes. There were, therefore, often fewer people in a category of stress than the simple addition of the numbers printed here indicates. Thus, for example, 99 clients reported economic problems to Napier, but they complained about 120 separate difficulties. (Discrepancies between figures mentioned in the text and the sums of the numbers given here are usually the result of the fact that cases were not counted twice in numbers that accompany generalizations.) Table C.1, which divides stresses by sex, includes one patient in the totals whose sex could not be ascertained.

Table C.1. *Stresses reported by Napier's patients by sex*

	Males (N = 263)		Females (N = 503)		Totals (N = 767)	
	N	%	N	%	N	%
Environmental perils						
Accident threatens self	1	0	8	2	9	1
child	1	0	1	0	2	0
others	1	0	0	0	1	0
Illness of self	19	7	35	7	54	7
of child	1	0	8	2	9	1
of spouse	6	2	5	1	11	1
of other	2	1	4	1	6	1
Death of spouse	9	3	33	7	42	5
of child	7	3	51	10	58	8
of parent	4	2	18	4	22	3
of other	4	2	15	3	19	2
Fire	2	1	7	1	9	1
Assault	8	3	3	1	11	1
Robbery	5	2	3	1	8	1
Attempted rape	0	0	4	1	4	1
Economic problems						
Death of stock	7	3	5	1	12	2
Debt	14	5	19	4	34	4
Poverty	3	1	12	2	15	2
Loss of job or lease	6	2	9	2	15	2
Lawsuit	7	3	7	1	14	2
Other economic problem	21	8	8	2	30	4
Generational						
Parents vs. children	9	3	15	3	24	3
Children vs. parents	21	8	11	2	32	4
Complaints re inheritance	7	3	2	0	9	1
Courtship						
Party in love	35	13	37	7	72	9
Love tiffs	15	6	44	9	59	8
Jilted	3	1	20	4	23	3
Seduced and abandoned	0	0	4	1	4	1
Premarital sex	8	3	5	1	13	2
Broken marital plan	7	3	12	2	19	2
Parental objection	6	2	15	3	21	3
"Friend's" objection	3	1	14	3	17	2
Employer's objection	1	0	2	0	3	1
Economic obstacle	5	2	10	2	15	2
Other obstacles	1	0	2	0	3	0
Loves former suitor	4	2	13	3	17	2

Table C.1 *(cont.)*

	Males (N = 263)		Females (N = 503)		Totals (N = 767)	
	N	%	N	%	N	%
Married vs. parents	4	2	4	1	8	1
Objects to child's marriage	2	1	3	1	5	1
Married to suit parents	2	1	3	1	5	1
Marital problem						
Spouse gives grief	3	1	22	4	25	3
Spouse "bad"	0	0	7	1	7	1
Couple argues	1	0	4	1	5	1
Spouse quarrelsome	3	1	23	5	26	3
Spouse doesn't "care"	1	0	5	1	6	1
Spouse adulterous	3	1	8	2	11	1
Sexual problem	1	0	3	1	4	1
Financial problem	0	0	19	4	19	2
Spouse misbehaves	0	0	5	1	5	1
Desertion	1	0	9	2	10	1
Other marital problem	11	4	39	8	50	7
Kin and neighbors						
Complaint re affines	3	1	14	3	17	2
Siblings, other kin	8	3	8	2	16	2
Law vs. kin	2	1	1	0	3	0
Other litigation	9	3	4	1	13	2
Conflict with female neighbor	2	1	8	2	10	1
Conflict with male neighbor	3	1	2	0	5	1
Conflict, sex unknown	5	2	10	2	15	2
Conflict re debt	2	1	2	0	4	1
Conflict re other	2	0	0	0	2	0
Slander re sex, self	1	0	6	1	7	1
Slander re sex, spouse	0	0	2	0	2	0
Slander re crime, self	6	2	4	1	10	1
Slander re crime, spouse	1	0	0	0	1	0
Other slander	0	0	9	2	9	1
Conflict with gentleman	2	1	1	0	3	0
Conflict with landlord	4	2	5	1	9	1
Conflict with official	1	0	0	0	1	0
Conflict between servants	0	0	3	1	3	0
Master vs. servant	12	5	3	1	15	2
Servant dissatisfied	4	2	0	0	4	1
Miscellaneous						
Too much study	23	9	4	1	27	4
Unclassifiable	6	2	4	1	10	1

APPENDIX D

Psychological symptoms of Napier's disturbed patients

Table D.1 lists the psychological symptoms of Napier's clients by sex. It is a record of the categories of mental disturbance I found in his notebooks as well as some miscellaneous information (e.g., "Symptoms described animistically"). This is raw data. I have not combined any categories except the most obvious synonyms. The unit of analysis is an episode of illness; when a client complained about the same problem repeatedly, I counted the symptom only once for each set of consultations without a gap of twelve months or more between visits. I assumed that a patient who returned more than a year later was probably suffering from a new affliction or a new episode of an old malady. A close study of separate episodes of illness involving the same person confirmed the assumption that there was little continuity between complaints made years apart. By grouping consultations into cases defined as episodes of illness the distortions caused by a single patient complaining many times about the same problem are minimized. But even using these assumptions, I could not make Viscount Purbeck's dozens of visits suitable for tabulation. His case was unique both in the number of times he met with Napier and the continuous nature of the tale the records about him tell. His problems are not included in this table. The sex of 5 clients could not be determined; their symptoms are included in the totals.

Table D.1. *Symptoms of mental disorder by sex*

Symptom	Males (N = 748)		Females (N = 1,286)		Totals (N = 2,039)	
	N	%	N	%	N	%
Mad	34	5	54	4	88	4
Lunatic	25	3	21	2	46	2
Mania	1	0	1	0	2	0
Frenzy	7	1	3	0	10	0
Melancholy	177	24	287	22	465	23
Mopish	160	21	187	15	347	17
Troubled in mind	257	34	458	36	717	35
Vexed	4	1	7	1	11	1
Discontent	9	1	48	4	57	3
Disquieted	10	1	24	2	34	2
Took grief	76	10	249	19	325	16
Took fright	43	6	120	9	163	8
Distracted	44	6	79	6	124	6
Light-headed	151	20	206	16	357	17
Raging	34	5	54	4	88	4
Furious	27	4	27	4	54	3
Frantic	62	8	63	5	126	6
Angry	8	1	15	1	23	1
Witless	19	3	28	2	47	2
Sottish	39	5	38	3	77	4
Senseless	36	5	75	6	112	5
Senses troubled	28	4	38	3	66	3
No memory	18	2	28	2	46	2
Unaware	3	0	3	0	6	0
Helpless	1	0	1	0	2	0
Can't follow his/her business	49	7	46	4	95	5
Quarrelsome	18	2	15	1	33	2
Stubborn	35	5	34	3	70	3
Suspicious	17	2	25	2	42	2
Threatens family member	17	2	14	1	31	2
Threatens others	4	1	0	0	4	0
Strikes	16	2	28	2	44	2
Struggles strongly	13	2	9	1	22	1
Broke the law	1	0	6	0	7	0
Tempted to kill spouse	5	1	7	1	12	1
Tempted to kill child	9	1	31	2	40	2
Tempted to kill child or self	0	0	20	2	20	1
Tempted to kill self	37	5	102	8	139	7
Just "tempted"	39	5	76	6	115	6

Table D.1 *(cont.)*

Symptom	Males (N = 748)		Females (N = 1,286)		Totals (N = 2,039)	
	N	%	N	%	N	%
Suicidal act	17	2	30	2	47	2
Attempted suicide	17	2	29	2	46	2
Harmed self	2	0	7	1	9	0
Tears clothes	14	2	19	1	33	2
Destroys own property	12	2	10	1	22	1
Religious preoccupation	23	3	32	2	55	3
Calls to God	10	1	13	1	23	1
Blasphemes	2	0	4	0	6	0
Refuses to pray	2	0	4	0	6	0
Apostate	5	1	16	1	21	1
Cannot pray or feel pious	15	2	21	2	36	2
Doubts own salvation	19	3	72	6	91	4
Guilt for sin	22	3	21	2	43	2
Tempted to blaspheme	12	2	15	1	27	1
Tempted to despair	4	1	16	1	20	1
Evil thoughts	24	3	55	4	79	4
Sexual urges	1	0	0	0	1	0
Sad	59	8	120	9	179	9
Grieving	22	3	85	7	107	5
Heartsick	0	0	4	0	4	0
Despair	24	3	63	5	87	4
Doubting	3	0	8	1	11	1
Fearful	81	11	202	16	283	14
Frets, cares	7	1	22	2	29	1
"Worldly"	11	1	11	1	22	1
Nervous gestures	12	2	15	1	27	1
Wandering	25	3	17	1	42	2
Solitary	23	3	21	2	44	2
Inactive	25	3	28	2	53	3
Weeps	21	3	80	6	101	5
Laughs	35	5	34	3	69	3
Sings, dances	14	2	17	1	31	2
Screams, cries	26	3	27	2	53	3
Raves	13	2	10	1	23	1
Idle talk	67	9	103	8	170	8
Too much talk	27	4	41	3	68	3
Too little talk	33	4	55	4	88	4
Refuses to talk	2	0	1	0	3	0
Curses	17	2	23	2	40	2
Sighs	1	0	24	2	25	1

Table D.1 *(cont.)*

Symptom	Males (N = 748)		Females (N = 1,286)		Totals (N = 2,039)	
	N	%	N	%	N	%
No appetite	34	5	55	4	90	4
Refuses food	4	1	6	0	10	0
Ravenous	6	1	12	1	18	1
Can't sleep	158	21	250	19	409	20
Wakes, starts	12	2	24	2	36	2
Symptoms worse at night	16	2	6	0	22	1
Religious change	4	1	7	1	11	1
Domestic change	1	0	3	0	4	0
Other change	3	0	5	0	8	0
No care for spouse	3	0	12	1	15	1
No care for child	1	0	23	2	24	1
Wants to leave home	0	0	7	1	7	0
Jealous	9	1	13	1	22	1
Fancies and conceits	73	10	88	7	162	8
Vision/perception of unnamed thing	8	1	23	2	31	2
Vision of Satan	7	1	9	1	16	1
Vision of man, woman	4	1	6	0	10	0
Flashes of light	3	0	5	0	8	0
Vision of animals	8	1	10	1	18	1
Voices	10	1	24	2	34	2
Tactile sensation	1	0	0	0	1	0
Other perceptions	7	1	12	1	19	1
Symptoms described animistically	8	1	35	3	43	2
Terrifying dream	21	3	41	3	63	3
Religious dream	2	0	5	0	7	0
Sexual dream	1	0	1	0	2	0
Outrageous	12	2	7	1	19	1
Self-accusing	2	0	8	1	10	0
Tempted to kill anybody	7	1	10	1	17	1
Doesn't know family	6	1	20	2	26	1
Runs	10	1	2	0	12	1
Drunk	14	2	8	1	22	1
Naked	7	1	2	0	9	0
Muses	13	2	13	1	26	1
Wants to die	4	1	6	0	10	0
Hates spouse	6	1	8	1	14	1
Leaps, starts	5	1	6	0	11	1
Godly	10	1	20	2	30	1

APPENDIX E

Cross tabulations of psychological symptoms

Tables E.1, E.2, and E.3 record the frequencies with which symptoms were found together in the same record of a consultation with Napier. This method of measuring the affinity between psychological symptoms minimizes the actual associations between them, because Napier did not re-record all of his client's complaints in every consultation. I used consultations rather than episodes of illness as the unit of analysis in these computations because the best indication that two symptoms were strongly linked in the minds of Napier and his informants was that they were actually written down at the same time. To simplify the computations, I have grouped together some problems touching on a single theme. Thus the category "all sadness" includes both "sad" and "grieving"; when both of these symptoms appeared in a single consultation, "all sadness" was counted only once.

Table E.1. *Symptoms of acute disorders*

Symptom	All disorders (N = 2,483)		Mad/ lunatic (N = 137)		Distracted (N = 134)		Light- headed (N = 372)	
	N	%	N	%	N	%	N	%
Mad	91	3.7	91	66.4	16	11.9	13	3.5
Lunatic	49	2.0	49	35.8	0	—	6	1.6
Melancholy	493	19.9	5	3.6	4	3.0	49	13.2
Mopish	377	15.2	14	10.2	13	9.7	60	16.1
Troubled in mind	794	32.0	15	10.9	21	15.7	94	25.3
Took grief	328	13.2	6	4.4	8	6.0	23	6.2
Took fright	168	6.8	6	4.4	5	3.7	25	6.7
Distracted	134	5.4	16	11.7	134	100.0	16	4.3
Light-headed	372	15.0	17	12.4	16	11.9	372	100.0
Raging	91	3.7	20	14.6	16	11.9	12	3.2
Furious	62	2.5	9	6.6	9	6.7	8	2.2
Frantic	131	5.3	24	17.5	12	9.0	38	10.2
Senseless	118	4.8	4	2.9	6	4.5	21	5.6
Can't follow business	100	4.0	3	2.2	3	2.2	18	4.8
Stubborn	74	3.0	9	6.6	7	5.2	16	4.3
Suspicious	45	1.8	1	0.7	3	2.2	9	2.4
Tempted to suicide	158	6.4	0	—	1	0.7	21	5.6
"Tempted"	132	5.3	1	0.7	4	3.0	15	4.0
Religious preoccupation	58	2.3	3	2.2	6	4.5	16	4.3
Doubts salvation	95	3.8	5	3.6	4	3.0	8	2.2
Evil thoughts	90	3.6	0	—	2	1.5	8	2.2
Sad	182	7.3	2	1.5	2	1.5	19	5.1
Grieving	107	4.3	1	0.7	2	1.5	7	1.9
Despair	97	3.9	0	—	9	6.7	9	2.4
Fearful	305	12.3	3	2.2	8	6.0	47	12.6
Wandering	43	1.7	2	1.5	7	5.2	16	4.3
Solitary	44	1.8	1	0.7	0	—	2	0.5
Inactive	53	2.1	1	0.7	3	2.2	9	2.4
Weeps	108	4.3	3	2.2	4	3.0	14	3.8
Laughs	78	3.1	12	8.8	8	6.0	20	5.4
Screams	54	2.2	2	1.5	8	6.0	8	2.2
Idle talk	175	7.0	9	6.6	19	14.2	57	15.3
Too much talk	75	3.0	12	8.8	15	11.2	30	8.1
Too little talk	92	3.7	2	1.5	8	6.0	20	5.4
Curses	46	1.9	3	2.2	5	3.7	9	2.4
Insomnia	434	17.5	28	20.4	26	19.4	110	29.6
Fancies and conceits	174	7.0	4	2.9	6	4.5	30	8.1
Frightening dreams	68	2.7	1	0.7	1	0.7	11	3.0
Mad/lunatic	137	5.5	137	100.0	16	11.7	17	4.6

Table E.1 (cont.)

Symptom	All disorders (N = 2,483)		Mad/ lunatic (N = 137)		Distracted (N = 134)		Light- headed (N = 372)	
	N	%	N	%	N	%	N	%
Grief/fright	482	19.4	12	8.8	13	9.7	45	12.1
All sensory	330	13.3	17	12.4	19	14.2	65	17.5
All hostility	143	5.8	11	8.0	10	7.5	30	8.1
All violence	89	3.6	14	10.2	14	10.4	13	3.5
All infanticidal	68	2.7	2	1.5	3	2.2	4	1.1
All harmful	158	6.4	18	13.1	16	11.9	23	6.2
All religious	293	11.8	11	8.1	14	10.4	50	13.4
All sadness	271	10.9	3	2.2	4	3.0	26	7.0
All moody	194	7.8	14	10.2	13	9.7	33	8.9
All loud	74	3.0	5	3.6	10	7.5	21	5.6
All domestic	75	3.0	10	7.3	5	3.7	16	4.3
All hallucinations	127	5.1	6	4.4	5	3.7	21	5.6

Table E.2. Symptoms of lesser disorders

Symptom	All disorders (N = 2,483)		Melancholy (N = 493)		Mopish (N = 377)		Troubled in mind (N = 794)	
	N	%	N	%	N	%	N	%
Mad	91	3.7	4	0.8	1	2.4	11	1.4
Lunatic	49	2.0	1	0.2	5	1.3	4	0.5
Melancholy	493	19.9	493	100.0	75	19.9	121	15.2
Mopish	377	15.2	75	15.2	377	100.0	72	9.1
Troubled in mind	794	32.0	121	24.5	72	19.1	794	100.0
Took grief	328	13.2	29	5.9	25	6.6	65	8.2
Took fright	168	6.8	25	5.1	16	4.2	50	6.3
Distracted	134	5.4	4	0.8	13	3.4	21	2.6
Light-headed	372	15.0	49	9.9	60	15.9	94	11.8
Raging	91	3.7	5	1.0	7	1.9	18	2.3
Furious	62	2.5	5	1.0	10	2.7	11	1.4
Frantic	131	5.3	8	1.6	14	3.7	22	2.8
Senseless	118	4.8	15	3.0	36	9.5	18	2.3

Table E.2 *(cont.)*

Symptom	All disorders (N = 2,483)		Melancholy (N = 493)		Mopish (N = 377)		Troubled in mind (N = 794)	
	N	%	N	%	N	%	N	%
Can't follow business	100	4.0	18	3.7	27	9.8	41	5.2
Stubborn	74	3.0	9	1.8	14	3.7	14	1.8
Suspicious	45	1.8	10	2.0	4	1.1	16	2.0
Tempted to suicide	158	6.4	27	5.5	14	3.7	62	7.8
"Tempted"	132	5.3	19	3.9	15	4.0	50	6.3
Religious preoccupation	58	2.3	7	1.4	6	1.6	22	2.8
Doubts salvation	95	3.8	26	5.3	14	3.7	40	5.0
Evil thoughts	90	3.6	19	3.9	9	2.4	42	5.3
Sad	182	7.3	75	15.2	34	9.0	54	6.8
Grieving	107	4.3	31	6.3	5	1.3	29	3.7
Despair	97	3.9	20	4.1	18	4.8	36	4.5
Fearful	305	12.3	97	19.7	35	9.3	101	12.7
Wandering	43	1.7	3	0.6	10	2.7	15	1.9
Solitary	44	1.8	18	3.7	13	3.4	8	1.0
Inactive	53	2.1	10	2.0	16	4.2	9	1.1
Weeps	108	4.3	31	6.3	19	5.0	28	3.5
Laughs	78	3.1	12	2.4	14	3.7	17	2.1
Screams	54	2.2	3	0.6	8	2.1	8	1.0
Idle talk	175	7.0	19	3.9	30	8.0	45	5.7
Too much talk	75	3.0	6	1.2	11	2.9	15	1.9
Too little talk	92	3.7	20	4.1	41	10.9	10	1.3
Curses	46	1.9	5	1.0	5	1.3	14	1.8
Insomnia	434	17.5	83	16.8	60	15.9	164	20.7
Fancies and conceits	174	7.0	57	11.6	13	3.4	71	8.9
Frightening dreams	68	2.7	14	2.8	3	0.8	21	2.6
Mad/lunatic	137	5.5	5	1.0	14	3.7	15	1.9
Grief/fright	482	19.4	54	11.0	39	10.3	113	14.2
All senses	330	13.3	54	11.0	105	27.9	66	8.3
All hostility	143	5.8	22	4.5	22	5.8	39	4.9
All violence	89	3.6	5	1.0	8	2.1	17	2.1
All infanticidal	68	2.7	9	1.8	3	0.8	27	3.4
All harmful	158	6.4	15	3.0	24	6.4	38	4.8
All religious	293	11.8	53	10.8	48	12.7	124	15.6
All sadness	271	10.9	101	20.5	38	10.1	77	9.7
All moody	194	7.8	42	8.5	36	9.5	46	5.8
All loud	74	3.0	4	0.8	9	2.4	11	1.4
All domestic	75	3.0	15	3.0	13	3.4	22	2.8
All hallucinations	127	5.1	14	2.8	15	4.0	48	6.0

Table E.3. *Symptoms of patients tempted to suicide and of patients with supernatural disorders*

Symptom	All disorders (N = 2,483)		Suicidal (N = 158)		Demoniacs[a] (N = 164)		Bewitched[a] (N = 293)		Religious symptoms (N = 293)	
	N	%	N	%	N	%	N	%	N	%
Mad	91	3.7	0	—	3	1.8	12	4.1	9	3.1
Lunatic	49	2.0	0	—	1	0.6	4	1.4	2	0.7
Melancholy	493	19.9	27	17.1	18	11.0	36	12.2	53	18.1
Mopish	377	15.2	14	8.9	19	11.6	46	15.6	48	16.4
Troubled in mind	794	32.0	62	39.2	68	41.5	104	35.4	124	42.3
Took grief	328	13.2	16	10.1	12	7.3	17	5.8	20	6.8
Took fright	168	6.8	12	7.6	6	3.7	22	7.5	17	5.8
Distracted	134	5.4	1	0.6	4	2.4	18	6.1	14	4.8
Light-headed	372	15.0	21	13.3	16	9.8	46	15.6	50	17.1
Raging	91	3.7	0	—	1	0.6	12	4.1	15	5.1
Furious	62	2.5	2	1.3	4	2.4	5	1.7	10	3.4
Frantic	131	5.3	4	2.5	7	4.3	12	4.1	14	4.8
Senseless	118	4.8	2	1.3	8	4.9	19	6.5	10	3.4
Can't follow business	100	4.0	7	4.4	10	6.1	15	5.1	12	4.1
Stubborn	74	3.0	0	—	3	1.8	5	1.7	8	2.7
Suspicious	45	1.8	5	3.2	1	0.6	10	3.4	3	1.0
Tempted to suicide	158	6.4	158	100.0	28	17.1	19	6.5	27	9.2
"Tempted"	132	5.3	8	5.1	30	18.3	19	6.5	29	9.9
Religious preoccupation	58	2.3	2	1.3	6	3.7	7	2.4	58	19.8
Doubts salvation	95	3.8	15	9.5	10	6.1	10	3.4	95	32.4
Evil thoughts	90	3.6	11	7.0	14	8.5	7	2.4	26	8.9
Sad	182	7.3	15	9.5	7	4.3	17	5.8	29	9.9
Grieving	107	4.3	2	1.3	4	2.4	10	3.4	13	4.4

Despair	97	3.9	13	8.2	13	7.9	8	2.7	32	10.9
Fearful	305	12.3	20	12.7	31	18.9	39	13.3	44	15.0
Wandering	43	1.7	1	0.6	4	2.4	3	1.0	5	1.7
Solitary	44	1.8	1	0.6	0	—	4	1.4	3	1.0
Inactive	53	2.1	2	1.3	3	1.8	5	1.7	0	—
Weeps	108	4.3	9	5.7	5	3.0	11	3.7	21	7.2
Laughs	78	3.1	1	0.6	2	1.2	5	1.7	5	1.7
Screams	54	2.2	1	0.6	4	2.4	12	4.1	11	3.8
Idle talk	175	7.0	6	3.8	6	3.7	24	8.2	21	7.2
Too much talk	75	3.0	0	—	2	1.2	10	3.4	7	2.4
Too little talk	92	3.7	1	0.6	4	2.4	17	5.8	13	4.4
Curses	46	1.9	3	1.9	4	2.4	11	3.7	12	4.1
Insomnia	434	17.5	27	17.5	27	16.5	61	20.5	60	20.5
Fancies and conceits	174	7.0	10	6.3	14	8.5	28	9.5	20	6.8
Frightening dreams	68	2.7	8	5.1	11	6.7	10	3.4	9	3.1
Mad/lunatic	137	5.5	0	—	4	2.4	16	5.4	11	3.8
Grief/fright	482	19.4	25	15.8	17	10.4	37	12.6	36	12.3
All senses	330	13.3	7	4.4	22	13.4	49	16.7	32	10.9
All hostility	143	5.8	6	3.8	5	3.0	15	5.1	13	4.4
All violence	89	3.6	0	—	4	2.4	8	2.7	13	4.4
All infanticidal	68	2.7	20	12.7	17	10.4	8	2.7	14	4.8
All harmful	158	6.4	15	9.5	25	15.2	19	6.5	28	9.6
All religious	293	11.8	27	17.1	46	28.0	34	11.6	293	100.0
All sadness	271	10.9	17	10.8	11	6.7	25	8.5	38	13.0
All moody	194	7.8	10	6.3	7	4.3	20	6.8	25	8.5
All loud	74	3.0	1	0.6	5	3.0	17	5.8	14	4.8
All domestic	75	3.0	5	3.2	4	2.4	11	3.7	10	3.4
All hallucinations	127	5.1	12	7.6	44	26.8	22	7.5	22	7.5

aIncludes all consultations with patients fearing harm by demons (148 cases) or witches (264 cases).

Notes

Preface

1 Michel Foucault, *Madness and Civilization*, trans. Richard Howard (New York, 1965), pp. 18–19. The English translation of this book should be compared with the revised French edition, *Histoire de la folie à l'âge classique* (Paris, 1972), pp. 20–1.
2 Foucault, *Madness and Civilization*, p. 39; *Histoire de la folie*, p. 53.
3 Foucault, *Madness and Civilization*, p. 47; *Histoire de la folie*, pp. 66–7.
4 For an interesting discussion of Foucault's attitudes toward the conventions of orthodox historiography, see Allan Megill, "Foucault, Structuralism and the Ends of History," *Journal of Modern History* 51 (1979): 451–503. Acting on the assumption that Foucault is bound by the rules of evidence and argument that constrain the fancies of ordinary historians, H. C. Erik Midelfort has exposed many of Foucault's errors in "Madness and Civilization in Early Modern Europe: A Reappraisal of Michel Foucault," Barbara Malament, ed. *After the Reformation: Essays in Honor of J. H. Hexter* (Philadelphia, 1980).
5 George Rosen has provided a more orthodox version of Foucault's thesis in *Madness in Society* (Chicago, 1968), Chaps. 4 and 5.

CHAPTER 1 *Insanity in early modern England*

1 The literature about culture and mental disorder is very large and very uneven. Among the works that stress the part played by society in defining and discovering mental abnormalities, well-known and interesting books include Erving Goffman, *Asylums* (Garden City, N.Y., 1961); Thomas Scheff, *Being Mentally Ill* (Chicago, 1966); Laurie Taylor, *Deviance and Society* (London, 1971); Ari Kiev, *Transcultural Psychiatry* (Harmonsworth, 1972). This perspective is criticized by Jane M. Murphy, "Psychiatric Labeling in Cross-Cultural Perspective," *Science* 191 (1976):1019–28. Two useful surveys of studies published prior to 1973 are Juris G. Draguns, "Psychopathology Across Cultures," *Journal of Cross-Cultural Psychology* 4 (1973):9–47, and Erwin Stengel, *Suicide and Attempted Suicide* (Harmondsworth, 1969), Chap. 6; for later publications see *Transcultural Psychiatric Review*. A recent study that strikes a balance between the excesses of the labeling theorists and their enemies and whose authors' views are similar to those presented here is G. M. Carstairs and R. L. Kapur, *The Great Universe of Kota: Stress, Change and Mental Disorder in an Indian Village* (London, 1976), esp. pp. 9–12.
2 A comprehensive anthology of selections from contemporary writings about insanity is Richard Hunter and Ida Macalpine, comps., *Three Hundred Years of Psychiatry 1535–1860* (London, 1963). For modern scholarship see Lawrence Babb, *The Elizabethan Malady* (East Lansing, Mich., 1951); Robert R. Reed, *Bedlam on the Jacobean Stage* (Cambridge, Mass., 1952); Bridget Gellert Lyons, *Voices of Melancholy* (New York, 1971); Louis B. Wright, *Middle-Class Culture in Elizabethan England* (London, 1935), pp. 588–92. The fundamental text, however, is

Robert Burton's great synthesis, *The Anatomy of Melancholy*, ed. Holbrook Jackson, 3 vols. (London, 1968).

3 I hope in future to publish the results of further research about the history of insanity and suicide in England after 1640. The assertions about that period made in this chapter are documented more extensively in the text below, and I have generally not repeated the later references here.

4 John Sym, *Lifes Preservative against self-killing* (London, 1637), Sig. A4ᵛ. See also S. E. Sprott, *The English Debate on Suicide* (La Salle, Ill., 1961).

5 For evidence of the increasing frequency of recorded suicide see Michael MacDonald, "The Inner Side of Wisdom: Suicide in Early Modern England," *Psychological Medicine* 7 (1977):566–7; P. E. H. Hair, "A Note on the Incidence of Tudor Suicide," *Local Population Studies*, No. 5 (1970):36–43; idem, "Deaths from Violence in Britain: A Tentative Secular Survey," *Population Studies* 25, No. 1 (1971):5–24; R. F. Hunnisett, ed., *Calendar of Nottinghamshire Coroners' Inquests, 1485–1558*, Thoroton Society, 25 (1969), passim; Peter Laslett, *The World We Have Lost*, 2nd ed. (London, 1971), pp. 145–7; Thomas R. Forbes, *Chronicle from Aldgate* (New Haven, 1971), pp. 171–2; Karla Oosterveen, "Deaths by Suicide, Drowning and Misadventure in Hawkshead, 1620–1700," *Local Population Studies*, No. 4 (1970):17–20; John Bellamy, *Crime and Public Order in England in the Later Middle Ages* (London, 1973), pp. 32–3.

6. Reed, *Bedlam on Stage*, pp. 16, 23–6; Hunter and Macalpine, *Psychiatry*, pp. 105–8; E. G. O'Donoghue, *The Story of Bethlehem Hospital* (London, 1914); Patricia Allderidge, "Management and Mismanagement at Bedlam, 1547–1633," in Charles Webster, ed., *Health, Medicine and Mortality in the Sixteenth Century* (Cambridge, 1979), pp. 152–69, esp. pp. 152–4, 158–60, 163.

7 William L. Parry-Jones, *The Trade in Lunacy* (London, 1972), Chaps. 1 and 2; Kathleen Jones, *A History of the Mental Health Services* (London, 1973), Chap. 1; Andrew T. Scull, *Museums of Madness: The Social Organization of Insanity in Nineteenth-Century England* (London, 1979).

8 Joel Hurstfield, *The Queen's Wards*, 2nd ed. (London, 1973), esp. pp. 49, 65, 72–6, 140, 243, and H. E. Bell, *An Introduction to the History and Records of the Court of Wards and Liveries* (Cambridge, 1953), esp. pp. 4, 6, 16, 102, 109, 128–32, 164, 199. The definitive work on lunacy in the Court of Wards is Richard Neugebauer, "Mental Illness and Government Policy in Sixteenth and Seventeenth Century England" (Ph.D. diss., Columbia University, 1976). A synopsis appeared as Richard Neugebauer, "Treatment of the Mentally Ill in Medieval and Early Modern England: A Reappraisal," *Journal of the History of the Behavioral Sciences* 14 (1978):158–69. I was unable to consult Dr. Neugebauer's thesis or his article until the manuscript of this book had been written. Our discussions of the Court of Wards are complementary, in part because Dr. Neugebauer was kind enough to discuss his work with me.

9 *A Commission with instructions and directions, granted by His Majestie to the Master and Counsaile of the Court of Wards and Liveries, For compounding for Wards, Ideots and Lunaticks* (London, 1617–18), pp. 11–12.

10 Bell, *Court of Wards*, pp. 130–1. A rapid reading of the Petition Books of the court confirms Bell's impression that the insane were usually committed to the care of their relatives or friends: Public Record Office, London (hereafter cited as PRO), Wards 9/214–220; Wards 10/27, esp., e.g., Wards 9/216, ff. 9, 58ᵛ; 9/218, ff. 133ᵛ, 154ᵛ.

11 Procedures in disputed cases are well illustrated in the documents pertaining to the lunacy of a rich Bedford lunatic, Edmund Francklin: Bedfordshire County Record Office, Francklin Papers, FN 1060–1084. See also Hurstfield, *Queen's Wards*, pp. 72–6; Bell, *Court of Wards*, pp. 131–2.

12 Bell, *Court of Wards*, pp. 128–30. Many seventeenth-century examples of inquisitions regarding lunacy survive among the records of the Petty Bag Office of Chancery and these are indexed in *Index of Inquisitions Preserved in the Public Record Office*, Lists and Indexes, Vol. 31 (1909), Vol. 33 (1909), and PRO, index 17612.

The informality that lay behind their standard phrases can be seen in the inquisition into the lunacy of Richard Pudsey. Lacking a formulary, the Oxfordshire jury described what they had heard about Pudsey's conduct and clearly put him to no special test or applied expert criteria: PRO, C142/718, f. 152.

13 Bell, *Court of Wards*, pp. 128, 131–2.
14 *An Act Touching Idiots and Lunatiques* (London, 1653).
15 Bell, *Court of Wards*, p. 164; *Calendar of State Papers, Domestic, Charles II, 1660–1661*, pp. 328–9; *Calendar of State Papers, Domestic, William and Mary, 1689*, pp. 19–20.
16 A. Fessler, "The Management of Lunacy in Seventeenth-Century England," *Proceedings of the Royal Society of Medicine* 49 (1956):901–7.
17 Michael Dalton, *The Countrey Iustice* (London, 1626), p. 98.
18 Lancashire County Record Office, QSO 2/31: I owe this reference to the kindness of Walter King. See also Fessler, "Management of Lunacy." Similar documents may be found in the printed sessions records of several counties, but it is impossible to judge from them if the law was uniformly enforced.
19 Christopher Hill, *Society and Puritanism* (New York, 1967), Chap. 12; John Pound, *Poverty and Vagrancy in Tudor England* (London, 1971); Sylvia S. Tollit, "The First House of Correction for the County of Lancaster," *Transactions of the Historical Society of Lancaster and Cheshire* 105 (1953):69–90.
20 Fessler, "Management of Lunacy," p. 904.
21 See esp. Wright, *Middle-Class Culture*, pp. 588–92; Babb, *Elizabethan Malady*; R. S. Roberts, "The Early History of the Import of Drugs into Britain," in F. N. L. Poynter, ed., *The Evolution of Pharmacy in Britain* (London, 1965).
22 Margaret Pelling and Charles Webster, "Medical Practitioners," in Webster, ed., *Health, Medicine and Mortality*; Keith Thomas, *Religion and the Decline of Magic* (New York, 1971), pp. 154–9, 177–252, 283–357; R. S. Roberts, "The Personnel and Practice of Medicine in Tudor and Stuart England," Part I, *Medical History* 6 (1962):363–82, and Part II, *Medical History* 8 (1964):217–34; Sir George Clark, *The Royal College of Physicians of London*, 2 vols. (Oxford, 1962–4); Christopher Hill, *Change and Continuity in Seventeenth-Century England* (Cambridge, Mass., 1975), Chap. 7; Charles Webster, *The Great Instauration: Science, Medicine, and Reform, 1626–1660* (New York, 1975), Chap. 4.
23 John Cotta, *A Short Discouerie of the vnobserued dangers of seueral sorts of ignorant and vnconsiderate Practisers of Physicke in England* (London, 1612), pp. 86, 88. Cf. Webster, *Great Instauration*, pp. 255–60; Clark, *College of Physicians*, 1:239–40, 246–9, 260–1.
24 Cotta, *Short Discouerie*, pp. 86, 94; Thomas, *Religion and Magic*, pp. 316–17.
25 Roberts, "Medicine," Pts. I and II; Clark, *College of Physicians*, Vol. 1.
26 Clark, *College of Physicians*, 1:146, 167–8, 199, 214, 216; A. L. Rowse, *Simon Forman: Sex and Society in Shakespeare's Age* (London, 1974), pp. 8–10, 32, 45–50, 56, 61, 154–5, 202–4, 250, 256, 288–9, 292, 296, 297.
27 Thomas, *Religion and Magic*, pp. 477–92.
28 John Bunyan, *Grace Abounding to the Chief of Sinners and Pilgrim's Progress*, ed. Roger Sharrock (London, 1966) p. 15.
29 Thomas, *Religion and Magic*, pp. 486–7.
30 See Chapter 4, pp. 170–2, and Chapter 5, pp. 223–6.
31 John Locke, *An Essay Concerning Human Understanding*, ed. A. C. Fraser, 2nd ed., 2 vols. (New York, 1959), 1:209–10; 2:528–9; Michael V. DePorte, *Nightmares and Hobbyhorses: Swift, Sterne, and Augustan Ideas of Madness* (San Marino, Calif., 1974), Chap. 1, esp. pp. 20–1; and Chapter 4, pp. 170–1. Locke himself mentioned melancholy as a cause of religious enthusiasm.
32 MacDonald, *Inner Side of Wisdom*; and Chapter 4, pp. 171–2.
33 See esp. *Report from the Select Committee on the Regulation of Madhouses in England, 1815, Parliamentary Papers, 1815*, 801; Parry-Jones, *Trade in Lunacy*, Chap. 8; Scull, *Museums of Madness*, pp. 73–82; Peter McCandless, "Insanity and Society: A Study of the English Lunacy Reform Movement, 1815–1870" (Ph.D. diss., University of Wisconsin–Madison, 1974), Chap. 1.

CHAPTER 2 *A healer and his patients*

1 Napier's papers are in the Bodleian Library, Oxford, and are part of the collection of Ashmole manuscripts: William H. Black, comp., *A Descriptive, Analytical and Critical Catalogue of the Manuscripts Bequeathed Unto the University of Oxford by Elias Ashmole* (Oxford, 1845), hereafter cited as *Ashmole Manuscripts*; W. D. Macray, *Index to the Catalogue of the Manuscripts of Elias Ashmole* (Oxford, 1866). The volumes containing Napier's medical notes are not sequentially numbered; they are listed in Macray's index.

2 Elias Ashmole, *Elias Ashmole (1617–1692): His Autobiographical and Historical Notes, his Correspondence, and Other Contemporary Sources Relating to his Life*, ed. C. H. Josten, 5 vols. (Oxford, 1966), 1: esp. 57–9, 84–5, 185–8, 209–10, 227, 235, 244, 262, 271, 284; 2:734, 1265–7, 1282; 3:1403, 1443, 1453, 1468; 4:1685, 1802, 1828–32, 1896; Frances Yates, *The Rosicrucian Enlightenment* (Boulder, Colo., 1972), esp. Chaps. 3 and 14; R. W. Hunt, "The Cataloguing of the Ashmolean Collections of Books and Manuscripts," *Bodleian Library Record* 4 (1952–3):162.

3 Biographies of three men who shared many of Napier's interests include A. L. Rowse, *Simon Forman: Sex and Society in Shakespeare's Age* (London, 1974); Derek Parker, *Familiar to All: William Lilly and Astrology in the Seventeenth Century* (London, 1975); Michael Hunter, *John Aubrey and the Realm of Learning* (New York, 1975), esp. Chap. 2. The last is an excellent analysis of the magical and scientific aspirations of these men.

4 Bodleian Library, Ashmole MS 213, f. 110 (hereafter cited as Ashml.); Ashml. 413, f. 63.

5 John Aubrey, *Aubrey's Brief Lives*, ed. Oliver Lawson Dick (Harmondsworth, 1972), pp. 78, 378–9; John Aubrey, *Three Prose Works*, ed. John Buchanan-Brown (Carbondale, Ill., 1972), pp. 86, 101–2. See also William Lilly, *History of His Life and Times* (London, 1715), pp. 52–4; Anthony Wood, *Athenae Oxonienses*, 4 vols. (London, 1815), 2: cols. 103–4. A list of theological queries to an angel similar to the one recalled by Aubrey may be found in Ashml. 237, f. 192^v.

6 Katherine Briggs, *Pale Hecate's Team* (London, 1962), p. 56; O. L. Dick in Aubrey, *Brief Lives*, p. 378.

7 Yates, *Rosicrucian Enlightenment*; Frances Yates, *Giordano Bruno and the Hermetic Tradition* (New York, 1964).

8 Keith Thomas, *Religion and the Decline of Magic* (New York, 1971), pp. 222–31.

9 Thomas, *Religion and Magic*, esp. Chaps. 8, 9, 12, 14–18, 22.

10 Peter French, *John Dee* (London, 1972), pp. 109–25. Napier owned Agrippa's book: Ashml. 407, f. 150; and he possessed works attributed to Lull: Ashml. 1480 (note his hand on art. I, f. 95^v). For his collection of hermetic and cabalistic manuscripts see Black, *Ashmole Manuscripts*; Ashml. 1730, f. 168; Ashml. 240, ff. 136–40^v; and the treatises in the hand of his assistant Gerence James, in British Library, Sloane MS 3826 ("Liber Salamonis" and "Liber Luna").

11 Sloane MS 3822, f. 24.

12 Rowse, *Simon Forman*, p. 33; Ashml. 407, f. 150; Ashml. 221, f. 51^v.

13 Lilly, *Life*, p. 101.

14 Lists of questions to be resolved by astrology or some supernatural means are scattered throughout the practice books; those that seem to have been used in séances include Ashml. 235, ff. 186^v–93; Ashml. 237, f. 192^v; Ashml. 223, ff. 192^v, 193^v, 194^v–5^v; Ashml. 222, ff. 194–7.

15 Yates, *Giordano Bruno*, p. 142.

16 Fugitive manuscripts concerning conjuring are among the Ashmole papers that found their way to the British Library; they include notes and copywork by Forman, Dee, Napier, and his assistants. Papers that Napier wrote or owned are in Sloane MSS 3822, 3826, 3679, 3846, 3854, and Additional MS 36674. Invocations and rituals involving angelic magic used by Napier are also in Ashml. 237, f. 190^v; Ashml. 1790, ff. 112–12^v, 113^v, 115. A parchment formula for invoking Raphael, folded and worn, is in Ashml. 244, ff. 130–2.

17 Ashml. 244, f. 131.

18 Thomas, *Religion and Magic*, p. 268.

19 "Goody Kent met me and Master Wallys [Napier's assistant] in the street and called us conjurers," Napier noted apprehensively in 1616: Ashml. 408, f. 28; Lilly remarks that he had many enemies but enjoyed the protection of Lord Wentworth, later the Earl of Cleveland, and the judgment appears to have been accurate: Lilly, *Life*, pp. 52, 55; Ashml. 414, f. 47. He prudently renewed his licenses to practice medicine when his reputation began to attract the attention of noblemen: Ashml. 222, f. 1^v; Ashml. 1293, now filed as Ashml. rolls 5 (1). See also Keith Thomas's brief observation about the religiosity and unlawfulness of Napier's activities: *Religion and Magic*, p. 379.

20 For Napier's biography and family see *Dictionary of National Biography* (hereafter cited as *DNB*), John Burke and John Bernard Burke, *Genealogical and Heraldic History of the Extinct and Dormant Baronetcies*, 2nd ed. (London, 1844), pp. 378–9, and Black, *Ashmole Manuscripts*, index s.v. "Napier." Richard, his father, and his brother used the alternative surname Sandy (or Sandie). This has caused some confusion about his education, the sources for which are Joseph Foster, comp., *Alumni Oxonienses* (1500–1714), 4 vols. (Oxford, 1892), 4:1310; Charles W. Boase, ed., *Registrum Collegii Exoniensis*, Oxford Historical Society, 26 (1894), p. 81; Andrew Clark, ed., *Register of the University of Oxford*, Vol. 2, Part II, Oxford Historical Society, 11 (1887), pp. 74, 99.

21 Lilly, *Life*, p. 53; Ashml. 213, f. 110. Napier's curates were Francis Shaxton, Robert Wallis (or Wallys), Ralph Ruddle, Gerence James, and Theodore Gravius. Wallys and James assisted Napier in his medical practice and became astrological physicians themselves; Gravius was a Bohemian alchemist; Ruddle achieved some prominence as a clergyman. See Bodleian Library, *Index of the Manuscripts of the Archdeaconry of Bucks*, Parish Register Transcripts, D/A/T 123; Henry Isham Longden, *Northampton and Rutland Clergy from 1500*, 15 vols. (Northampton, 1940), 7:225; Black, *Ashmole Manuscripts* index s.v. "Richard Napier" and the name of each curate.

22 The improvements to the rectory are discussed in Royal Commission on Historical Monuments (England), *An Inventory of the Historical Monuments in Buckinghamshire*, 2 vols. (London, 1913), 2:128. Napier arranged to purchase the parsonage for £200 in 1610 and in that same year his brother became the owner of the advowson; *Victoria County History* (hereafter cited as *VCH*), *Bucks.*, 4:391, and Ashml. 215, f. 60^v. A draft note settling Napier's landed property on the younger Richard survives, but it does not indicate the extent or value of the lands: Ashml. 1730, f. 235. The fiscal misadventures of Sir Richard may be followed in the Uthwatt papers, Buckinghamshire County Record Office, D/U/1.

23 Aubrey, *Three Prose Works*, p. 102.

24 William Gadstone first appears as Napier's financial manager in 1610 (Ashml. 239, f. 132) and he was still conducting his business in 1631 (Ashml. 232, f. 475). The quotation is from the former citation. Napier's fees are recorded unsystematically in practice books written before Gadstone took over. A normal range of 6–18d and instances of gratis cases may be observed in, e.g., Ashml. 202 (practice notes for 1600).

25 Ashml. 408, f. 155^v.

26 Ashml. 413, ff. 12 and 227.

27 Napier was first approached about treating Purbeck in 1620 (Ashml. 414, f. 192), but entreaties began in earnest two years later (Ashml. 231, f. 184^v; Ashml. 223, ff. 49^v, 93). Purbeck became his patient in June 1622 and was with Napier for extended periods in 1622, 1624, and 1631. The scandal is described in two potboilers, and there is much their authors overlooked in Napier's notes and elsewhere: [Thomas Longueville], *The Curious Case of Lady Purbeck: A Scandal of the XVIIth Century* (London, 1909); Laura L. Nosworthy, *The Lady of Bleeding Heart Yard: Lady Elizabeth Hatton, 1578–1646* (New York, 1936).

28 Ashml. 410, ff. 81, 83.

29 Ashml. 1730, ff. 203–3ᵛ, 212–3ᵛ.
30 Ashml. 414, f, 47. The chancellor may have been either Baron Verulam (Francis Bacon) or Bishop John Williams.
31 Ashml. 1730, ff. 203–3ᵛ, 212–3ᵛ.
32 Ashml. 1730, f. 227.
33 See, e.g., Ashml. 1279, f. 2 ff.; Ashml. 238, ff. 218ᵛ–19; Ashml. 1473, ff. 452–6, 529.
34 Ashml. 413, f. 4; Ashml. 402, f. 28; Ashml. 212, f. 256.
35 See Chapter 5, pp. 220–2 for Napier's attitudes toward laymen he suspected of Puritanism.
36 Ashml. 1730, ff. 180–1ᵛ, 182–3, 199–200ᵛ.
37 Ashml. 1730, ff. 180ᵛ–1.
38 Ashml. 213, f. 148; Ashml. 416, f. 203; *DNB*.
39 Ashml. 414, f. 15ᵛ; Ashml. 1730, f. 217.
40 Ashml. 220, f. 40ᵛ. For Twisse see *DNB*.
41 Ashml. 231, f. 116ᵛ; Ashml. 1148, ff. 203–28ᵛ.
42 Cf. French, *John Dee*, Chaps. 4 and 5.
43 Ashml. 242, ff. 187–90. The treatise is in several fragments: Ashml. 204, ff. 50–64ᵛ; Ashml. 242, ff. 137–8ᵛ; Ashml. 242, ff. 187–96. Napier probably composed the work at Simon Forman's request, but plans to publish it apparently were never carried out: Ashml. 240, f. 103.
44 J. Sears McGee, *The Godly Man in Stuart England* (New Haven, 1976), pp. 71–5; the quotation is on p. 72.
45 McGee, *Godly Man*, pp. 72–3.
46 Sloane MS 3822, ff. 64–7ᵛ.
47 Ashml. 1730, ff. 207–7ᵛ.
48 Ashml. 1730, ff. 207–7ᵛ.
49 Thomas, *Religion and Magic*, pp. 318, 354–5, 367–71; Allan Chapman, "Astrological Medicine," in Charles Webster, ed., *Health, Medicine and Mortality in the Sixteenth Century* (Cambridge, 1979); Carroll Camden, Jr., "Elizabethan Astrological Medicine," *Annals of Medical History* 2 (1930):217–26.
50 Thomas, *Religion and Magic*, p. 369; for Thornborough, see *DNB*; Ashml. 415, f. 15ᵛ; Ashml. 416, f. 49; Ashml. 1730, f. 217 (Williams); Ashml. 416, f. 203 (Peterborough); Ashml. 217, f. 133ᵇ (Abbot).
51 Thomas, *Religion and Magic*, pp. 371–7.
52 Thomas, *Religion and Magic*, pp. 354–5; Bernard S. Capp, *Astrology and the Popular Press: English Almanacs, 1500–1800* (London, 1979).
53 Ashml. 226, f. 3; Rowse, *Simon Forman*, p. 151.
54 Rowse, *Simon Forman*, pp. 150–6; see also Ashml. 175, passim, and Ashml. 182, arts. 2,3.
55 Lilly, *Life*, p.53; Ashml. 240, ff. 104–4ᵛ.
56 Lilly, *Life*, p. 53.
57 Ashml. 213, ff. 170–1.
58 Ashml. 1501, art. 5, ff. 5–6ᵛ. Napier's views about the importance of accurate information regarding his patients' symptoms are also illustrated by Ashml. 1730, ff. 202, 205, and Ashml. 232, f. 298.
59 Thomas, *Religion and Magic*, pp. 305–22; Black, *Ashmole Manuscripts*, describes the collections of all these astrologers.
60 This is admittedly a very subjective judgment. It is based on a survey of the casebooks in the British Library's Sloane manuscripts and the printed examples. Some physicians, such as Sir Theodore de Mayerne, were quite meticulous and are obvious exceptions to this generalization: Theodore de Mayerne, *Opera Medica*, ed. J. Browne (London, 1703). See Simon Forman's textbook of astrological physic for an explicit demand that adepts keep careful records and consult them to improve their medical skills: Ashml. 363, ff. 2–4, esp. 3ᵛ.
61 George Atwell, *An Apology, Or, Defense of the divine art of Natural Astrology* (London, 1660), pp. 26–7.

62 When his nephew, James Evington, wrote to him anxious to learn the secrets of astrology, Napier reprimanded him for his interest in such vain pursuits and advised him to abandon all thought of astrological studies; he was not a proselytizer and taught astrological medicine to just two or three men during his long career: Ashml. 240, f. 126.

63 Michael Shepherd, Brian Cooper, Alexander C. Brown, and Graham Kalton, *Psychiatric Illness in General Practice* (London, 1966), pp. 16–17.

64 Lilly, *Life*, pp. 53–4.

65 Ashml. 196, f. 103. For Worcester see E. R. C. Brinkworth, "The Laudian Church in Buckinghamshire," *University of Birmingham Historical Journal* 5 (1955–6):38; Ashml. 217, f. 31. It should also be noted, however, that at the height of his fame he treated the Puritan Earl of Bedford and his wife and that he was a medical confidant of his niece's husband, Sir Thomas Myddelton, the younger, a future Presbyterian and Parliamentarian: Ashml. 1730, ff. 202, 205; Ashml. 211, ff. 146, 514 (Bedford).

66 See Chapter 5, pp. 220–2.

67 Among Napier's patients, prominent Catholics and recusant families included the Countess of Buckingham, Viscount Purbeck, the Digbys, the Dormers, the Mordaunts, and the Temples.

68 Cf. John G. Howells and N. Livia Osborn, "The Incidence of Emotional Disorder in a Seventeenth-Century Medical Practice," *Medical History* 14 (1970):192–8. In this study of the casebook of Dr. John Hall (1575–1635) the authors arrive at a much higher incidence of mental disorder than the rates indicated in Napier's practice notes. They do not share my timidity about classifying a great many ambiguous conditions as symptoms of mental disorder.

69 See Chapter 5, under "Demons, witches, and madmen."

70 Thomas, *Religion and Magic*, pp. 11–12, 248–9; Napier's fees were about the same as those Thomas found wizards and cunning folk charging. For popular reactions to the high prices normally charged by physicians and revolutionary alternatives, see Christopher Hill, *Change and Continuity in Seventeenth-Century England* (Cambridge, Mass., 1975), Chap. 7, and Charles Webster, *The Great Instauration: Science, Medicine, and Reform, 1626–1660* (New York, 1975), Chap. 4.

71 George Lipscomb, *The History and Antiquities of Buckingham*, 4 vols. (London, 1847), 4:227.

72 Ashml. 363, f. 4^v; cf. Sloane MS 99, f. 4^v.

73 Lewis Bayly, *The Practice of Piety*, 31st ed. (London, 1633), pp. 49–61.

74 Robert Burton, *The Anatomy of Melancholy*, ed. Holbrook Jackson, 3 vols. (London, 1968), 1:172, 210–11, 414–19; Stanley W. Jackson, "Unusual Mental States in Medieval Europe, I. Medical Syndromes of Mental Disorder: 400–1100 A.D.," *Journal of the History of Medicine* 27 (1972):275.

75 Burton, *Anatomy of Melancholy*, 1:242–5; Duchess of Newcastle, *CCXI Sociable Letters* (London, 1664), p. 71 (I owe this reference to Sara Mendelson); Lawrence Babb, *The Elizabethan Malady* (East Lansing, Mich., 1951), Chaps. 4–7.

76 Burton, *Anatomy of Melancholy*, 1:39. Notice the range of conditions described as madness, mania, and distraction in the contemporary sources anthologized in Richard Hunter and Ida Macalpine, comps., *Three Hundred Years of Psychiatry 1535–1860* (London, 1963), pp. 1–275. See also Babb, *Elizabethan Malady*, Chap. 2.

77 Convenient reviews of the sociology and epidemiology of mental disorder are Ransom J. Arthur, *An Introduction to Social Psychiatry* (Harmondsworth, 1971); Roger Bastide, *The Sociology of Mental Disorder*, trans. Jean McNeil (London, 1972); Ari Kiev, *Transcultural Psychiatry* (Harmondsworth, 1972); Michael Shepherd et al., *Psychiatric Illness in General Practice* (London, 1966), Chap. 1; Morton Beiser, "Psychiatric Epidemiology," in *The Harvard Guide to Modern Psychiatry*, ed. Armand M. Nicholi, Jr. (Cambridge, Mass., 1978), pp. 607–26.

78 For a discussion of melancholy see Chapter 4, under "Melancholy: the crest of courtier's arms." Appendix D lists all the psychological symptoms of Napier's disturbed clients by sex.

79 The worst comprehensive study of women and mental illness is the biggest and best known, Phyllis Chesler, *Women and Madness* (New York, 1974); one of the best is a short and scholarly piece, Walter Gove and Jeanette Tudor, "Adult Sex Roles and Mental Illness," *American Journal of Sociology* 78 (1973):812–25.

80 Shepherd et al., *Psychiatric Illness*, pp. 164–6.

81 Shepherd et al., *Psychiatric Illness*, pp. 16–17.

82 For Napier's views about women see Ashml. 1473, f. 529; Ashml. 1730, f. 216ᵛ.

83 Rowse, *Simon Forman*, Chap. 5; Forman's diaries and practice books, Ashml. 234, 226, 195, 219, 236, and 411, passim; Thomas, *Religion and Magic*, pp. 316–17; anonymous astrological casebook, Ashml. 330.

84 Roger Thompson, *Women in Stuart England and America* (London, 1974), pp. 31–35; Paul Slack and Peter Clark, *English Towns in Transition, 1500–1700* (New York, 1976), pp. 87–8; Charles Phythian-Adams, *Desolation of a City: Coventry and the Urban Crisis of the Late Middle Ages* (Cambridge, 1979), pp. 199–200; Peter Laslett, "Mean Household Size in England Since the Sixteenth Century," in Peter Laslett and Richard Wall, eds., *Household and Family in Past Time* (Cambridge, 1972), p. 145.

85 Conditions in these villages are discussed later in this chapter, pp. 61–7.

86 The sample years were 1600, 1610, 1620, and 1630; the sex ratios for those years were, respectively, 71.0, 70.8, 80.6, and 87.8.

87 Napier treated 1,267 cases of mental disorder among women over 14; 284 (22.4%) of them suffered from gynecological or obstetrical illnesses. For other contemporary physicians' preoccupation with female diseases see Anonymous Medical Practice Book, Sloane MS 461, ff. 15, 45, 77, 78ᵛ, 83; Anonymous Compilation of Medical Records (mostly concerning gynecological afflictions), 1600–20, Sloane MS 63, ff. 2–34; "On the Diseases of Women" (seventeenth century), Sloane MS 421, art. A., ff. 2–25ᵛ; Howells and Osborn, "Incidence of Emotional Disorder."

88 Carol Z. Wiener suggested this argument to me, and she has demonstrated the influence of sex roles on violent crime in her "Sex Roles and Crime in late Elizabethan Hertfordshire," *Journal of Social History* 8 (1975):38–60.

89 Edward Jorden, *A briefe discourse of a disease Called the Suffocation of the Mother* (London, 1603); Ilza Veith, *Hysteria: The History of a Disease* (Chicago, 1965), Chap. 7. Most historians of psychiatry identify hysteria and "mother," but Napier employed the term to describe conditions marked by discomfort in the region of the womb or menstrual cramps; seldom did he note psychiatric symptoms or any of the dramatic signs of hysteria in such cases.

90 Gerrard Winstanley, *The Law of Freedom and Other Writings*, ed. Christopher Hill (Harmondsworth, 1973), pp. 59, 296.

91 Bayly, *Practice of Piety*, pp. 57–60; see Chapter 3, under "Misfortune and mental disorder."

92 Demographic studies of infant and childhood mortality during the period include E. A. Wrigley, "Mortality in Pre-Industrial England: The Example of Colyton, Devon, Over Three Centuries," *Daedalus* 92, No. 2 (1968):546–80; Ursula M. Cowgill, "Life and Death in the Sixteenth Century in the City of York," *Population Studies* 21 (1967):53–62; T. R. Forbes, *Chronicle from Aldgate* [London] (New Haven, 1971), pp. 70–1; Lawrence Stone, *The Crisis of the Aristocracy* (Oxford, 1965), pp. 166–74; R. E. Jones, "Infant Mortality in Rural North Shropshire, 1561–1810," *Population Studies* 20 (1976):305–17; Roger Schofield and E. A. Wrigley, "Infant and Child Mortality in England in the Late Tudor and Early Stuart Period," in Webster, *Health, Medicine and Mortality*. For the proportion of children in the population see Peter Laslett, *The World We Have Lost*, 2nd ed. (London, 1971), pp. 108–9; D. V. Glass, "Two Papers on Gregory King," in D. V. Glass and D. E. C. Eversley, eds., *Population in History* (London, 1965), pp. 180–3, 204–16; John Pound, *The Norwich Census of the Poor*, Norfolk Record Society 40 (1971):17; and the discussion of the effects of rates of fertility and mortality on age structures in E. A. Wrigley, *Population and History* (New York, 1969), pp. 8–10, 23–8.

93 Quoted in Paul Slack, "Mirrors of Health and Treasures of Poor Men: The Uses of the Vernacular Medical Literature of Tudor England," in Webster, *Health, Medicine and Mortality*, p. 267.

94 Adam Martindale, *The Life of Adam Martindale*, Chetham Society, o.s., 4 (1845):214–15; Ralph Josselin, *The Diary of Ralph Josselin, 1616–1683*, ed. Alan Macfarlane, British Academy Records of Social and Economic History, n.s. 3 (London, 1976):113–14, 202–4, 205, 567, 568. For childhood diseases see Lawrence Stone, *The Family, Sex and Marriage in England, 1500–1800* (London, 1977), pp. 75–9; Forbes, *Aldgate*, p. 103; Alan Macfarlane, *Witchcraft in Tudor and Stuart England* (New York, 1971), pp. 162–3; E. Poeton, "The Midwives Deputie," Sloane MS 1954, ff. 99^v–142^v.

95 Shepherd et al., *Psychiatric Illness*, p.28.

96 The three youngest children were Robert Summerly (2), Mary Ellys (3), and Henry Goodfellow (3). Summerly was "simple and mopish" and wasting away. His parents thought he was bewitched: Ashml. 214, f. 317. Ellys had a congested chest, and Napier thought that a prank by other children who threatened to hang her might have made her sick with fright: Ashml. 207, f. 124^v. Goodfellow was "full of melancholy and careth for no company nor delight"; he also had acute abdominal pains: Ashml. 409, f. 116. The symptoms of Summerly and Goodfellow could have been caused by roundworm infestation, a common childhood malady. None of Napier's patients under ten was mad.

97 Thus none of the sixteenth-century Londoners killed by "thought" (anxiety), according to one parish register, was under twenty: Forbes, *Aldgate*, p. 103. Thomas Phaire's contemporary list of children's diseases includes nightmares but not lunacy, anxiety, or gloom; Ivy Pinchbeck and Margaret Hewitt, *Children in English Society*, 2 vols. (London, 1970), 1:5.

98 M. P. Tilley, *A Dictionary of Proverbs in England in the Sixteenth and Seventeenth Centuries* (Ann Arbor, Mich., 1950), p. 98; Bayly, *Practice of Piety*, p. 49; A. M. Platt and B. L. Diamond, "The Origins and Development of the 'Wild Beast' Concept of Mental Illness and Its Relation to Theories of Criminal Responsibility," *Journal of the History of the Behavioral Sciences* 2 (1966):366–7. See Bartholomaeus Anglicus, *De Proprietatibus Rerum* (London, 1535), ff. lxxvii^v and lxxxiiii (*sic*) for an influential medical pronouncement about the mental powers of children.

99 Thomas Nashe, *The Unfortunate Traveller and Other Works*, ed. J. B. Steane (Harmondsworth, 1972), p. 211; Tilley, *Proverbs*, p. 98.

100 H. E. Bell, *An Introduction to the History and Records of the Court of Wards and Liveries* (Cambridge, 1953), pp. 128–32.

101 Keith Thomas, "Age and Authority in Early Modern England," *Proceedings of the British Academy* 62 (1976):224–5.

102 John Earle, *Microcosmographie* (? 1627; reprint ed., Leeds, 1966), p. 2.

103 Hunter and Macalpine, *Psychiatry*, p. 182.

104 William Shakespeare, *The Complete Works*, ed. G. B. Harrison (New York, 1952), *Lear* act 1, sc. 1, lines 298–303.

105 Burton, *Anatomy of Melancholy*, 1:210; Thomas, "Age and Authority," pp. 42–3.

106 Ashml. 194, f. 286 (Booth). See also Ashml. 238, f. 8 (Hutton).

107 Ashml. 193, f. 126^v (Foukes); Ashml. 235, f. 107 (Whitlock); Ashml. 235, f. 117^v (Bichmoe); Ashml. 238, f. 83 (Broket); Ashml. 231, f. 64 (Booth).

108 Glass, "Two Papers on Gregory King," pp. 181–2, 211–15. Keith Thomas reminds me that old people were less mobile than young, but because Napier's patients often used intermediaries, the effects of immobility could have been remedied.

109 Thomas, "Age and Authority," pp. 238–44; Thomas, *Religion and Magic*, pp. 563–4; John Pound, *Poverty and Vagrancy in Tudor England* (London, 1971), p. 26.

110 Thomas, "Age and Authority," p. 245.

111 Ashml. 231, f. 64 (Booth); Ashml. 238, f. 83 (Broket); Ashml. 235, f. 117^v (Bichmoe); Ashml. 232, f. 232 (Evens).

112 Ashml. 229, f. 249 (Write).

113 Shepherd et al., *Psychiatric Illness*, pp. 88–9; Gove and Tudor, "Adult Sex Roles and Mental Illness," pp. 812–25.
114 Church of England, *The Two Books of Homilies* (Oxford, 1859), p. 505.
115 E. P. Thompson, *The Making of the English Working Class* (Harmondsworth, 1969), pp. 9–11, 939.
116 For appellations of status and social structure see Laslett, *World We Have Lost*, pp. 38–9; Lawrence Stone, "Social Mobility in England, 1500–1700," *Past and Present*, No. 33 (1964):17–21; Thomas Wilson, *The State of England . . . 1600*, ed., F. J. Fisher (London, 1936), p. 17.
117 This is far from being a comprehensive list of Napier's influential patients; some of the churchmen he knew are mentioned earlier in this chapter, p. 22. Many of his most notable clients are noticed in Black, *Ashmole Manuscripts*, and in Ashml. 423, ff. 60–60ᵛ, 62–73. The people and families mentioned in the text are noticed in *DNB*; G. E. Cockayne, ed., *Complete Peerage of England, Scotland, Ireland*, 13 vols., rev. ed. (London, 1910–49); *VCH, Buckinghamshire, Bedfordshire, Northamptonshire* (incomplete); G. Baker, *History and Antiquities of the County of Northampton*, 2 vols. (London, 1822–41); and the records of the heralds' visitations of Northamptonshire, Buckinghamshire, and Bedfordshire, *Harleian Record Society*, Vols. 19, 58, 87. References to them in Napier's manuscripts are too numerous to mention in a single note; citations will be provided on request.
118 For fees ranging from 6–18d, see Ashml. 202, 221, 228, 404, passim. There were often variations in charges, and fees of two and four shillings are not unusual in these early volumes. For examples of lowered and forgiven fees see Ashml. 404, f. 36, and Ashml. 228, f. 111. Charges included medicines. The nobility paid much more, Lord Scrope handing over £100 on one occasion: Ashml. 405, f. 213; charges usually included lodging for the patient and a servant or two during treatment.
119 Cicely Howell, "Stability and Change, 1300–1700," *Journal of Peasant Studies* 2 (1975):479, for wage rates in nearby Leicestershire.
120 Christopher Hill, Introduction to Winstanley, *Law of Freedom*, p. 25; P. A. J. Pettit, "The Economy of the Northamptonshire Royal Forests" (D. Phil. diss., Oxford University, 1959), p. 310; Joan Thirsk, "The Farming Regions of England," in Joan Thirsk, ed., *The Agrarian History of England and Wales, IV, 1500–1640* (Cambridge, 1967), pp. 236–7.
121 Pettit, "Royal Forests," p. 310.
122 Stone, *Aristocracy*, Chap. 3; Alan Everitt, "Social Mobility in Early Modern England," *Past and Present*, No. 33 (1966):56–73; idem, *Change in the Provinces* (Leicester University, Department of English Local History, Occasional Papers, 2nd Ser., 1, 1969), pp. 37–8.
123 Bastide, *Mental Disorder*, pp. 78–103, esp. p. 100; Morton Beiser, "Psychiatric Epidemiology," in *Harvard Guide to Modern Psychiatry*, pp. 609–26, esp. pp. 620–2.
124 Patients' dwellings could be located in 1,724 cases, and the percentages represent proportions of locatable cases.
125 Hundreds within about ten miles included Newport, Buckingham, Cottesloe, and Ashendon in Buckinghamshire; Redbournstoke, Wylly, and Manshead in Bedfordshire; and Cleley, Towcester, Green's Norton, Wymersley, and Fawsley in Northamptonshire and they were the patients' homes in 924 cases. Extending the range to about fifteen miles includes the Bedfordshire hundred of Stodden and the Northamptonshire hundreds of King's Sutton, Norbottle Grove, Spelhoe, Hamfordshoe, and Higham Ferrers and adds cases to the total of 1,077.
126 P. A. J. Pettit, *The Royal Forests of Northamptonshire*, Northamptonshire Record Society Publications, 23 (1968), Chap. 7, Table 23, and Appendix 4.
127 A. Norman Groome, "Higham Ferrers Elections in 1640," *Northamptonshire Past and Present* 2, No. 5 (1958):243; Peter Laslett and John Harrison, "Clayworth and Cogenhoe," in H. E. Bell and R. L. Ollard, eds., *Historical Essays Presented to David Ogg* (London, 1963), p. 176.

128 The yearly incidence of mental disorder in Napier's practice is given in Appendix B. No correlations between short-term changes in economic conditions (measured by price fluctuations for agricultural and industrial goods) and the rate of consultations for mental disorder could be demonstrated. For a presentation of the data and some speculations see Michael MacDonald, "Madness and Healing in Seventeenth-Century England" (Ph.D. diss., Stanford University, 1979), pp. 112–17.

129 The complex pattern of omissions from Napier's case notes, gaps caused by the destruction of manuscripts, and Napier's own habits of record keeping, make it very difficult to chart the movements in his case loads accurately. The moving average of all clients' consultations presented in Figure 2.3 is based on estimates derived from a survey of Napier's business in even numbered years. Carol Dickerman and I counted the number of medical consultations with Napier during those years, and I then adjusted four of the figures to compensate for missing records. The adjustments were made with seasonal fluctuations in Napier's work load in mind and were very conservative. Whether the apparent slump in Napier's business between 1608 and 1614 evident in Figure 2.3 represents a real phenomenon or merely measures the loss of unusual numbers of records is not clear. The manuscripts for that period are unusually jumbled, and there is some reason to suspect that Napier kept parallel notebooks that have perished.

130 Among the most interesting exchanges between Napier and Digby are Ashml. 174, ff. 75–9; Ashml. 213, ff. 25, 73^v–4; Ashml. 240, f. 131; Ashml. 406, f. 306; Ashml. 194, f. 189. For contacts with the Dormers see, e.g., Ashml. 409, ff. 41^v, 110^v, 148, 193^v; Ashml. 199, f. 89; Ashml. 414, ff. 54^v, 165; Ashml. 203, ff. 127^v, 185, 191, 193^v, 198, 200–25, passim. See *DNB*, s.v. "Kenelm Digby" and "Robert Dormer."

131 Joan Thirsk, "Seventeenth-Century Agriculture and Social Change," in Paul S. Seaver, ed., *Seventeenth-Century England* (New York, 1975), pp. 72–110.

132 *VCH, Bucks.*, 4:275–6, 477–8; Oliver Ratcliff, *The History of Antiquities of the Newport Pagnell Hundreds* (Olney, 1900), p. 389.

133 Thirsk, "Seventeenth-Century Agriculture," pp. 79–80; idem, *Agrarian History*, pp. 241–2 and Table 2; A. C. Chibnall, *Sherington: Fiefs and Fields of a Buckinghamshire Village* (Cambridge, 1965), Chap. 22 and pp. 190–204.

134 Pettit, *Royal Forests*, pp. 141–8, 162–3, and Table 20, p. 144.

135 Hill in Winstanley, *Law of Freedom*, p. 25; Thirsk, "Seventeenth-Century Agriculture," p. 155, n. 5; idem, *Agrarian History*, pp. 232–7; Edwin F. Gay, "The Midland Revolt and the Inquisitions of Depopulation of 1607," *Transactions of the Royal Historical Society*, 2nd ser. 18 (1904), 195–244.

136 Ashml. 222, f. 45^v (Hust).

137 Ashml. 213, f. 67^v (Stonell). Robert Lucas was turned out of his holding because he was too mentally disturbed to work; he probably could not pay his rent, Ashml. 233, ff. 5^v, 6, 41^v.

138 Ashml. 196, f. 56^v (Deanes).

139 Pettit, *Royal Forests*, Chap. 7, Tables 20, 23, 24.

140 Ashml. 223, f. 167 (Scravington); Ashml. 233, f. 105 (Bell). See also Ashml. 409, f. 79 (Colman); Ashml. 200, ff. 238^v–9 (Page); Ashml. 218, ff. 157^v–8 (Allyn); and notes 143–5.

141 The bookbinder who assembled Napier's manuscripts used many lists of loans as endpapers in the volumes of his medical practice. His credit was extended to people of all social standings and trades, and loans ranged from hundreds of pounds to his brother, Robert, to a few shillings to his neighbors: see, e.g., Ashml. 409, f. 201 (Napier); Ashml. 199, f. 193^v (Britten). The records of the repayment of his loans make it very plain that Napier did not charge interest. Thus Goodman Evens, the town peddler, borrowed 40s in May 1620 and repaid the same amount in April 1621, Ashml. 414, f. 224^v; Ashml. 233, f. 96^v; see also Ashml. 198, ff. 1–1^v; Ashml. 220, f. 192; Ashml. 408, f. 183^v; Ashml. 220, f. 186^v; Ashml. 213, f. 178; Ashml. 194, f. 28. The point is an important one, because Napier had no religious objection to charging interest; the return he got from lending to his friends and neighbors was paid in goodwill rather than hard

cash. For Napier's views about usury see Ashml. 1730, ff. 156–7ᵛ. For some general remarks about credit and debt among English villagers, see Alan Macfarlane, *Reconstructing Historical Communities* (Cambridge, 1977), pp. 159–60.

142 Alan Everitt, "The Marketing of Agricultural Produce," in Thirsk, *Agrarian History*, pp. 567–8.

143 Ashml. 193, f. 325ᵛ (Holman); Ashml. 405, f. 39 (Houston). Cf. Ashml. 228, f. 59ᵛ (Vurny); Ashml. 227, f. 121ᵛ (Collins); Ashml. 224, f. 228ᵛ (Bassington).

144 Ashml. 213, f. 6 (Bonfield). For other instances of family ties strained by problems arising from indebtedness see Ashml. 217, f. 103ᵛ (White); Ashml. 413, f. 61 (Kingman); Ashml. 217, f. 135 (Harnesse); Ashml. 409, f. 109 (Skynner).

145 For economic miscalculations among Napier's indebted clients see Ashml. 224, f. 218ᵛ (Hart); Ashml. 402, f. 173ᵛ (Linsee); Ashml. 404, f. 124ᵛ (Missenton); Ashml. 223, f. 80 (Pilkinton). For misfortunes of the kinds mentioned see Ashml. 218, f. 82, Ashml. 402, f. 170 (Birchmore); Ashml. 223, f. 32ᵛ (Belgrave); Ashml. 232, f. 17 (Hull); Ashml. 197, f. 15ᵛ (Beely); Ashml. 220, f. 176 (Palmer); Ashml. 402, f. 111 (Wels); Ashml. 213, f. 78ᵛ (Norrish); Ashml. 218, f. 27; Ashml. 217, f. 18ᵛ (Lovell); Ashml. 213, f. 18 (Hangor). Some people were ruined by other people's bad debts for which they had provided security: Ashml. 203, f. 228 (Russell); Ashml. 408, f. 109 (Robarts).

146 Thomas, *Religion and Magic*, Chap. 1 and passim.

147 Bastide, *Mental Disorder*, pp. 128–38.

148 E. R. C. Brinkworth, "A Study of the Visitation Books of the Archdeaconry of Buckingham, 1633–1637" (B. Litt. thesis, Oxford University, 1948), pp. 155–6; C. W. Foster, ed., *The State of the Church in the Reigns of Elizabeth and James I*, Lincoln Record Society 23 (1926), pp. cxvi–cxxv, 863.

149 Paul S. Seaver, *The Puritan Lectureships* (Stanford, 1970), pp. 234–5.

150 Elizabeth J. I. Allen, "The State of the Church in the Diocese of Peterborough, 1601–1642" (B. Litt. thesis, Oxford University, 1972), pp. 124–30; *A Paper on Puritans in Northamptonshire Dated 16 July 1590* [John Taylor, ed.] (Northampton, 1878), a reprint of British Library, Lansdowne MS 64, f. 51; Patrick King, "The Seventeenth Century 'Census' of Cogenhoe," *Northamptonshire Past and Present* 3, No. 6 (1965):272.

151 King, " 'Census' of Cogenhoe," p. 272; Laslett and Harrison, "Clayworth and Cogenhoe," p. 176; Groome, "Higham Ferrers Elections," pp. 243–4.

152 E. R. C. Brinkworth, "The Laudian Church in Buckinghamshire," *University of Birmingham Historical Journal* 5 (1955–6), 56; Foster, *State of the Church*, p. xcv; *DNB* for families named.

153 John H. Raach, *A Directory of English Country Physicians, 1603–1643* (London, 1962), pp. 96–7, 111.

154 Lilly, *Life*, p. 54; John Cotta, *A Short Discouerie of the vnobserued dangers of seuerall sorts of ignorant and vnconsiderable Practisers of Physicke in England* (London, 1612), pp. 89–94, and idem, *The Infallible, trve and Assvred Witch: or, the Second Edition of the Tryall of Witchcraft, Shewing the Right and Trve Methode of Discouerie* (London, 1624), p. 75. (This passage denounces those who profess "the erecting of figures," and someone has written "Dr. Napper" in the margin of the Bodleian Library copy; the handwriting resembles William Lilly's.)

155 Bastide, *Mental Disorder*, p. 100.

156 The fullest theoretical account of this perspective is Thomas Scheff, *Being Mentally Ill: A Sociological Theory of Mental Illness* (Chicago, 1966); cf. the cogent criticisms and the evidence presented by Jane M. Murphy, "Psychiatric Labeling in Cross-cultural Perspective," *Science* 191 (1976): 1019–28.

CHAPTER 3 *Stress, anxiety, and family life*

1 See, e.g., Erich Fromm, *The Fear of Freedom* (London, 1960), Chap. 3; Robert Mandrou, *Introduction to Modern France, 1500–1640*, trans. R. E. Hallmark (New York, 1976), pp. 208–54; Lynn White, Jr., "Death and the Devil," in Robert S. Kinsman, ed., *The Darker Vision of the Renaissance* (Berkeley, 1974), pp. 25–46.

2 Alan Macfarlane, *Witchcraft in Tudor and Stuart England* (New York, 1970); Keith Thomas, *Religion and the Decline of Magic* (New York, 1971), esp. Chaps. 1–3, 14–18, 21–22; David Levine and Keith Wrightson, "The Social Context of Illegitimacy in Early Modern England" (Paper presented to the Cambridge Group for the History of Population and Social Structure, 1975); Peter Laslett and Karla Oosterveen, "Long-term Trends in Bastardy in England, 1561–1960," *Population Studies* 27 (1973):225–86; S. E. Sprott, *The English Debate on Suicide* (La Salle, Ill., 1961); P. E.H. Hair, "A Note on the Incidence of Tudor Suicide," *Local Population Studies* 5 (1970):36–43, and "Deaths from Violence in Britain: A Tentative Secular Survey," *Population Studies* 25 (1971):5–24; Joel Samaha, *Law and Order in Historical Perspective* (New York, 1974); Anthony Fletcher, *Tudor Rebellions* (London, 1968); M. E. James, "The Concept of Order and the Northern Rising of 1569," *Past and Present*, No. 60 (1973):49–83; Michael Walzer, "Puritanism as a Revolutionary Ideology," *History and Theory* 3 (1963): 59–90; idem, *The Revolution of the Saints* (New York, 1969), pp. 200–10, 309, 313; Lawrence Stone, *The Causes of the English Revolution* (London, 1972), p. 113.

3 Morris Palmer Tilley, *A Dictionary of the Proverbs in England in the Sixteenth and Seventeenth Centuries* (Ann Arbor, Mich., 1950), p. 515.

4 William Drage, *A Physical Nosonomy* (London, 1665), p. 67. For some comparable lists see Robert Burton, *The Anatomy of Melancholy*, ed. Holbrook Jackson, 3 vols. (London, 1968), 1:357–9; Robert Yarrow, *Soveraigne Comforts for a trovbled conscience* (London, 1634), pp. 29–30; Robert Bolton, *Instructions For a Right comforting Afflicted Consciences*, 2nd ed. (London, 1635), pp. 198–9; John Sym, *Lifes Preservative against self-killing* (London, 1637), pp. 211–17; Joseph Blagrave, *Blagrave's Astrological Practice of Physick* (London, 1671), p. 184. For a discussion of the problems listed by these writers in the lives of autobiographers of humble social standing see Bernard S. Capp, *The Fifth-Monarchy Men* (London, 1972), pp. 94–7.

5 The ratios express the number of females per hundred males. For further discussion of sex ratios and comparisons see Chapter 2, under "Sex."

6 Richard W. Hudgens, "Personal Catastrophe and Depression," in B. S. Dohrenwend and B. P. Dohrenwend, eds., *Stressful Life Events: Their Nature and Effects* (New York, 1974); the other essays in this collection are also useful and provide a spectrum of opinion about the problem. There is another way in which patients reporting stresses were like the other patients in the practice: When they suffered from mental disorders, their symptoms were like those of disturbed clients who mentioned no stress (except that they naturally suffered from more "grief" and "fright" symptoms explicitly associated with troubling or traumatic events).

Psychological symptoms most commonly reported by mentally disturbed and distress patients (in percent)

	All mentally disturbed (N = 2,039)	Distressed patients (N = 767)
Troubled in Mind	35	33
Mopish	17	18
Melancholy	23	16
Fearful	14	13

Note: Omits Trauma ("griefs" and "frights"). The terminology is explained in Chapter 4.

7   Lawrence Stone, *The Family, Sex and Marriage in England 1500–1800* (London, 1977), p. 552.
8   Thomas Wright, *The Passions of the Minde in generall* (London, 1604), p. 40.
9   This rather pessimistic view of domestic relations during the early modern period was first advanced by Philippe Ariès in his celebrated *Centuries of Childhood*, trans. Robert Baldick (New York, 1962). The most important treatments of family life in England from this perspective are Edward Shorter, *The Making of the Modern Family* (New York, 1975), and especially, Stone, *Family, Sex and Marriage*, pp. 221–69, 665–66. Shorter and Stone both share Ariès's belief that domestic relations among all classes were emotionally impoverished during our period, although their arguments differ from his and from each other's in important particulars.
    The effort to discern changing patterns of sentiment within the family is particularly significant historiographically, because most scholars now believe that structurally the typical family unit has undergone little change since the early modern era. Peter Laslett and Richard Wall, eds., *Household and Family in Past Time* (Cambridge, 1972), Introduction, Chaps. 1–4; Peter Laslett, *Family Life and Illicit Love in Earlier Generations* (Cambridge, 1977), Chap. 1; Lutz K. Berkner, "The Stem Family and the Developmental Cycle of the Peasant Household: An Eighteenth-Century Austrian Example," *American Historical Review* 77 (1972):398–418; review of Laslett and Wall, *Times Literary Supplement*, 4 May 1973, pp. 485–7; Jean-Louis Flandrin, *Families in Former Times*, trans. Richard Southern (Cambridge, 1979), Chap. 2. Lawrence Stone, *The Crisis of the Aristocracy* (Oxford, 1965), p. 589; David Hey, *An English Rural Community: Myddle Under the Tudors and Stuarts* (Leicester, 1974), pp. 214–15; Margaret Spufford, *Contrasting Communities: English Villagers in the Sixteenth and Seventeenth Centuries* (Cambridge, 1974), pp. 114–16.
10 Thomas Becon, "The Sick Mannes Salue," in *Prayers and Other Pieces of Thomas Becon*, ed. John Ayre, Parker Society 4 (1844), pp. 89–90.
11 Spufford, *Contrasting Communities*, p. 321.
12 Thomas, *Religion and Magic*, Chap. 1; Alan Macfarlane, *The Family Life of Ralph Josselin* (Cambridge, 1970) pp. 170–1; Paul Slack, "Some Aspects of Epidemics in England, 1485–1640" (D. Phil. diss., Oxford University, 1972), p. 11. Examples of astrological "accidents" may be found in Bodleian Library, Ashmole MSS (hereafter cited as Ashml.), 174, ff. 75–9 (Sir Kenelm Digby), and Ashml. 423, f. 97 (Thomas Napier); many other such lists are noted by William H. Black, comp., *A Descriptive, Analytical and Critical Catalogue of the Manuscripts Bequeathed Unto the University of Oxford by Elias Ashmole* (Oxford, 1845). Ronald Finucane, "The Use and Abuse of Medieval Miracles," *History* 60 (1975):1–10 is excellent.
13 Thomas, *Religion and Magic*, Chap. 4; Macfarlane, *Ralph Josselin*, Chap. 11. E. P. Thompson charges that Josselin's providential beliefs make his testimony about the anxieties of living in a very dangerous world suspect: "Anthropology and the Discipline of Historical Context," *Midland History* 1, No. 3 (1972):41–55. His criticism is rendered untenable by J. Sears McGee, *The Godly Man in Stuart England* (New Haven, 1976), Chap. 2.
14 Peter Laslett, *The World We Have Lost*, 2nd ed. (London, 1971), pp. 96–8; Thomas Forbes, *Chronicle from Aldgate* (New Haven, 1971), Chap 4, esp. p. 103; Andrew B. Appleby, "Nutrition and Disease: The Case of London, 1550–1750," *Journal of Interdisciplinary History* 6 (1975):1–22; Charles Webster, ed., *Health, Medicine and Mortality in the Sixteenth Century* (Cambridge, 1979), Chaps. 1, 2, 4; Thomas McKeown, *The Modern Rise of Population* (London, 1976).
15 Ashml. 216, f. 47ᵛ (Stoe).
16 Richard Baxter, *The Practical Works*, ed. William Orme, 23 vols. (London, 1830), 3:324–5; 17:254–7; Stone, *Family, Sex and Marriage*, p. 215; Bolton, *Right comforting*, pp. 198–200; Richard Greenham, *The Workes* (London, 1601), p. 27.
17 Adam Martindale, *The Life of Adam Martindale*, ed. Richard Parkinson, Chetham Society, o.s., 4:108.
18 Thomas Fuller, *The Holy and the Profane States* (Boston, 1864), pp. 52–3.

19 Ashml. 201, f. 68.
20 Burton, *Anatomy of Melancholy*, 1:357–9.
21 Laslett, *Family Life*, Chap. 1; Flandrin, *Families in Former Times*, pp. 65–74; Peter Clark, "Migration in England during the Late Seventeenth and Early Eighteenth Centuries," *Past and Present*, No. 83 (1979):57–90; Lawrence Stone, "The Rise of the Nuclear Family," in Charles Rosenberg, ed., *The Family in History* (n.p. [Philadelphia], 1975); Stone, *Family, Sex and Marriage*, pp. 146–8.
22 Stone, "Nuclear Family"; M. E. James, *Family, Lineage and Civil Society* (Oxford, 1974), pp. 19–29, 102–3, 178–80, 189; Christopher Hill, *Society and Puritanism in Pre-Revolutionary England*, 2nd ed. (New York, 1967), Chap. 13; Clark, "Migration in England," p. 81. Kathleen Davies in "The Sacred Condition of Equality – How Original Were Puritan Doctrines of Marriage?" (*Social History*, No. 5 [1977], pp. 563–80) questions the importance of popular Puritan writers, but Anthony Fletcher finds that among the Sussex gentry in the early seventeenth century Puritans held "the most advanced ideas about marriage and courtship" and that they valued intimacy, romance, and domestic happiness: *A County Community in Peace and War: Sussex 1600–1660* (London, 1975), pp. 31–4.
23 Macfarlane, *Ralph Josselin*, pp. 153–79.
24 Thomas Nashe, *The Terrors of the Night* in his *The Unfortunate Traveller and Other Works*, ed. J. B. Steane (Harmondsworth, 1972), p. 211.
25 Lawrence Stone, "The Domestic Revolution," *Times Literary Supplement*, 28 May 1976, p. 637; Stone, *Aristocracy*, pp. 589–94; M. J. Tucker, "The Child as Beginning and End: Fifteenth and Sixteenth Century English Childhood," in Lloyd deMause, ed., *The History of Childhood* (New York, 1974), pp. 229–57; Lawrence Stone, "The Massacre of the Innocents," *New York Review of Books*, 14 November 1974, pp. 25–31; Ivy Pinchbeck and Margaret Hewitt, *Children in English Society*, 2 vols. (London, 1969), 1:7.
26 Ariès, *Centuries of Childhood*, pp. 38–40.
27 Shorter, *Modern Family*, Chap. 5, esp. pp. 170, 172.
28 Stone, *Family, Sex and Marriage*, pp. 64–73, 161–78, 470–80, 679.
29 Wright, *Passions of the Minde*, p.7. See also Thomas Hobbes, *The English Works*, ed. William Molesworth, 11 vols. (London, 1845), 3:16.
30 *Lord Nottingham's Chancery Cases*, ed. D. E. C. Yale, 2 vols., Selden Society, 79 (1961–2), 21:894–5. See also Chapter 2, pp. 42–4.
31 Heinrich Bullinger, *The Decades of Henry Bullinger*, ed. Thomas Harding, 4 vols., Parker Society (Cambridge, 1849–52), 1:405–6. Cf. Hugh Latimer, *Works*, vol. 1, *Sermons*, ed. George Elwes Corrie, Parker Society (Cambridge, 1844), pp. 252–3.
32 Thomas Becon, *The Catechism with Other Pieces*, ed. John Ayre, Parker Society (Cambridge, 1844), pp. 347–9. Cf. William Perkins, *A Golden Chaine* [and other treatises] (Cambridge, 1600), p. 72.
33 Samuel Clarke, *The Lives of sundry Eminent Persons in this Later Age* (London, 1683), p. 68.
34 William Paulet, *The Lord Marques Idlenes* (London, 1586), pp. 55, 83–4. Cf. Richard Capel, *Tentations*, 4th ed. (London, 1650), pp. 198–9.
35 Ashml. 212, f. 58 (Gostick).
36 Ashml. 406, f. 64.
37 Ashml. 214, f. 353 (Foster). Other examples of women grieved by the loss of infants and small children may be given: "infant," Ashml. 239, f. 152 (Browne); "nine days old," Ashml. 224, f. 130^v (Burlye); two weeks old, Ashml. 232, f. 442 (Somers); a babe in arms, Ashml. 198, f. 74 (Williams). Samuel Pepys, ever vigilant of social proprieties, arched his eyebrows when a woman who had lost a baby in childbirth invited her cronies to her house less than a fortnight later: *The Diary of Samuel Pepys*, vol. 1, *1660*, eds. Robert Latham and William Matthews (London, 1970), p. 252. The testimonies of two humble women disturbed by the deaths of children are in Henry Walker, *Spirituall Experiences of sundry Beleevers* (London, 1653), pp. 26, 68.
38 Ashml. 416, f. 403 (Wynfield); Ashml. 407, f. 67 (Ellis); Ashml. 415, f. 101

(Craftes). See also Ashml. 416, f. 369 (Angin); Ashml. 415, f. 107ᵛ (Kent); Ashml. 216, f. 229ᵛ (Cope); Ashml. 218, f. 198ᵛ (Richardson); Ashml. 228, f. 265 (Harrys); Ashml. 228, f. 274ᵛ (Porter); Ashml. 211, f. 137 (Gould); Ashml. 211, f. 52 (Woadle). All the patients in these cases were women; all of them were physically ill.

39 Ashml. 239, f. 152 (Browne). See also, e.g., Ashml. 174, f. 374 (anonymous); Ashml. 404, f. 274ᵛ (Longville); Ashml. 217, f. 117 (Rheade); Ashml. 414, f. 96 (Warner); Ashml. 202, f. 8ᵛ (Smith); Ashml. 197, f. 19ᵛ (Fawnes). See also Thomas, *Religion and Magic*, p. 317.
40 Ashml. 233, f. 57ᵛ (Nueman); Ashml. 406, f. 67 (Plotte).
41 Ashml. 217, f. 115ᵛ (Crawley).
42 Ashml. 211, f. 268 (Rowly).
43 Ashml. 232, f. 107 (Goodcheape); Ashml. 404, f. 289ᵛ (Morton). Commenting on a case that occurred in 1668, Chief Justice Hale argued that if a woman accused of infanticide had no motive for killing her child, had not concealed the death, and was honest and virtuous, the jury might acquit her by reason of *temporary* insanity induced by the rigor of childbirth and sleeplessness. In this instance it would seem that the crime itself was taken virtually to be proof of insanity. Nigel Walker, *Crime and Insanity in England*, 2 vols. (Edinburgh, 1968), 1:127.
44 See, e.g., the case of Katherine Smith, Ashml. 229, f. 125ᵛ. Napier recorded 25 consultations with patients who blamed witches or demons for infanticidal urges.
45 Keith Wrightson, "Infanticide in Earlier Seventeenth-Century England," *Local Population Studies* No. 15 (1975):10–21. Cf. Barbara A. Hanawalt, "Childrearing among the Lower Classes of Late Medieval England," *Journal of Interdisciplinary History* 8 (1977):1–22.
46 Ashml. 215, f. 187ᵛ (Clark).
47 Ashml. 402, f. 113 (Faldoe); see also the case of Ann Wilson, deranged by the fear that medicine had harmed her unborn child and unable to love and nurture it after its birth: "since cannot love her child nor follow her business" (Ashml. 410, f. 25; Ashml. 406, f. 116; Ashml. 194, f. 317).
48 Ashml. 410, f. 59 (Koburne).
49 Ashml. 239, f. 179 (Savil). Cf. Walker, *Spirituall Experiences*, pp. 35–6.
50 Ralph Josselin, *The Diary of Ralph Josselin, 1616–1683*, ed. Alan Macfarlane, British Academy Records of Social and Economic History, n.s. 3 (London, 1976):113–14, 202–4, 205, 567, 568; note in particular Josselin's account of the death of his eight-year-old daughter, Mary, her large funeral, and his neighbors' sympathy (pp. 202–4), and also his plea in 1673: "God hath taken five of ten; Lord let it be enough, and spare that we may recover strength" (p. 568). (Cf. Macfarlane, *Ralph Josselin*, pp. 165–6.) Martindale, *Life*, p. 109; Simonds D'Ewes, *The Autobiography and Correspondence*, ed. James O. Halliwell, 2 vols. (London, 1845), 2:44–6.
51 Ashml. 240, f. 97; cf. Thomas, *Religion and Magic*, p. 329.
52 Ashml. 1458, f. 119; see also ff. 129–30ᵛ.
53 Ashml. 215, f. 225ᵛ; Ashml. 193, f. 245. An earlier letter to Napier about Sir Robert's sick children well illustrates the complexities of evidence concerning attitudes toward children. Its author, Valentine Lawrence, reports that Sir Robert's daughter Sara suffers extremely from "epileptical fits" and that her brother has died. The attending nurse is weary of Sara's fits and wishes she would die; but at the same time the servants are reluctant to inform the absent parents about the crisis at home for fear of "smaying" them. Thus the same document displays both the callous fatalism of a nurse and an apprehensive assumption of parental concern: Ashml. 170, f. 150.
54 Stone, *Aristocracy*, pp. 591–5; idem, "Nuclear Family"; idem, *Family, Sex and Marriage*, pp. 159–91.
55 Wrightson, "Infanticide," p. 11; Carol Z. Wiener, "Sex Roles and Crime in Late Elizabethan Hertfordshire," *Journal of Social History* 8 (1975):57n.

56 Cf. Stone, *Family, Sex and Marriage*, pp. 405–80.

57 Peter Laslett calculates that almost one-third of the households in England before
the Industrial Revolution contained servants at a given point in time. Because the
prosperity of the household no doubt waxed and waned, depending upon the
ages and economic fortunes of the couple at its nucleus, the figures extracted
from statistic listing are lower than the true proportion of families that employed
servants at one time or another. The implication of this observation is that only
cottagers and wage laborers are likely not to have shared their homes with a
servant at some point. The statistics Laslett presents also suggest that a majority
of men and women spent some time in service before they married; this is certainly true for women. Because he fails to stipulate whether he counted apprentices as servants – a legitimate equation from many perspectives – the role of
unrelated young people in the family and the place of living away from home in
the lives of most people may be understated even by these computations. Laslett,
Family Life, pp. 29–35, 45–6, 72–4; Laslett, *World We Have Lost*, pp. 72–3. Cf.
Charles Phythian-Adams, *Desolation of a City: Coventry and the Urban Crisis of the
Late Middle Ages* (Cambridge, 1979), Chaps. 20, 22.

58 Sir Thomas Smith, *De Republica Anglorum* (1565; reprint., Cambridge, 1906), p.
138.

59 C. B. Macpherson's assertion that servants and laborers were socially degraded
for the same reason (i.e., because by selling their labor they had alienated their
birthright) obscures an important point. The contractual obligations assumed by
servants were more thorough, durable, and degrading than those assumed by
laborers. Servants sold their *obedience* for a long period of time (usually a year);
laborers sold their *labor* for relatively short periods of time (a day or a week). As
Smith's remark shows, the categories may have been linked in the minds of
contemporaries when they thought about the kinds of people who owed obedience to heads of households, but they knew that the two conditions were not
identical. See C. B. Macpherson, *The Political Theory of Possessive Individualism*
(Oxford, 1962), pp. 17, 282–3, and Keith Thomas, "The Levellers and the Fran-
chise," in G. E. Aylmer, ed. *The Interregnum* (London, 1972), pp. 70–8.

60 Gordon Schochet, "Patriarchalism, Politics and Mass Attitudes in Stuart England," *Historical Journal* 12 (1969):415–19; idem, *Patriarchalism in Political
Thought* (New York, 1975), pp. 65–71, 73, 82, 85–6.

61 Quoted in Levin L. Schücking, *The Puritan Family*, trans. Brian Battershaw
(New York, 1970), pp. 56–7.

62 Schücking, *Puritan Family*, pp. 96–102; Chilton Latham Powell, *English Domestic
Relations, 1487–1653* (1917; reprint ed., New York, 1972), pp. 106, 127, 129,
234–42; William Perkins, *The Works of William Perkins*, ed. Ian Breward
(Abingdon, Berks., 1970), pp. 431–6.

63 Ashml. 181, f. 21 (Tuckwell); Ashml. 229, f. 93 (Wood); Ashml. 415, f. 224, and
Ashml. 216, f. 15 (Fisher). Cf. Ashml. 413, f. 212 (Ingold); Ashml. 406, f. 363
(Ravensden); Ashml. 413, f. 22ᵛ (Bays).

64 Ashml. 415, f. 224; Ashml. 216, f. 15 (Fisher).

65 Ashml. 239, ff. 81ᵛ, 86, 86ᵛ, 90, 127, 158ᵛ, 173ᵛ, 181.

66 Stone, "Nuclear Family," pp. 36–49; Stone, *Family, Sex and Marriage*, p. 167,
and, more generally, pp. 163–71.

67 See, e.g., Jocelyn Dunlop and R. D. Denman, *English Apprenticeship and Child
Labour: A History* (New York, 1912), pp. 185–9; Carl Bridenbaugh, *Vexed and
Troubled Englishmen* (London, 1967), pp. 90–1; John Cordy Jeaffreson, *Middlesex
County Records*, 4 vols. (London, 1886–92), 2:14, 39, 47, 100, 101; 3:23, 176, 209,
210, 230, 231, 239, 294, 318, 328, 364; F. G. Emmison, *Elizabethan Life: Disorder*
(Chelmsford, 1970), pp. 155–6.

68 Ashml. 198, f. 139ᵛ, and Ashml. 196, f. 114ᵛ (Osburne).

69 Ashml. 227, f. 112 (Cardwell). Em Smalbones told Napier she was sick and
grieved because her husband was compelled to explain at the assizes his role in
the death of their maidservant: Ashml. 203, f. 247ᵛ (Smalbones). For other ex-

amples of abused servants see: Ashml. 218, f. 124 (Gothwell); Ashml. 230, f. 136ᵛ (Evans); Ashml. 222, f. 84ᵛ (Scot).

70 Ashml. 410, f. 117 (Burton). For other. examples of servants seduced by their masters see Ashml. 218, f. 124 (Gothwell); Ashml. 413, f. 212 (Ingold); Ashml. 406, ff. 78, 81ᵛ (Norman); Ashml. 202, f. 58 (Burtch); Ashml. 214, f. 136 (Homes); Ashml. 227, f. 169 (anonymous); Bridenbaugh, Vexed and Troubled, p. 90; Keith Wrightson, "The Puritan Reformation of Manners with Special Reference to the counties of Lancashire and Essex, 1640–1660" (Ph.D. diss., Cambridge University, 1973), pp. 60–1; Stone, Family, Sex and Marriage, pp. 642–3, 646–7; G. R. Quaife, Wanton Wenches and Wayward Wives: Peasants and Illicit Sex in Early Seventeenth Century England (London, 1979), pp. 72–3.

71 Ashml. 402, f. 169ᵛ (?Fenkes).

72 Ashml. 228, f. 22ᵛ (Gilbert).

73 Pinchbeck and Hewitt discuss the emergence in the early eighteenth century of the recognition that better legislation was necessary to afford redress to abused servants and apprentices: Children, 1:247, 248–50. See also Bridenbaugh, Vexed and Troubled, pp. 90–1 and n. 15; Ashml. 410, f. 117 (Burton).

74 Ashml. 409, f. 109 (Skynner).

75 The most severe punishments seem not to have been exercised. The desperate measure of slavery was rapidly repealed two years after its enactment; and the Statute of Artificers (1563) provided merely for the recapture and imprisonment of runaways until they find "sufficient surety well and honestly to serve their masters." C. S. L. Davies, "Slavery and the Protector Somerset; the Vagrancy Act of 1547," Economic History Review, 2nd ser. 19 (1966):533–49, esp. 533–6, 541–5; The Statutes at Large, From the First Year of King Edward I to the End of the Reign of Queen Elizabeth (London, 1770), p. 543 (5 Eliz. Cap. 4, Sec. 47); John Pound, Poverty and Vagrancy in Tudor England (London, 1971), pp. 41–2; W. D. Holdsworth, A History of English Law, 13 vols., 3rd ed. (London, 1923), 4:383–94; Frank Aydelotte, Elizabethan Rogues and Vagabonds (Oxford, 1913), pp. 62–3, 68–9.

76 Ashml. 201, f. 151a (Smyth). Three of Napier's patients who ran away from their masters were considered mentally unsound: Ashml. 196, f. 149 (Robinson); Ashml. 406, f. 78 (Norman); Ashml. 196, f. 20ᵛ (Pen).

77 Stone, Family, Sex and Marriage, pp. 180–94, 270–320; Shorter, Modern Family, pp. 3–21, 138–61.

78 Ashml. 198, ff. 116ᵛ, 146; see also ff. 87ᵛ, 99ᵛ, 146ᵛ, and Ashml. 196, f. 140 (Travell).

79 Ashml. 406, f. 21ᵛ (May).

80 William Shakespeare, As You Like It, act 4, sc. 1, lines 94–108.

81 John Aubrey, Aubrey's Brief Lives, ed. O. Dick (Harmondsworth, 1972), pp. 215–16; Ashml. 182, f. 77 (Malins). For other men who killed themselves (or tried to) because of unrequited love see Ashml. 410, f. 80; Ashml. 405, f. 10 (Walker); Ashml. 405, f. 224 (Norman); John Evelyn, The Diary of John Evelyn, ed. E. S. de Beer, 6 vols. (Oxford, 1955), 4:71.

82 Burton, Anatomy of Melancholy, 3:153. See also Lawrence Babb, The Elizabethan Malady (East Lansing, Mich., 1951), Chap. 6; William Ramesey, The Gentleman's Companion (London, 1672), pp. 193–5.

83 Becon, Catechism, p. 355.

84 Ashml. 231, f. 112ᵛ (Fossy). Cf. Ashml. 202, f. 9ᵛ (Nichols).

85 Ashml. 196, f. 35 (Winch).

86 Ashml. 202, f. 6ᵛ (Knight).

87 Ashml. 237, f. 70 (Faldo).

88 Edwin Sandys, The Sermons, ed. John Ayre, Parker Society (Cambridge, 1842), p. 281; see also pp. 50–1, 325–6. Cf. Andrew Boorde, The Breuiary of healthe (London, 1552), p. lxii.

89 Wrightson, "Puritan Reformation of Manners," pp. 57, 60–2; Quaife, Wanton Wenches, pp. 59–64.

90 Ashml. 230, f. 128ᵛ, and Ashml. 235, f. 5ᵛ (Walker). See also Ashml. 202, f. 42 (Ams); Ashml. 215, f. 21 (Blundell); Ashml. 407, f. 20ᵛ (Davye); Ashml. 182, f. 116ᵛ (Nichols); Ashml. 220, f. 55 (Earell); Ashml. 237, f. 56 (Batheler).

91 Levine and Wrightson, "Illegitimacy," pp. 24, 29–30; Wrightson's study of 66 cases of bastardy in Lancashire, 1626–40, and 64 cases in Essex, 1627–60, shows that defendants in 13 of the Lancashire and 17 of the Essex cases mentioned private promises to marry, "Puritan Reformation of Manners," p. 57. See also Elizabeth J. I. Allen, "The State of the Church in the Diocese of Peterborough, 1601–1642" (B. Litt. thesis, Oxford University, 1972), p. 7.

92 Christopher Hill, *The World Turned Upside Down* (Harmondsworth, 1975), p. 320.

93 Levine and Wrightson, "Illegitimacy."

94 Drage, *Physical Nosonomy*, pp. 202–3.

95 The tale is told briefly by Stone in *Aristocracy*, p. 596, and in lurid detail in [Thomas Longueville], *The Curious Case of Lady Purbeck: A Scandal of the XVIIth Century* (London, 1909) and Laura L. Nosworthy, *The Lady of Bleeding Heart Yard: Lady Elizabeth Hatton, 1578–1646* (New York, 1936). See also *Dictionary of National Biography*, s.v. "John Villiers." Of the many references to Purbeck's case in Napier's notes, these are the most revealing: Ashml. 218, f. 190ᵛ; Ashml. 402, ff. 22, 52, 105ᵛ, 120, 184ᵛ; Ashml. 410, f. 83.

96 Stone, *Aristocracy*, p. 661.

97 Ashml. 218, f. 230; Ashml. 413, f. 4 (Myles). Other examples in Ashml. 193, f. 140 (D. Smith); Ashml. 202, ff. 9ᵛ, 11 (Nichols); Ashml. 404, f. 265 (Moore); Ashml. 233, f. 93ᵛ (Wyllisan); Ashml. 405, f. 304ᵛ (Madge); Ashml. 202, f. 205 (Rive); Ashml. 217, f. 98 (Bendish); Ashml. 238, f. 161 (Butler).

98 Ashml. 405, f. 64 (Lane). See also Marquis of Halifax (George Savile), *Halifax: Complete Works*, ed. J. P. Kenyon (Harmondsworth, 1969), pp. 271, 277; Ruth Spalding, *The Improbable Puritan: A Life of Bulstrode Whitelocke* (London, 1975), pp. 38–42, 50–51; Alice Thornton, *The Autobiography of Mrs. Alice Thornton*, Surtees Society 62 (1973):61–2, 77. Cf. Ramesey, *Gentleman's Companion*, p. 195.

99 Stone, *Aristocracy*, Chap. 11; Walzer, *Revolution of Saints*, pp. 193–5.

100 See, e.g., William Gouge, *Of Domesticall Duties* (London, 1622), pp. 196–8.

101 Lucy Hutchinson, *Memoirs of Colonel Hutchinson* (London, 1968), p. 51. See also Macfarlane, *Ralph Josselin*, p. 95.

102 Stone, *Aristocracy*, pp. 594–600, 609–12.

103 Halifax, *Works*, pp. 271, 277.

104 Ashml. 215, f. 21 (Blundell).

105 Ashml. 415, f. 164 (Clarke); cf. Ashml. 402, f. 46ᵛ (Fulwood).

106 Ashml. 215, f. 62 (Alworth); Ashml. 222, f. 96 (Geary). Cf. Ashml. 197, f. 9 (Julian).

107 Ashml. 414, ff. 36, 38, 120ᵛ, 124ᵛ, 130ᵛ, and esp. 187 (Fettiplace). Cf. William Salmon, *Iatrica: Seu praxis Medendi. The Practice of Curing Diseases* (London, 1694), p. 777.

108 Ashml. 228, f. 191ᵛ (Longe). See also Ashml. 235, f. 29 (Morgan), and two cases identical to Longe's described by Wrightson, "Reformation of Manners," p. 62.

109 For examples of women who married against their friends' will, all of whom were tormented by guilt and fear, see Ashml. 404, f. 305ᵛ (Harryson); Ashml. 415, f. 226ᵛ (Lankaster); Ashml. 218, f. 190 (Osburne); Ashml. 404, f. 193 (Stoneher).

110 John Spencer, *A Discourse of Divers Petitions* (London, 1641), pp. 77–8.

111 Laslett, *Family Life*, pp. 71–3; Peter Clark, "The Migrant in Kentish Towns, 1580–1640," in Peter Clark and Paul Slack, eds., *Crisis and Order in English Towns, 1500–1700* (London, 1972), pp. 124, 129, 134–5; E. A. Wrigley, "A Simple Model of London's Importance in Changing English Society and Economy, 1650–1750," *Past and Present*, No. 37 (1967):esp. 45–55.

112 Ashml. 405, f. 224ᵛ (Sir R. Chitwood's miller).

113 Ashml. 415, f. 222ᵛ (Stafford).

114 Stone, "Nuclear Family"; idem, *Family, Sex and Marriage*, pp. 4–9, 102–5, 123–218; Macfarlane, *Ralph Josselin*, Chaps. 7–10.
115 William and Malleville Haller, "The Puritan Art of Love," *Huntington Library Quarterly* 5 (1941–2):235–72; Stone, *Aristocracy*, Chap. 11; Stone, "Nuclear Family," pp. 49–57; Walzer, *Revolution of Saints*, pp. 193–6; Davies, "Sacred Equality."
116 Keith Thomas, "The Double Standard," *Journal of the History of Ideas* 20 (1959):195–216; Stone, *Aristocracy*, pp. 662–71. Dr. Carol Wiener has found that in Elizabethan Hertfordshire men were punished more severely in bastardy cases than women, "Punishment of Parents of Bastards in Late-Elizabethan Hertfordshire" (paper presented to the Berkshire Conference on the History of Women, 1974).
117 Powell, *Domestic Relations*, p. 8 and Chap. 3; Thomas, "Double Standard," pp. 200–01; Stone, *Family, Sex and Marriage*, pp. 195–202, 216–18.
118 Stone, "Nuclear Family," p. 53; idem, *Family, Sex and Marriage*, pp. 151–218; Keith Thomas, "Women and the Civil War Sects," in Trevor Aston, ed., *Crisis in Europe, 1560–1660* (Garden City, N.Y., 1967). For a contrasting point of view see Alice Clark, *The Working Life of Women in the Seventeenth Century* (1919; reprint ed., London, 1968), and more recently, Louise A. Tilly, Joan W. Scott, and Miriam Cohen, "Women's Work and European Fertility Patterns," *Journal of Interdisciplinary History* 6 (1976):454.
119 Paulet, *Marques Idlenes*, p. 85. For other contemporary literature about women see Louis B. Wright, *Middle-Class Culture in Elizabethan England* (London, 1964), Chaps. 7, 8, 13; Powell, *Domestic Relations*, pp. 101–68, passim; D. M. Stenton, *The English Woman in History* (London, 1957), Chaps. 3, 6, and esp. pp. 108–9; Gouge, *Domesticall Duties*, pp. 16–30; Keith Thomas, "Woman and Sects," p. 44.
120 Ashml. 415, f. 201ᵛ (Taylor). See also Ashml. 404, f. 262ᵛ (Gilberte); Thomas, *Religion and Magic*, p. 528; E. P. Thompson, " 'Rough Music': le charivari anglais," *Annales, E.S.C.* 27 (1972):285–312; Wiener, "Sex and Crime."
121 Allen, "Diocese of Peterborough," p. 65; Thomas, *Religion and Magic*, pp. 528–9, 530; J. S. Cockburn, ed., *Crime in England 1550–1800* (London, 1977), p. 57; R. A. Marchant, *The Church Under the Law* (London, 1969), p. 219. See also *Three Elizabethan Domestic Tragedies*, ed. Keith Sturgess (Harmondsworth, 1969), p. 182
122 Church of England, *The Two Books of Homilies* (Oxford, 1859), p. 505.
123 Ashml. 202, f. 21ᵛ (Abrahall).
124 Ashml. 404, f. 181ᵛ, and also Ashml. 404, ff. 178ᵛ, 114ᵛ, Ashml. 202, f. 181ᵛ (Rawlins).
125 Ashml. 228, f. 30 (Easton).
126 Stenton, *English Woman*, Chaps. 2, 4; Roger Thompson, *Women in Stuart England and America* (London, 1974), pp. 162–4. Examples of wealthy women who managed to secure their property from their husbands' meddling may be found in Ashml. 227, f. 134, and at Buckingham County Record Office, D/U/1/3.
127 Ashml. 404, f. 262 (?Gilborte).
128 Quoted in Hey, *Myddle*, p. 214.
129 Cf. Clark, *Working Life of Women*; Macfarlane, *Ralph Josselin*, pp. 106–9.
130 Ashml. 406, f. 113ᵛ (Robinson).
131 Ashml. 235, ff. 37, 37ᵛ (?Pedder); Ashml. 239, f. 110ᵛ (Maryot).
132 Ashml. 404, f. 141ᵛ (Ladimore); Ashml. 198, f. 104 (Chaplyn); Stone, *Aristocracy*, pp. 662–8; Alan Macfarlane, "The Regulation of Marital and Sexual Relationships in Seventeenth Century England, with Special Reference to the County of Essex" (M. Phil. thesis, London School of Economics, 1968), p. 129; Ashml. 202, f. 5 (Fisher), for a man married to an adulterous wife; Wrightson, "Puritan Reformation of Manners," p. 45.
133 John Pound, ed., *The Norwich Census of the Poor*, Norfolk Record Society, 40 (1971):95 (table), which shows that 3.2% of the Norwich poor were deserted women. Paul Slack, "Vagrants and Vagrancy in England, 1598–1664," *Economic*

History Review, 2nd ser. 27 (1974):366–7. Examples of women deserted by their husbands may be found in Ashml. 222, f. 97ᵛ; Ashml. 223, f. 133 (Jones); Ashml. 239, f. 45ᵛ (Thomson); Ashml. 405, f. 214ᵛ (Rands); Ashml. 405, f. 42 (Greene).

134 The true extent of separation and divorce is difficult to determine. Legally, divorce was almost impossible to obtain, particularly for women: Powell, *Domestic Relations*, pp. 861–70; C. S. G. Gibson, "Marriage Breakdown and Social Class in England and Wales Since the Reformation" (Ph.D. diss., University of London, 1972), p. 7; Thomas, "Double Standard," pp. 200–1; Halifax, *Works*, pp. 277–8. On the other hand, there is some evidence that separations and divorces did occur on all social levels: Stone, *Aristocracy*, pp. 655–6; Hill, *World Upside Down*, p. 320; Powell, *Domestic Relations*, Chap. 3, esp. pp. 66, 83; Walzer, *Revolution of Saints*, pp. 195–6; F. G. Emmison, *Elizabethan Life: Morals and the Church Courts* (Chelmsford, 1973), pp. 3, 39, 164–8 (seventeen cases of suit for divorce, five or six times successful); Ashml. 202, ff. 42, 53 (Gladstone); Ashml. 202, f. 163 (Bury) (two cases of "divorce" followed by remarriage noted by Napier).

135 E. R. C. Brinkworth, "A Study of the Visitation Books of the Archdeaconry of Buckingham, 1633–1637 (B. Litt. thesis, Oxford University, 1947), pp. 138–9; Marchant, *Church Under Law*, p. 219; Emmison, *Church Courts*, pp. 161–4, 167–8; Hill, *Society and Puritanism*, p. 305; Elias Ashmole, *Elias Ashmole, 1617–1692*, ed. C. H. Josten, 5 vols. (Oxford, 1966), 1:108–9.

136 Ashml. 229, ff. 192ᵛ, 195ᵛ (Harvey); Ashml. 181, f. 75 (?Hutton).

137 Emmison, *Church Courts*, p. 162; Ashml. 409, f. 4ᵛ (Edwards).

138 Philip Julius, Duke of Stettin-Pomerania, quoted in Thomas, *Religion and Magic*, p. 528.

139 Jeremy Taylor, *The Marriage Ring*, in his *Discourses on Various Subjects*, 3 vols. (Boston, 1816), 1:344–5, 351.

140 Church of England, *Two Books of Homilies*, pp. 510–11.

141 Ashml. 407, f. 46 (Podder); Ashml. 228, f. 231 (Spencer). See also Ashml. 193, f. 367ᵛ; Ashml. 229, ff. 73ᵛ, 114, 177ᵛ (Sanford); Ashml. 229, f. 154 (Lene); Ashml. 239, f. 194ᵛ (Chapman); Ashml. 414, f. 115 (Ordway); Ashml. 409, f. 124 (Rush).

142 Ashml. 224, f. 335 (Sussex). For other instances of apparent sexual incompatibility see Ashml. 405, f. 267ᵛ (Coals); Ashml. 235, ff. 122, 125 (Skynner); Ashml. 237, f. 19 (Ignoram); and esp. Ashml. 413, ff. 64–64ᵛ, the case of Mistress Elizabeth Barkeley, of whom Napier remarks: "Her husband did not much relish her, nor come to her . . . She did love him exceedingly, and was jealous." In the cases of 9 men and 13 women, disturbed clients were said to be jealous, evidently without cause; and in 11 other cases, the distress of 3 women and 8 men was attributed to the actual adultery of their spouses.

143 Ashml. 414, f. 92 (Nueman). See also Ashml. 218, f. 236ᵛ (Prescot); Ashml. 414, f. 49ᵛ (Parry); Ashml. 193, ff. 314ᵛ–15 (Tyrringham).

144 Relevant examples are Ashml. 228, f. 228 (Wels); Ashml. 224, f. 218ᵛ (Hart); Ashml. 216, f. 97ᵛ (Soule); Ashml. 404, fragment pinned to f. 30ᵇ (Earell); Ashml. 228, f. 4 (Blundell).

145 Ashml. 233, f. 93ᵛ (Wyllison); Ashml. 416, f. 197 (Selbee).

146 Quoted in Davies, "Sacred Equality," p. 568. For Shorter's views, see *Modern Family*, pp. 54–65.

147 Thomas, *Religion and Magic*, p. 17; Spufford, *Communities*, pp. 116–18; Stone, *Aristocracy*, pp. 168, 589–91, 619–23.

149 Ashml. 202, f. 112ᵛ (Laurence); see also Pinchbeck and Hewitt, *Children*, 1:13, 63; Stone, *Aristocracy*, p. 591.

150 Ashml. 233, f. 143ᵛ, and Ashml. 220, f. 40 (Lancton). Good examples of women whose grief outweighed any financial problems caused by their husbands' deaths are at Ashml. 227, f. 128ᵛ (Rider); Ashml. 416, f. 245 (Redman); Ashml. 227, f. 209ᵛ (Peacock); Ashml. 404, f. 253ᵛ (Warwick). Nor were the severely disturbed the only patients who suffered because of their husbands' deaths: Three instances of physically ill women who were bereaved are Ashml. 228, f. 216 (Raynolds);

Ashml. 202, f. 4ᵛ (Haddon); Ashml. 197, f. 112ᵛ (Mistress Fayre). An interesting example of official acceptance of the idea that a spouse's death could cause insanity is in *Calendar of the Patent Rolls, Elizabeth I*, Vol. 3, *1563–1566* (London, 1960), p. 322.

151 Ashml. 218, f. 149ᵛ (Flesher); Ashml. 230, f. 354ᵛ, Ashml. 233, ff. 5ᵛ, 6, 41ᵛ, Ashml. 42, f. 121 (Lucas); Ashml. 405, f. 103ᵛ (Games); Ashml. 200, f. 239 (Page) are particularly illuminating. All together, 9 cases of mental disorder involving men and 33 involving women were attributed to their spouses' deaths.

152 Spalding, *Impossible Puritan*, pp. 42, 44.

153 Stone, *Aristocracy*, pp. 589–600, 609–23, 649–71, esp. p. 660; Macfarlane, *Ralph Josselin*, pp. 106–10; Fletcher, *County Community*, pp. 31–4; Hutchinson, *Memoirs*, pp. 11–13, 34–6. Alan Macfarlane in collaboration with Sarah Harrison and Charles Jardine, *Reconstructing Historical Communities* (Cambridge, 1977), pp. 177–80.

154 Macfarlane, *Ralph Josselin*, Chap. 10.

155 Schochet, "Patriarchalism," p. 429.

156 Thomas, *Religion and Magic*, pp. 527–8; Samaha, *Law and Order*, pp. 36–7, 41–94, passim.

157 Slack, "Vagrants," pp. 364–5; A. L. Beier, "Vagrants and the Social Order in Elizabethan England," *Past and Present*, No. 64 (1974):3–29; A. L. Beier and J. F. Pound, "Debate: Vagrants and the Social Order," *Past and Present*, No. 71 (1976):126–34. Samaha and Cockburn note that although the rate of felonies increased late in Elizabeth's reign, the totals during its last decades were swollen chiefly by thefts, not by murders, infanticides, suicides, manslaughters, or rapes (Samaha, *Law and Order*, pp. 18–94, esp. pp. 18–21; Cockburn, *Crime in England* Chaps. 2, 5, 6, esp. pp. 52–71).

158 Ashml. 224, f. 172 (Nameless); another attempt to procure an abortifacient from Napier is at Ashml. 227, f. 169. For suicides because of pregnancy see Public Record Office, London, Star Chamber 8/2/41, f. 1; Oliver Heywood, *His Autobiography, Diaries, Anecdote and Event Books*, ed. J. Horsfall Turner, 4 vols. (Bingley and Brighouse, 1881–5), 3:197; Public Record Office, London, King's Bench 9/755, f. 247; John Aubrey, "Observations," in *Three Prose Works*, ed. John Buchanan-Brown (Carbondale, Ill., 1972), p. 352.

159 Ashml. 193, f. 337 (Mallet).

160 Ashml. 409, f. 109 (Skynner); Ashml. 200, f. 108ᵛ (Lockley).

161 Ashml. 182, f. 107ᵛ (Barnwell); Ashml. 182, ff. 46ᵛ–47 (Smith); Ashml. 224, f. 187ᵛ; Ashml. 233, f. 49ᵛ, and Ashml. 414, f. 107 (Browne). See also Thomas, *Religion and Magic*, pp. 530–1, 544, 551–2; G. L. Kittredge, *Witchcraft in Old and New England* (1929; reprint ed., New York, 1972), pp. 47, 236.

162 Thomas, *Religion and Magic*, Chap. 17; Macfarlane, *Witchcraft*, Chaps. 12, 15, and 16; Cockburn, *Crime in England*, Chap. 3.

163 Ashml. 223, f. 29ᵛ (Woddle).

164 Ashml. 409, f. 60ᵛ (Payne); Ashml. 231, f. 178ᵛ (Buckingham); Ashml. 415, f. 178ᵛ (Clark).

165 Ashml. 410, f. 196 (Steaphens); Ashml. 218, f. 21ᵛ (Yeady); Ashml. 217, f. 164 (Fontayne); Ashml. 223, f. 177ᵛ (Cocken).

166 For widows see Ashml. 220, f. 126ᵛ; Ashml. 220, f. 66; Ashml. 235, f. 57ᵛ; Ashml. 414, f. 9; Ashml. 218, f.125ᵛ; and two cases involving the physically deformed are Ashml. 199, f. 99 (Whitten); Ashml. 217, f. 63ᵛ (Shepherd).

167 Ashml. 213, f. 76ᵛ (Smyth).

168 Forbes, *Aldgate*, p. 106; Stone, *Aristocracy*, pp. 590, 619, and Fig. 16; E. A. Wrigley, "Mortality in Pre-Industrial England: The Example of Colyton, Devon, Over Three Centuries," *Daedalus* 97, No. 2 (1968):547. Cf. T. Forbes, "Mortality Books for 1820 to 1849 from the Parish of St. Bridge, Fleet Street, London," *Journal of the History of Medicine* 27 (1972):22.

169 One example was Agnes Olny whose delivery was so badly botched by a clumsy midwife that "she ever after continued lame and could not hold her water": Ashml. 221, f. 50.

170 The man was Mark Wells: Ashml. 406, f. 14. For women who expressed fear about bearing children see Ashml. 215, f. 15 (Nixon); Ashml. 193, f. 265 (Orpyn); Ashml. 202, f. 65ᵛ (Page); Ashml. 404, f. 59 (Palmer).

171 For examples of women anxious because of barrenness see Ashml. 181, f. 93; Ashml. 197, f. 19ᵛ; Ashml. 239, f. 152; Ashml. 228, f. 214; Thomas, *Religion and Magic*, p. 317. A woman mocked for having no children was Mary Gilberte, Ashml. 404, f. 262 (?Gilborte).

172 Macfarlane, *Ralph Josselin*, pp. 85, 150, 151; Margaret Hoby, *Diary of Lady Margaret Hoby, 1599–1605*, ed. D. M. Meads (Boston, 1930), p. 63; Ashml. 193, f. 67ᵛ (Aussoppe). See also Ashml. 193, f. 203 (Lene) and Ashml. 207, f. 113ᵛ (Fisher) for mental disturbances attributed to solitary or disrupted deliveries. See also P. Willughby, *Observations in Midwifery* (London, 1863), pp. 273–5.

173 Ashml. 224, ff. 124ᵛ, 171 (Bower); Ashml. 198, ff. 53, 76, 83 (Baneberry); Ashml. 230, f. 26 (Boddington); Ashml. 227, f. 119 (Whitting); Ashml. 414, f. 200ᵛ (Cock).

174 Cockburn, *Crime in England*, Chap. 6; Stone, *Family, Sex and Marriage*, pp. 93–102. For examples of witchcraft accusations that followed from feuds see Ashml. 217, f. 133ᵇᵛ (Stoe); Ashml. 404, f. 15ᵛ (Walkynden); Ashml. 201, f. 42 (Leaper); Ashml. 214, f. 117 (Flack); Ashml. 232, f. 347 (Hipwell); Ashml. 409, unfoliated (Payne).

175 Ashml. 232, f. 345 (Smith).

176 Ashml. 238, f. 159 (Brytton).

177 Ashml. 202, f. 192ᵛ (Gondone).

178 Ashml. 239, f. 84ᵛ (Clively).

179 Ashml. 228, f. 18 (Welhed).

180 Macfarlane, *Ralph Josselin*, Chap. 10.

181 Ashml. 119, f. 97ᵛ (Bale).

182 Macfarlane, *Witchcraft*, pp. 169–70; Thomas, *Religion and Magic*, pp. 546–69. Witchcraft accusations, both among Napier's patients and among Essex villagers, were not uncommonly made by a member or members of a family on behalf of the victim. When a child, for example, was believed to have been bewitched, the injury was felt to have been inflicted upon the *family*, and the accusation was made by the parents: Macfarlane, *Witchcraft*, pp. 162–3. Cf. Paul Boyer and Stephen Nissenbaum, *Salem Possessed* (Cambridge, Mass., 1974), pp. 143–51.

183 There were just 9 such cases, and 4 of them were mentioned to Napier by disturbed wives.

184 If the literature of the Elizabethan and Jacobean periods were approached from this perspective, historians and literary critics alike might find fresh insights in familiar and much abused texts. Some comedy in particular could be interpreted as culturally cathartic, as mythic reconciliations of psychological conflicts that changing social circumstances sharpened during the period. This strategy would enable readers to negotiate beyond both the crude literalism that leads a Peter Laslett to repudiate literature and the stratospheric structuralism that prompts a Northrop Frye to neglect history. The extremes are illustrated in Laslett, *World We Have Lost*, pp. 84–112, and Northrop Frye, *A Natural Perspective* (Toronto, 1965).

CHAPTER 4 *Popular stereotypes of insanity*

1 Burton, *The Anatomy of Melancholy*, ed. Holbrook Jackson, 3 vols. (London, 1968), 1:397, 408.

2 Thomas Scheff, *Being Mentally Ill* (Chicago, 1966); Erving Goffman, *Asylums* (Garden City, N.Y., 1961), Chap. 3.

3 Bodleian Library, Ashmole MSS (hereafter cited as Ashml.), 222, f. 96ᵛ (Stiles).

4 Scheff, *Being Mentally Ill*; Ari Kiev, *Transcultural Psychiatry* (Harmondsworth, 1972), pp. 56–77; Harold Garfinkel, *Studies in Ethnomethodology* (Englewood

Cliffs, N.J., 1967); G. M. Carstairs and R. L. Kapur, *The Great Universe of Kota: Stress, Change and Mental Disorder in an Indian Village* (London, 1976), pp. 11–12. Cf. Gregory Bateson, *Steps Towards an Ecology of Mind* (London, 1973), pp. 167–250. For contrasting approaches see Dorothea C. Leighton, John S. Harding, David B. Macklin, Allister M. Macmillan, and Alexander H. Leighton, *The Character of Danger* (New York, 1963), and Jane Murphy, "Psychiatric Labeling in Cross-Cultural Perspective," *Science* 191 (1976):1019–28.

5 Wilkie Collins, *The Moonstone*, ed. J. I. M. Stewart (Harmondsworth, 1966), pp. 425–6.

6 A full list of the symptoms tabulated is provided in Appendix D.

7 These observations are not significantly affected by the sex ratio among mentally disturbed patients. Cross tabulations by sex of all the symptoms discussed here are given in Appendix D.

8 Burton, *Anatomy of Melancholy*, 1:408.

9 See Chapter 5, under "Demons, witches, and madmen," for a discussion of diabolical possession in Napier's practice.

10 Robert R. Reed, *Bedlam on the Jacobean Stage* (Cambridge, Mass., 1952), esp. 29–33. Examples of the other types mentioned may be found in Gamini Salgado, ed., *Cony-Catchers and Bawdy-Baskets* (Harmondsworth, 1972), pp. 108–9; Jack Lindsay, ed., *Loving Mad Tom: Bedlamite Verses of the XVI and XVII Centuries* (London, 1927); Thomas Nashe, *The Unfortunate Traveller and Other Works*, ed., J. B. Steane (Harmondsworth, 1971), pp. 52, 80, 211, 232; Charles Hindley, ed., *The Roxburghe Ballads*, 2 vols. (London, 1874), 2:286, 436; Enid Welsford, *The Fool: His Social and Literary History* (Garden City, N.Y., 1961). A measure of the importance of madness in drama may be taken by tracing the many references to the word and its synonyms in the works of some major playwrights. See, e.g., Martin Spevack, *A Complete and Systematic Concordance to the Works of Shakespeare*, 6 vols. (Hildesheim, Germany, 1968–70), 4:466, 1038–40; 5:1994, 1996, 2004–5; Charles Crawford, *A Concordance to the Works of Thomas Kyd* (Vaduz, Liechtenstein, 1963), p. 247, and idem, *The Marlowe Concordance* (Vaduz, Liechtenstein, 1963), pp. 772–3.

11 Reed, *Bedlam on Stage*, pp. 16, 23–6.

12 See, e.g., Star Chamber MSS (hereafter cited as STAC) 8/1/6, 7; STAC 8/2/5, 6, 26, 41, 42; STAC 8/3/4, 10; Edwin Harbin Bates [alias Bates Harbin], ed., *Quarter Sessions Records for the County of Somerset*, 3 vols., Somerset Record Society, 23, 24, 28 (1907–12), 1:99–100, 228; 2:100; S. C. Ratcliff, and H. C. Johnson, eds., *Warwick County Records: Quarter Sessions Order Book*, 5 vols. (Warwick, 1937), 3:57.

13 *Oxford English Dictionary*, s.v. "Bedlam"; Ashml. 200, f. 212 (Miller).

14 Morris P. Tilley, *A Dictionary of the Proverbs in England in the Sixteenth and Seventeenth Centuries* (Ann Arbor, Mich., 1950), proverbs indexed s.v. "mad," "madness," "madman."

15 Salgado, *Cony-Catchers*, pp. 62, 108–9; Lindsay, *Loving Mad Tom*; William Shakespeare, *King Lear* in *The Complete Works*, ed. G. B. Harrison (New York, 1952). All subsequent citations to Shakespeare are from this edition.

16 Napier was careless about indicating when his patients were represented by intermediaries. He does record the presence of representatives (usually near kin or friends) in about 10% of all cases of mental disorder. The figures for acute insanity are much higher: 30% for lunacy, 20% for madness, and 20% for distraction. These are certainly underestimates.

17 "Mad" and "lunatic" were exact synonyms in Napier's vocabulary of mental disorder, and he employed them interchangeably. He wrote both words in the notes for one consultation only three times in a total of 140 consultations for madness and lunacy. Because the pattern of symptoms associated with both were identical, it would have been redundant to label a patient's distress with both terms.

18 Michael Dalton, *The Countrey Iustice*, 3rd ed. (London, 1626), p. 243, see also pp. 235, 267 for suicide and larceny. Nigel Walker, *Crime and Insanity in En-*

gland, 2 vols. (Edinburgh, 1968), 1: Chaps. 1 and 2; cf. Charles Gross, ed., *Select Cases from the Coroner's Rolls, A.D. 1265–1413,* Selden Society, 9 (1895): 46–7.

19 John Cordy Jeaffreson, *Middlesex County Records,* 4 vols. (London, 1887–8), 2:182; 3:170, 236, 291, 368; J. S. Cockburn, ed., *Calendar of Assize Records, Sussex Indictments, Elizabeth I* (London, 1975), pp. 35, 314; F. G. Emmison, *Elizabethan Life: Morals and the Church Courts* (Chelmsford, 1973), pp. 83, 160, 168, 283–4, 301.

20 Harbin Bates, *Quarter Sessions Somerset,* 1:99–100, 223–4; 2:71–2; 3:125–6; A. Fessler, "The Management of Lunacy in Seventeenth Century England," *Proceedings of the Royal Society of Medicine* (1956):903; Ratcliff and Johnson, *Warwick County Records,* 49:267. As might be expected, preventive detention was sometimes abused, and sane people found themselves imprisoned because of false testimony by their enemies: see, e.g., *Acts of the Privy Council, 1629–1630* (London, 1960), 45:143; Harbin Bates, *Quarter Sessions Somerset,* 1:227.

21 See Public Record Office, London (hereafter cited as PRO), Wards 9/216, s.v. "James Stroud," and D. E. C. Yale, ed., *Lord Nottingham's Chancery Cases,* Selden Society, 73 (1954):16–17, for typical disputes. Richard Neugebauer, "Mental Illness and Government Policy in Sixteenth and Seventeenth Century England" (Ph.D. diss., Columbia University, 1976), pp. 47–8. Richard Hunter and Ida Macalpine (*Three Hundred Years of Psychiatry 1535–1860* [London, 1963], pp. 64–5, 70) have collected some exceptional instances of expert testimony, and perhaps it was more common to seek the advice of physicians when charges of witchcraft were involved; Keith Thomas, *Religion and the Decline of Magic* (New York, 1971), p. 537.

22 Salgado, *Cony Catchers,* pp. 62, 108–9.

23 Ratcliff and Johnson, *Warwick County Records,* 3:267. See also *Acts of the Privy Council, 1630–1631* (London, 1964), 46:108; Historical Manuscript Commission, *Report 9, Salisbury Papers,* 19, p. 177.

24 H. E. Bell, *An Introduction to the History and Records of the Court of Wards and Liveries* (Cambridge, 1953), p. 128.

25 Ashml. 194, f. 189 (Sanders); Ashml. 215, f. 212 (Lelan).

26 Ashml. 175, f. 62^v (Marcum); Ashml. 211, f. 306 (Barton). See also Ashml. 405, f. 345 (Randall); Ashml. 229, ff. 192^v, 195^v; Ashml. 203, f. 172 (Harvey); Ashml. 408, f. 169^v (Hitchcock); Ashml. 229, f. 154 (Lane); Ashml. 181,.f. 75 (Hutton); Ashml. 197, f. 11^v (Hooton); Ashml. 214, f. 137 (Parker); Ashml. 200, f. 25 (Seaton); Ashml. 416, f. 197 (Selbee); Ashml. 194, f. 317 (Wilson); Ashml. 414, f. 73^v (Darling); Ashml. 405, f. 78^v (Fish).

27 Ashml. 406, f. 171 (Hixon).

28 Emmison, *Church Courts,* p. 163, and also pp. 161–2.

29 Ashml. 232, f. 414 (Bateman). For other examples see Ashml. 235, f. 107 (Whitlock); Ashml. 407, f. 20^v (Davye); Ashml. 223, f. 170^v (Meanes); Ashml. 214, f. 353 (Morish); Harbin Bates, *Quarter Sessions Somerset,* 1:88; B. Howard Cunnington, ed., *Records of the County of Wilts* (Devizes, 1932), p. 94; Fessler, "Management of Lunacy," p. 902.

30 Ashml. 224, f. 8 (anonymous).

31 Ashml. 233, f. 86^v (Hatley). See also Ashml. 222, f. 89 (Tiplady); Ashml. 408, f. 165 (Sanders); Ashml. 201, ff. 160, 161, 186, 230.

32 Ashml. 217, f. 166 (Lane).

33 Ashml. 402, f. 170 (Birchmore).

34 Ashml. 404, f. 104^v (Peach); Ashml. 218, f. 69^v (Broughton).

35 Ashml. 233, f. 86^v (Hatley); Ashml. 215, f. 122^v (Meadowes). Other cases of adults who were believed to be mentally abnormal because they defied their parents are in Ashml. 416, f. 195 (Langkton); Ashml. 227, f. 33 (Chapman); Ashml. 194, f. 269 (anonymous); Ashml. 237, f. 89^v (Bosse). A man wrote to the astrologer John Booker in 1654 complaining that his son would "not be ruled by anybody" and asking whether it was best to transport him to Virginia. Booker thought that the son was suffering from a "spice of melancholy" and recom-

mended that marrying a virgin would cure him faster than a trip to Virginia: Ashml. 174, ff. 411–13.

36 Ashml. 413, f. 119ᵛ (Stoe); Ashml. 406, ff. 370, 372 (Bateson); Ashml. 207, f. 55ᵛ (Miller).

37 See Chapter 3, pp. 81–5.

38 Cockburn, *Assize Records, Sussex Indictments*, p. 35; Oliver Heywood, *His Autobiography, Diaries, Anecdote and Event Books*, ed. J. Horsfall Turner, 4 vols. (Bingley and Brighouse, 1881–5), 3:193.

39 Harbin Bates, *Quarter Sessions Somerset*, 3:305. See also Ashml. 409, f. 4ᵛ (Edwards); Ashml. 232, f. 442 (Wilkinson).

40 Ashml. 235, f. 9 (Maryot); Ashml. 214, f. 172 (Hanson).

41 Ashml. 194, f. 101; Ashml. 238, ff. 28, 76 (Baker). Cf. Ashml. 215, f. 106ᵛ (Straker); Ashml. 198, f. 158 (Tilcock).

42 Thomas Smith, *De Republica Anglorum* (1565; reprint., Cambridge, 1906), pp. 31–41; Lawrence Stone, "Social Mobility in England, 1500–1700," *Past and Present*, No. 33 (1966):16–55.

43 Ashml. 227, f. 61 (Collins); Ashml. 237, f. 119 (Mann). See also Ashml. 224 f. 56ᵛ, and Ashml. 244, f. 57ᵛ (Woulse).

44 John Spencer, *A Discourse of Divers Petitions* (London, 1641), p. 75; Hunter and Macalpine, *Psychiatry*, p. 104.

45 M. W. Barley, "Rural Housing in England," in Joan Thirsk, ed., *The Agrarian History of England and Wales, IV, 1500–1640* (Cambridge, 1967), pp. 721, 735, 749; W. G. Hoskins, "The Rebuilding of Rural England, 1570–1640," *Past and Present*, No. 4 (1953):50, and idem, *The Midland Peasant* (London, 1957), pp. 285–6, 291, 297. See also Fernand Braudel, *Capitalism and Material Life, 1400–1800*, trans. Miriam Kochan (New York, 1973), pp. 214–15.

46 The social and psychological expressiveness of dress is discussed in Mary Ellen Roach and Joanne Bubolz Eicher, eds., *Dress, Adornment and the Social Order* (New York, 1965); Lawrence Stone, *The Crisis of the Aristocracy* (Oxford, 1965), pp. 562–6, Braudel, *Capitalism and Material Life*, and Phillis Cunnington and Catherine Lucas, *Occupational Costume in England: From the Eleventh Century to 1914* (London, 1967), are pertinent historical works. A first-century reference to madmen tearing or shredding their clothing is in Gregory Zilboorg, *A History of Medical Psychology* (New York, 1967), p. 75.

47 C. H. Williams, ed., *English Historical Documents, 1485–1558* (London, 1967), pp. 249–52.

48 Burton, *Anatomy of Melancholy*, 1:105–6.

49 Church of England, *The Two Books of Homilies* (London, 1859), pp. 308–19; Philip Stubbes, *The Anatomie of Abuses* (London, 1583), pp. 16–94.

50 Cunnington and Lucas, *Occupational Costume*; H. D. Traill, ed., *Social England*, 6 vols. (New York, 1895), 3:385–90.

51 Roy Strong, *The English Icon: Elizabethan and Jacobean Portraiture* (London, 1969), p. 35; see also pp. 21, 36–7, 352–4; Bridget Gellert Lyons, *Voices of Melancholy* (London, 1971), p. 22.

52 Burton, *Anatomy of Melancholy*, 2:236.

53 Judith Neaman, *The Suggestion of the Devil* (Garden City, N.Y., 1975).

54 Ashml. 410, f. 29ᵛ (Knot). See also Ashml. 224, f. 56ᵛ (Woulse); Ashml. 196, f. 128ᵛ (Muns).

55 Ashml. 414, f. 210 (Katelin).

56 Ashml. 200, f. 212 (Miller). See also Ashml. 416, f. 351 (Wats).

57 Ashml. 402, f. 75 (Savage); Ashml. 224, f. 358 (Nueman).

58 Fessler, "Management of Lunacy," p. 903. See also Hunter and Macalpine, *Psychiatry*, p. 123 (quoting Daniel Oxenbridge, 1642), and Ashml. 199, f. 139 (Piddington); Ashml. 416, f. 192 (Allen); Ashml. 238, f. 61 (Hatton); Ashml. 212, f. 31 (Jackson); Ashml. 215, f. 225 (Dorle); Ashml. 227, f. 216 (Harrell); Ashml. 198, f. 135 (Shorland).

59 The simple clothes of farm laborers were worth between 5% and 12% of their total wealth. Richard Napier spent £3 6s. to outfit an apprentice with two sets of

clothing in 1615, a sum that suggests it would have taken a builder about thirty days to earn enough for a complete set of apparel. Alan Everitt, "Farm Labourers," in Thirsk, *Agrarian History*, pp. 449–50, 864; Ashml. 196, f. 147.

60 Spencer, *Discourse of Divers Petitions*, pp. 75–6.

61 PRO C 142/718, m. 152.

62 Ashml. 230, f. 177 (Smith).

63 STAC 8/1/7, f. 1; STAC 8/3/4, f. 3; STAC 8/3/10, f. 1; STAC 8/2/46.

64 Thomas Rogers Forbes, *Chronicle from Aldgate: Life and Death in Shakespeare's London* (New Haven, 1971), p. 31; David G. Hey, *An English Rural Community: Myddle Under the Tudors and Stuarts* (Leicester, 1974), p. 46. For later examples see Leon Radzinowicz, *A History of English Criminal Law and Its Administration from 1750*, 4 vols. (New York, 1948), 1:195–7.

65 Examples of efforts to spare families from the consequences of suicide verdicts may be found in STAC 8/1/29, 32, 35, 38, 39, 40, 41; STAC 8/2/42, 46; STAC 8/3/38, f. 1. Royal officials apparently permitted some survivors to buy back confiscated properties at a favorable price, STAC 8/3/13, f. 2.

66 Edmund Wingate, *Justice Revived* (London, 1661), pp. 66, 81; John Sym, *Lifes Preservative against self-killing* (London, 1637), p. 159.

67 Dalton, *Countrey Iustice*, pp. 235, 243; Wingate, *Justice Revived*, p. 88; Sym, *Lifes Preservative*, p. 172; STAC 8/1/6, f. 5; STAC 8/3/14, f. 2. Cf. Heinrich Bullinger, *The Decades of Henry Bullinger*, ed. Thomas Harding, Parker Society, 4 vols. (Cambridge, 1850), 2:414–15.

68 Of the suicides recorded for Bedfordshire, Buckinghamshire, and Northamptonshire between 1597 and 1644, 58% (154) left no goods at all; 43% (66) of the male suicides had no property to seize. The recorded occupations of these people were humble: a yeoman and 29 laborers, 37 spinsters, 7 husbandmen, 3 servants, a netmaker, a rough mason, a freemason, an apprentice, a shoemaker, a tinker, a hostler, a weaver, a bricklayer, an innkeeper, a butcher's wife, and a shepherd's wife are mentioned in the surviving inquests. PRO KB 9/692–826. For a rare reference to a suicide note see STAC 8/3/10, f.2.

69 For a discussion of the problems of establishing premeditation from circumstantial evidence and the ways that they were solved see Michael MacDonald, "The Inner Side of Wisdom: Suicide in Early Modern England," *Psychological Medicine* 7 (1977):566–72. John Sym provides a description of the "signs of self-murder" in *Lifes Preservative*, pp. 259–61.

70 Susan Snyder, "The Left Hand of God: Despair in Medieval and Renaissance Tradition," *Studies in the Renaissance* 12 (1965):49, 50–7; Thomas, *Religion and Magic*, pp. 473–7; R. R. Hunnisett, ed., *Calendar of Nottinghamshire Coroners' Inquests, 1485–1558*, Thoroton Society, 25 (1969):xxv; STAC 8/3/10, f. 2; John Bunyan, *Grace Abounding to the Chief of Sinners and Pilgrim's Progress*, ed. Roger Sharrock (London, 1966), p. 232; Nehemiah Wallington, "A record of the Mercies of God," London, Guildhall Library MS 204, pp. 1–10 (I owe this reference to the kindness of Paul Seaver). Other important discussions of the Devil's role in tempting men to despair and suicide are Edmund Spenser, *Books I and II of the Faerie Queen*, ed. Robert Kellogg and Oliver Steele (New York, 1965), p. 187; Sym, *Lifes Preservative*, pp. 246–50; Burton, *Anatomy of Melancholy*, 3:395–408. See also Jean-Claude Schmitt, "Le suicide au moyen âge," *Annales, E.S.C.* 21 (1976):3–27.

71 Ashml. 217, f. 67 (Hayford).

72 Ashml. 414, f. 194ᵛ (Toe); Ashml. 199, ff. 11, 28 (Toe); Ashml. 218, f. 42ᵛ (Southan).

73 Ashml. 215, f. 298ᵛ (Lea). For cases of other patients who saw or heard the Devil or other evil spirits urge them to commit suicide, see Ashml. 404, f. 289ᵛ (Morton); Ashml. 227, f. 57 (Neale); Ashml. 227, f. 94ᵛ (Chalice); Ashml. 409, f. 83ᵛ (Payne). The experiences of these people confirm John Sym's remark that the "visible apparition of the Devil, speaking to and persuading a man to kill himself" often accompanied suicidal gloom: *Lifes Preservative*, p. 246.

74 Ashml. 239, f. 179 (Savil); Ashml. 230, f. 99ᵛ (Kent). Similar beliefs are described in language close to the clients' own words in Ashml. 203, f. 35ᵛ (Copket); Ashml. 229, f. 39ᵛ (Houghton); Ashml. 235, f. 114ᵛ (Bichmoe); Ashml. 203, f. 226ᵛ (Shepherd); Ashml. 213, f. 18ᵛ (Page); Ashml. 196, f. 180ᵛ (Franklin); Ashml. 201, f. 15 (Athew).

75 Essex County Record Office, Terling Parish Register, p. 1 (I owe this reference to Keith Wrightson); Forbes, *Chronicle from Aldgate*, p. 165.

76 Thomas, *Religion and Magic*, pp. 469–77.

77 Hobbes stated the difficulty clearly; see *The English Works*, ed. W. Molesworth, 11 vols. (London, 1840), 6:88–9. Cf. John Foxe, *The Acts and Monuments of John Foxe*, ed. George Townsend, 8 vols. (New York, 1965), 6:715.

78 Burton, *Anatomy of Melancholy*, 1:390.

79 Burton, *Anatomy of Melancholy*, 1:431; see also 1:390, 416, 431–9; 2:113; 3:187, 287, 408. Lawrence Babb, *The Elizabethan Malady* (East Lansing, Mich., 1951), pp. 33, 36.

80 The best discussions of suicide in drama are Theodore Spencer, *Death and Elizabethan Tragedy* (New York, 1960), pp. 141, 158–79, 218, 233, 251, 252; Clifford Leech, "Le Dénouement par le suicide dans la tragédie élisabethaine et jacobéenne," in *La Théâtre tragique*, ed. Jean Jacquot (Paris, 1962), pp. 179–89; Curtis B. Watson, *Shakespeare and the Renaissance Concept of Honor* (Princeton, 1960), pp. 117–23, 341–5; Mark Stavig, *John Ford and the Traditional Moral Order* (Madison, Wisc., 1968), pp. 141, 158, 162, 163.

81 Of 493 melancholy patients, 27 were suicidal; 62 of 794 patients who were "troubled in mind" wanted to kill themselves; 6.4% of all consultations for mental disorder involved suicidal compulsions. Cf. Hunter and Macalpine, *Psychiatry*, p. 226.

82 See Appendix E, Table E3 for the frequencies of the symptoms associated with suicidal behavior. A clerical approach to the problem is in Sym, *Lifes Preservative*, pp. 247–8.

83 Bartholomaeus Anglicus, *De Proprietatibus rerum* (London, 1535), p. lxxxvii; Penelope B. R. Doob, *Nebuchadnezzar's Children: Conventions of Madness in Middle English Literature* (New Haven, 1974), p. 113.

84 John Aubrey, *Aubrey's Brief Lives*, ed. Oliver Lawson Dick (Harmondsworth, 1972), pp. 215–16. (For an interpretation of Falkland's moods and actions that denies they were suicidal see *Selections from Clarendon*, ed. G. Huehns [London, 1968], pp. 58–61.)

85 Burton, *Anatomy of Melancholy*, 1:439. See also Hunter and Macalpine, *Psychiatry*, p. 28. Other writers remarked that violent madmen endangered their own lives as well as those of others. Thus Andrew Boorde reported the case of one Mychell, a lunatic who slew his wife, his sister-in-law, and himself, and warned against leaving potential instruments of death in the hands of confined madmen, lest they kill themselves: *A Compendyous Regiment or Dyetary of Helth*, ed. F. J. Furnivall, Early English Text Society, Extra Series, 10 (1870):298; cf. Hunter and Macalpine, *Psychiatry*, pp. 13, 113.

86 STAC 8/42/2.

87 STAC 8/3/10, ff. 1–2. See also STAC 8/1/7; STAC 8/2/6, f. 1 (now filed with STAC 8/3/43); STAC 8/3/4, f. 3; STAC 8/2/26, f. 1.

88 STAC 8/3/10, f. 1. See also STAC 8/2/42, f. 1; STAC 8/3/4, f. 2.

89 STAC 8/3/14, f. 2.

90 STAC 8/1/6, f. 5.

91 STAC 8/1/6, ff. 2ᵛ, 3.

92 Nicholas Culpeper, *Culpeper's School of Physick* (London, 1659).

93 Ashml. 230, f. 71 (Cras); cf. Ashml. 410, f. 129ᵛ (Deemer).

94 Ashml. 215, f. 294ᵛ (Ashton). See also Ashml. 415, f. 189 (Musgrave); Ashml. 410, f. 20 (Hixon); Ashml. 222, f. 35ᵛ (Walker).

95 Ashml. 414, f. 57 (Browne).

96 Ashml. 230, f. 141 (Fisher).

97   Ashml. 224, f. 65 (Iremonger); Ashml. 233, f. 50ᵛ (Turney).
98   Ashml. 222, f. 146ᵛ (Perkins).
99   Ashml. 227, f. 216 (Hurrell). Among Napier's mentally disturbed clients, 40 cursed and 68 talked too much and too fast.
100 Ashml. 214, f. 73 (Grave). See also Ashml. 230, f. 156 (Cuts).
101 John Archer, *Every Man his own Doctor* (London, 1673), p. 127.
102 Tilley, *Proverbs*, p. 14.
103 Hunter and Macalpine, *Psychiatry*, pp. 55–8, esp. p. 56.
104 Ashml. 402, f. 27 (Hustwate).
105 Matthew H. Peacock, "Certificates of Alleged Cures of Lunacy by John Smith, of Wakefield, in 1615," *Yorkshire Archaeological Journal* 16 (1902):254–5.
106 Ashml. 194, f. 239 (Akens).
107 C. L. Barber, *Shakespeare's Festive Comedy* (Cleveland, 1966), Chaps. 9 and 10; Neaman, *Suggestion of the Devil*, pp. 52–3, 56, 134–6, 141, 143, 181; Christopher Hill, *The World Turned Upside Down* (Harmondsworth, 1975), pp. 39–50. Other examples of mad wanderers are in Ashml. 416, f. 388 (Taylour); Ashml. 323, f. 40 (Lyster); Ashml. 232, f. 16 (Hopkins).
108 Fessler, "Management of Lunacy," p. 903.
109 Ashml. 237, f. 108 (Baker).
110 Ashml. 207, f. 113ᵛ (Fisher). See also Ashml. 198, f. 60 (Cello).
111 Ashml. 224, f. 228ᵛ (Bassington).
112 Fessler, "Management of Lunacy," p. 903.
113 William George Smith and Janet E. Heseltine, comps., *The Oxford Dictionary of English Proverbs*, 2nd ed., ed. Paul Harvey (Oxford, 1966), p. 396.
114 Ashml. 222, f. 51ᵛ (Burges); Ashml. 408, f. 46ᵛ (Payne). Cf. Ashml. 222, f. 35ᵛ (Walker).
115 Bodleian Library, MS Bodley 154, ff. 2ᵛ–3.
116 Ashml. 412, f. 124ᵛ (Tyler); Ashml. 227, f. 27 (Morgan); Ashml. 200, f. 212 (Harbart); Ashml. 239, f. 29ᵛ (Adams); Ashml. 237, f. 80ᵛ (Lovet). For other examples of senseless raving see Ashml. 408, f. 58ᵛ (Alice Harvey); Ashml. 200, f. 18ᵛ (Piggot); Ashml. 223, f. 142 (Cooper); Ashml. 200, f. 70 (Clark); Ashml. 207, f. 69ᵛ (Gulliver); Ashml. 402, f. 75 (Savage).
117 Thomas, *Religion and Magic*, pp. 469–77.
118 Ashml. 235, f. 116ᵛ (Olive); Ashml. 213, f. 18ᵛ (Page); Ashml. 196, f. 151 (Peach); Ashml. 414, f. 104ᵛ (Peach).
119 Ashml. 408, f. 58ᵛ (Harvey); Ashml. 196, f. 131ᵛ (Hodell).
120 Ashml. 214, f. 145 (Rose).
121 Ashml. 198, f. 186 (Simpson); Ashml. 211, f. 197 (Kelly). For other instances in which damnation seemed immediate and inevitable see Ashml. 182, f. 209ᵛ (Richardson); Ashml. 415, f. 162ᵛ (Sparle); Ashml. 405, f. 33 (Clarke); Ashml. 232, f. 122 (Hale); and Ashml. 193, f. 180 (Butcher).
122 Ashml. 182, f. 209ᵛ (Richardson); Ashml. 199, f. 126 (Godfrey); Ashml. 222, f. 96ᵛ (Stiles).
123 Ashml. 201, f. 15 (Athew); Ashml. 196, f. 180ᵛ (Franklin).
124 George Trosse, *The Life of the Reverend Mr. George Trosse*, ed. A. W. Brink (Montreal, 1974), p. 93.
125 Alice Thornton, *The Autobiography of Mrs. Alice Thornton*, Surtees Society, 62 (1875):50–3, esp. 52.
126 Elias Ashmole, *Elias Ashmole (1617–1692)*, ed. C. H. Josten, 5 vols. (Oxford, 1966), 2:457, n. 5.
127 Cockburn, *Assize Records, Sussex Indictments*, pp. 156–7.
128 John Jewel, *The Works*, ed. John Ayre, Parker Society, 4 vols. (Cambridge, 1845–50), 3:359.
129 John Graunt, *Natural and Political Observations . . . Upon the Bills of Mortality* (London, 1662), p. 20 and table following p. 74.
130 Burton, *Anatomy of Melancholy*, 1:140. Cf. Hunter and Macalpine, *Psychiatry*, pp. 14, 27.
131 Heywood, *Autobiography*, 4:31–2.

132 Ashml. 193, f. 224ᵛ (Burser).
133 Ashml. 200, f. 237 (Page); cf. Ashml. 239, f. 88 (Snowe); Ashml. 194, f. 146 (Clark); Ashml. 222, ff. 95ᵛ, 96, 102ᵛ (Shatbolt); Ashml. 239, f. 146ᵛ (Whyting); Ashml. 220, f. 4 (Caynee); Ashml. 220, f. 159ᵛ (Thomson).
134 Shakespeare, *King Lear*, act 3, sc. 4, lines 108–10.
135 Records concerning the lunacy of 28 lunatics from Bedforshire, Buckinghamshire, and Northamptonshire may be found in PRO, Wards 9/197, 214–20, 551; Wards 18/27 and Wards 511, 3, 30, and 44. Two wards treated by Napier possessed lands worth only £6 and £12 10s. and another from the area was worth just £10 16s.: Wards 5/3/1122, Wards 5/1/974, and Wards 5/3/1015. No records of pauper lunatics for the region have survived. I am grateful to Richard Neugebauer for helping me locate these records.
136 This estimate is based on crude population density figures in H. C. Darby, *A New Historical Geography of England* (Cambridge, 1973). I am grateful to John Chavez for providing this calculation.
137 Victor Harris, *All Coherence Gone* (Chicago, 1949), pp. 39–40; see also pp. 93–108, 112–14, 139–40. Joseph Hall, *Heaven Upon Earth, and Characters of Vertves and Vices*, ed. Rudolf Kirk (New Brunswick, N.J., 1948), p. 102.
138 Burton, *Anatomy of Melancholy*, 1:120–1.
139 Burton, *Anatomy of Melancholy*, 1:410.
140 Joseph Hall, *Works*, 12 vols. (Oxford, 1839), 6:20–1; Thomas Wright, *The Passions of the Minde in generall* (London, 1604); Thomas Hobbes, *Leviathan*, ed. C. B. Macpherson (Harmondsworth, 1971), pp. 139–140; Lily B. Campbell, *Shakespeare's Tragic Heroes* (New York, 1968).
141 Babb, *Elizabethan Malady*; Lyons, *Voices of Melancholy*; Noel Brann, "The Renaissance Passion of Melancholy" (Ph.D. diss., Stanford University, 1965); Louis B. Wright, *Middle-Class Culture in Elizabethan England* (London, 1964), pp. 581–2.
142 John B. Bamborough, *The Little World of Man* (London, 1951), pp. 108–9; Babb, *Elizabethan Malady*, pp. 74, 78; John Earle, *Microcosmos* (1627; reprint., Leeds, 1966), p. 85; Burton, *Anatomy of Melancholy*, 1:242.
143 Napier had used technical language often in the first years he practiced; in 1624 he began employing novel terms, such as "melancholy adust," which are stressed by Burton: Ashml. 227, f. 106ᵛ. He owned a copy of *Anatomy of Melancholy*, which he lent to Mr. George Myles in 1625: Ashml. 224, f. 239ᵛ.
144 See Chapter 2, pp. 49–53.
145 Ashml. 413, f. 149, and Ashml. 218, ff. 161ᵛ, 189ᵛ (Spencer); see also Ashml. 231, f. 165 (Mrs. Hanger).
146 Ashml. 409, f. 115 (Price). For similar cases see Ashml. 212, f. 504 (Mr. Roger Hacket for his wife); Ashml. 409, f. 110ᵛ (Lady Dormer for her son); Ashml. 416, f. 135 (Sir Edmund Osborne, Bt., for his brother).
147 Ashml. 405, f. 80 (Evans). See also under Napier's report of a letter Lady Hazelrigge's husband (?Sir Arthur Hesilrige) wrote to him about his wife in 1630: Ashml. 194, f. 45 (Hazelrigge); Lady Westmoreland's report about Robert Maddison (1627): Ashml. 227, f. 117.
148 Some socially prestigious patients were thought to be particularly susceptible to melancholy. Lady Katherine Dyer, for instance, was "subject to melancholy passions": Ashml. 222, f. 92. See also Ashml. 181, f. 167 (Dorrington, gentlewoman); Ashml. 230, f. 347ᵛ (Digby, Sir Everrard's sister).
149 Babb, *Elizabethan Malady*, pp. 42–7; Basil Clarke, *Mental Disorder in Earlier Britain* (Cardiff, 1975), p. 226.
150 Nashe, *Traveller and Other Works*, p. 218.
151 Ashml. 413, f. 51 (Rice).
152 Ashml. 194, f. 436 (Horne); cf. Ashml. 237, f. 91ᵛ (Dalie). See also Burton on melancholy jealousy, *Anatomy of Melancholy*, 3:257–311.
153 Ashml. 416, f. 295 (Davys).
154 Ashml. 218, f. 112ᵛ (Iremonger); Ashml. 198, f. 146 (Trevell); Ashml. 416, f. 388 (Taylour); Ashml. 222, f. 139 (Norwich).

155 Thomas, *Religion and Magic*, Chap. 18, esp. p. 578.
156 Ashml. 201, f. 183 (Ekins).
157 Ashml. 410, f. 195 (Ringe).
158 Thomas, *Religion and Magic*, pp. 131–40, 144–6; Hill, *World Upside Down*, Chap. 13.
159 Phillip Harth, *Swift and Anglican Rationalism* (Chicago, 1961), pp. 103–11; John F. Sena, "Melancholic Madness and the Puritans," *Harvard Theological Review* 66 (1973):293–309.
160 Ashml. 402, f. 74 (Mydlemore); Ashml. 235, f. 125ᵛ (Laurenc).
161 Thomas, *Religion and Magic*, pp. 144–6. The letters of some sixteenth-century enthusiasts who were supposed to be deluded by the authorities are in the Burghley papers, British Library, Lansdowne MS 42, item 76 and MS 99, items 3, 4, 9–22, 25–31, 37, 56, 82. The diagnoses scribbled on them are anachronistic; they seem to have been made by John Strype.
162 Nashe, *Traveller and Other Works*, p. 217; see also pp. 216–18; Burton, *Anatomy of Melancholy*, 1:159–60; Bamborough, *Little World of Man*, pp. 30, 36–41, 45–6, 47, 53, 62, 87, 89, 98–9, 105, 106; Babb, *Elizabethan Malady*, passim, esp. pp. 42–7.
163 See, e.g., Ashml. 407, f. 144ᵛ (Norwoode); Ashml. 220, f. 49 (Spencer); Ashml. 237, f. 54ᵛ (Morgayne); Ashml. 211, f. 453 (Joicelyn).
164 Ashml. 224, f. 231ᵛ (Adams); cf. Nashe, *Traveller and Other Works*, p. 216.
165 See, e.g., Ashml. 231, f. 38ᵛ (Watts).
166 Burton, *Anatomy of Melancholy*, 1:385 ("They fear where there is no ground for fear, they are alarmed about trifles") and pp. 385–9 generally for melancholy fears.
167 Ashml. 200, f. 220 (Horne); Ashml. 416, f. 197 (Selbee); Ashml. 216, f. 17 (Musgrave); Ashml. 194, f. 379 (Knit); Ashml. 407, f. 65ᵃ (Pearson).
168 Ashml. 414, f. 14 (Glover).
169 Ashml. 194, f. 317 (Wilson).
170 Ashml. 224, f. 148ᵛ (Ball).
171 Ashml. 412, f. 124 (Kimball); Ashml. 211, f. 344 (Fouke); Ashml. 412, f. 153 (Collins). For other miscellaneous examples of melancholy fearfulness or excessive anxiety see Ashml. 409, f. 115 (Price); Ashml. 223, f. 101ᵛ (Edwards); Ashml. 237, f. 62 (Evans); Ashml. 238, f. 26ᵛ (Freeman); Ashml. 221, f. 46ᵛ (Hill); Ashml. 239, f. 140 (Ereswell); Ashml. 237, f. 74 (Mathew).
172 Wright, *Passions of the Minde*, pp. 273–8.
173 Burton, *Anatomy of Melancholy*, 1:337; Stephen Bradwell's remarks about plague in Hunter and Macalpine, *Psychiatry*, p. 111; Campbell, *Shakespeare's Tragic Heroes*, Chaps. 6 and 15; and Chapter 3.
174 *Oxford English Dictionary*, s.v. "grief."
175 Burton, *Anatomy of Melancholy*, 1:389.
176 Strong, *English Icon*, pp. 352–4.
177 Ashml. 215, f. 23 (Chayne).
178 Ashml. 238, f. 42 (Stiff).
179 Quoted in Babb, *Elizabethan Malady*, p. 105; see pp. 102–10 generally.
180 Ashml. 233, f. 143ᵛ (Lancton). Other good cases of melancholic grief are at Ashml. 211, f. 292 (Ripell); Ashml. 405, f. 111ᵛ (Mats); Ashml. 224, f. 143ᵛ (Markham); Ashml. 405, f. 80 (anonymous gentleman); Ashml. 218, f. 149ᵛ (Flesher).
181 Ashml. 218, f. 149ᵛ (Flesher). See also Ashml. 416, f. 135.
182 Ashml. 211, f. 306 (Barton); Ashml. 222, f. 86 (Gregory); Ashml. 217, f. 64ᵛ (March); Ashml. 218, f. 241 (Newell).
183 Burton, *Anatomy of Melancholy*, 1:395–6.
184 Ashml. 224, f. 23 (Experience). See also Ashml. 410, f. 139 (Palmer); Ashml. 416, f. 135 (Osburne); Ashml. 407, f. 187ᵛ (Hazelwood); Ashml. 194, f. 45 (Hazelrigge).
185 Archer, *Every Man His Own Doctor*, pp. 119–20.
186 Ashml. 235, f. 120 (Kings); Ashml. 230, f. 132ᵛ (Askue). For other examples of mopish patients with melancholic problems see Ashml. 410, ff. 64–5ᵛ (Barker);

Ashml. 414, f. 215 (Hunt); Ashml. 413, f. 137ᵛ (Deacon); Ashml. 416, f. 31 (Wapell); Ashml. 408, f. 92 (Glover); Ashml. 231, f. 185ᵛ (Fletcher); Ashml. 232, f. 236 (Lady Fyrnet); Ashml. 215, f. 91 (Martyn); Ashml. 218, f. 223 (Leaventhrope).

187 Ashml. 232, f. 125 (Hector); see also Ashml. 220, f. 22 (Smith); Ashml. 198, f. 44 (Amples); Ashml. 221, f. 112 (Filde); Ashml. 196, f. 4ᵛ (Pen); Ashml. 207, f. 199ᵛ (Pampion); Ashml. 329, ff. 105–6 (Pars); Ashml. 413, f. 222 (Browne).

188 For examples of mopish patients who were unable to perform their usual business see Ashml. 239, f. 104 (Hall); Ashml. 239, f. 32ᵛ (Emmerton); Ashml. 227, f. 109 (Eastwick); Ashml. 408, unnumbered f. between ff. 143–5 (Fossie); Ashml. 232, f. 29 (Hull); Ashml. 233, f. 5ᵛ (Lucas); Ashml. 194, f. 298 (Rabins); Ashml. 213, f. 122 (anonymous).

189 See, e.g., Ashml. 229, f. 159ᵛ (Dobs); Ashml. 229, f. 251 (Greene); Ashml. 193, f. 203 (Lea); Ashml. 196. f. 136ᵛ (Nichols); Ashml. 212, f. 187 (Norish); Ashml. 239, f. 39 (Poling); Ashml. 232, f. 371 (Coates); Ashml. 238, f. 138ᵛ (Sheplye); Ashml. 211, f. 393 (Edridge).

190 Stanley W. Jackson, "Galen – On Mental Disorders," *Journal of the History of the Behavioral Sciences* 5 (1969):376; Hunter and Macalpine, *Psychiatry*, pp. 25, 44.

191 William Battie, *A Treatise on Madness*, ed. Richard Hunter and Ida Macalpine (London, 1962), pp. 5, 38–40, 67.

192 *The Tempest*, act 5, sc. 1, lines 237–40. Cf. *Henry V*, act 3, sc. 7, lines 142–4.

193 *Hamlet*, act 3, sc. 1, lines 78–81.

194 Ashml. 233, ff. 5ᵛ–6 (Lucas).

195 R. W. Southern, *The Making of the Middle Ages* (New Haven, 1969), p. 176.

196 The European background of the concept of melancholy is discussed by Babb, *Elizabethan Malady*, and by Brann, "Renaissance Passion of Melancholy." Continental ideas about other forms of mental disorder are also mentioned by them and by P. M. Laignel-Lavestine and Jean Vinchon, *Les Maladies de l'esprit et leurs médecins du XVIᵉ au XIXᵉ siècle* (Paris, 1930); Oskar Diethelm and Thomas F. Hefferman, "Felix Platter and Psychiatry," *Journal of the History of Behavioral Sciences* 1 (1965):10–23; Stanley W. Jackson, "Unusual Mental States in Medieval Europe. I. Medical Syndromes of Mental Disorder: 400–1100 A.D.," *Journal of the History of Medicine*, 27 (1972):262–97; Franz G. Alexander and Sheldon T. Selsnick, *The History of Psychiatry* (New York, 1966).

197 Doob, *Nebuchadnezzar's Children*, Chap. 1; Penelope B. R. Doob, "Ego Nabugodonoser: A Study of Conventions of Madness in Middle English Literature" (Ph.D. diss., Stanford University, 1969); Judith S. Neaman, "The Distracted Knight: A Study of Insanity in the Arthurian Romances" (Ph.D. diss., Columbia University, 1968).

198 Schmitt, "Le Suicide au moyen âge," *Annales, E.S.C.* 31 (1976):3–5; Snyder, "Left Hand of God," pp. 49, 50–7.

199 Smith and Heseltine, *Oxford Dictionary of Proverbs*, p. 395.

200 William Fleetwood, *The Relative Duties of Parents and Children, Husbands and Wives, Masters and Servants . . . With Three more [sermons] upon the Case of self-murther* (London, 1715), p. 477.

201 Heywood, *Autobiography*, 3:195.

202 Guildhall Library MS 204, p. 5.

203 Ashml. 235, f. 117 (Olive); Ashml. 213, f. 18ᵛ (Page); Ashml. 196, f. 151 (Peach); Ashml. 404, f. 105 (Peach); Ashml. 223, f. 124ᵛ (Persivall).

204 Hall, *Works*. 8:88.

205 Ashml. 216, f. 198 (Hearne).

206 Ashml. 233, f. 57ᵛ (Neuman). Examples of similar thoughts after bereavements are Ashml. 200, f. 43 (Harrold); Ashml. 200, ff. 238ᵛ–9 (Page); Ashml. 198, f. 150ᵛ (Lawrence); Ashml. 224, f. 51 (Peacock).

207 Ashml. 414, f. 54 (Darling).

208 Ashml. 200, f. 177ᵛ (Mercer).

209 Ashml. 229, ff. 268, 269 (Berring).

210 Ashml. 414, f. 55ᵛ (Gregory). For other expressions of religious gloom see

Ashml. 405, f. 104ᵛ (Hill); Ashml. 413, f. 104ᵛ (Spenloe); Ashml. 407, f. 64ᵛ (K. Smith); Ashml. 214, f. 242 (Dea); Ashml. 200, f. 187 (Turner); Ashml. 239, f. 99 (?Rusford); Ashml. 218, f. 35 (Wyndgate); Ashml. 216, f. 188ᵛ (Tomkins); Ashml. 404, f. 150ᵛ (Croutche).

211   William Haller, *The Rise of Puritanism* (New York, 1957), p. 33 and Chap. 4 generally; Owen C. Watkins, *The Puritan Experience* (London, 1972), p. 168; William Perkins, *A Golden chaine* [and other treatises] (Cambridge, 1600), pp. 657–63, 667; Richard Capel, *Tentations*, 4th ed. (London, 1650), pp. 192–4; Thomas Wilson, *Saints by Calling* (London, 1620), pp. 30, 42–3, 166–7, 195–205; Thomas Wilson, *A Sermon of the Spirituall Combat* in his *Jacob's Ladder* (London, 1611); Arthur Hildersham, quoted in David Stannard, "Death and Dying in Puritan New England," *American Historical Review* 78 (1973):1311; Samuel Clarke, *Lives of sundry Eminent Persons* (London, 1683), pp. 70–1.

212   Thomas Adams, *The Works*, 3 vols. (Edinburgh, 1861), 1:254–93.

213   Hall, *Works*, 8:115; see also pp. 173–4, 256–60.

214   Ashml. 201, f. 119ᵛ (Buttres).

215   Ashml. 237, f. 68ᵛ (Pendred). See also Ashml. 211, f. 219 (Woodward); Ashml. 218, f. 82 (Burchmore); Ashml. 198, f. 139ᵛ (Osburne); Ashml. 202, f. 208 (Farmer); Ashml. 224, f. 136ᵛ (Allen); Ashml. 230, f. 12ᵛ (Blackwell).

216   Ashml. 200, f. 108 (Hall). See also Ashml. 200, f. 163 (Buck); Ashml. 402, f. 49ᵛ (Moore); Ashml. 217, f. 166 (Lane); Ashml. 229, f. 27 (Seer); Ashml. 227, f. 11ᵛ (Clayton); Ashml. 213, f. 67ᵛ (Stonell).

217   Burton, *Anatomy of Melancholy*, 1:199–201.

218   Sym, *Lifes Preservative*, pp. 247–8.

219   Harth, *Swift and Anglican Rationalism*, pp. 103–11; Sena, "Melancholic Madness"; Truman Guy Steffan, "The Social Argument against Enthusiasm," *Studies in English*, 21 (Austin, Texas, 1941), pp. 39–63; George Rosen, "Enthusiasm: 'a dark lanthorn of the spirit,' " *Bulletin of the History of Medicine* 42 (1968):393–421; Michael V. DePorte, *Nightmares and Hobbyhorses: Swift, Sterne, and Augustan Ideas of Madness* (San Marino, Calif., 1974), pp. 33, 37–43, 58, 65; Jackson I. Cope, *Joseph Glanvill, Anglican Apologist* (St. Louis, 1956), pp. 30–2, 40–1, 53–8, 65, 73–9, 83, 146–7, 157, 159–65; George Williamson, "The Restoration Revolt against Enthusiasm," *Studies in Philology* 30 (1933):571–603.

220   Thomas Church, *Remarks on the Reverend Mr. John Wesley's last journal* (London, 1745), p. 68; Theophilus Evans, *The History of Modern Enthusiasm*, 2nd ed. (London, 1757), pp. 130–3; George Lavington, *The Enthusiasm of the Methodists and Papists compared*, 3 parts in 2 vols. (London, 1754), Pt. 3:23–69, esp. 36, 38, 54–5, 59, 65–9; Ronald Paulson, *Hogarth's Graphic Works*, 2 vols., rev. ed. (New Haven, 1970), 1:247–9; 2: pl. 232. Lavington was an inconsistent rationalist, who also charged Wesley with witchcraft: *Enthusiasm of Methodists*, Pt 3:30, 37–8, 44–5, 56, 58, 158–98.

221   See, e.g., Lavington, *Enthusiasm of Methodists*, Pt. 3:16; Evans, *History of Modern Enthusiasm*, p. 127; Joseph Trapp, *The Nature, Folly, Sin, and Danger of being Righteous over-much*, 2nd ed. (London, 1739), esp. pp. 39–49; John Langehorne, *Letters on religious retirement, melancholy, and enthusiasm* (London, 1762), esp. pp. 14–15, 19, 59–67; Henry Stebbing, *A sermon on the new birth* (London, 1739), esp. pp. 13–17; Church, *Remarks on Wesley's journal*, pp. 67–76; Samuel Johnson, *A dictionary of the English language* (London, 1755), s.v. "Enthusiasm."

222   Battie, *Treatise on Madness*, pp. 5–6; John Ferriar, *Medical Histories and Reflections*, 3 vols. (London, 1795), 2:85; Dennis Leigh, *The Historical Development of British Psychiatry, Volume 1, 18th and 19th Century* (New York, 1961), pp. 44–6, 59–60. The traditionalist John Monro resisted the argument that madness was necessarily based on delusion: see John Monro, *Remarks on Dr Battie's Treatise on Madness*, ed. Richard Hunter and Ida Macalpine, in Battie, *Treatise on Madness*, pp. 3–7.

223   Capel, *Tentations*, pp. 193–4; Arthur Hildersham quoted in Stannard, "Death and Dying," p. 1311; Perkins, *Golden chaine*, p. 667; Wilson, *Saints by Calling*, pp. 30, 42–3, 111–12, 142, 145–6, 166–7; Clarke, *Lives of sundry Persons*, pp. 70–1; Watkins, *Puritan Experience*, pp. 9–10, 13.

224 *Oxford English Dictionary*, s.v. "Suicide"; Schmitt, "Suicide au moyen âge," pp. 4–5, 21, n. 18.
225 Charles Moore, *A full inquiry into the subject of Suicide*, 2 vols. (London, 1790), 1:323–4; John Wesley, *Works*, 14 vols. (Grand Rapids, Mich., 1958–9), 12:481.
226 Radzinowicz, *English Criminal Law*, 1:217. For eighteenth-century attitudes toward suicide see Derek Jarrett, *England in the Age of Hogarth* (London, 1974), pp. 206, 210–11, 219–21; Hunter and Macalpine, *Psychiatry*, pp. 342–6, 351–3, 402–10; Roland Bartel, "Suicide in Eighteenth-Century England, The Myth of a Reputation," *Huntington Library Quarterly* 23 (1959–60):145–58; S. E. Sprott, *The English Debate on Suicide* (La Salle, Ill., 1961), Chap. 4; Oswald Doughty, "The English Malady of the Eighteenth Century," *Review of English Studies* 2 (1926):257–69.
227 W. R. Ward, *Religion and Society in England* (London, 1972), pp. 47, 78–9; James Obelkevich, *Religion and Rural Society: South Lindsey, 1825–1875* (Oxford, 1976), Chap. 6; J. F. C. Harrison, *The Second Coming: Popular Millenarianism 1780–1850* (New Brunswick, N.J., 1979).

CHAPTER 5 *Psychological healing*

1 See, e.g., Robert Burton, *The Anatomy of Melancholy*, ed. Holbrook Jackson, 3 vols. (London, 1968), 1:178; Joseph Blagrave, *Blagrave's Astrological Practice of Physick* (London, 1671), p. 184.
2 Burton, *Anatomy of Melancholy*, 1:357.
3 Cf. Burton, *Anatomy of Melancholy*, 1:206–8.
4 Burton, *Anatomy of Melancholy*, 1:178.
5 Penelope B. R. Doob, *Nebuchadnezzar's Children: Conventions of Madness in Middle English Literature* (New Haven, 1974), Chap. 2.
6 George Fox, *George Fox's 'Book of Miracles,'* ed. Henry J. Cadbury (Cambridge, 1948), p. 92. See also John Foxe, *The Acts and Monuments*, ed. George Townsend, 8 vols. (London, 1853–70; reprint ed., New York, 1965), 1:89; 4:419; 8:634, 635, 636, 639–40, 642, 646, 648–9, 670; Thomas Beard, *The Theatre of God's iudgements*, 6th ed. (London, 1618), pp. 60, 65–6, 87–8, 306–17, 572–82; William Perkins, *A Golden chaine* [and other treatises] (Cambridge, 1600); p. 22; Burton, *Anatomy of Melancholy*, 1:132–3; A. W. Brink's Introduction to his edition of George Trosse, *The Life of the Reverend Mr. George Trosse* (Montreal, 1974), pp. 17–20; Keith Thomas, *Religion and the Decline of Magic* (New York, 1971), pp. 93–4.
7 Bodleian Library, Ashmole MSS (hereafter cited as Ashml.), 402, f. 30 (Gaph).
8 The best description of medical practice in Tudor and Stuart England is Margaret Pelling and Charles Webster, "Medical Practitioners," in Charles Webster, ed., *Health, Medicine and Mortality in the Sixteenth Century* (Cambridge, 1979), pp. 165–235. The variety of medical healing is richly illustrated in Thomas, *Religion and Magic*, pp. 8–14, 177–211, 275–7, 286–7, 290, 295, 300, 305–6, 316–17, 330, 332–4, 354–5, 378–80, 536–8, 546, 649–50, 657–60. Standard sources focused mainly on the physicians, surgeons, and apothecaries are Paul H. Kocher, *Science and Religion in Elizabethan England* (San Marino, Calif., 1953), Chaps. 6, 10–13; George Clark, *A History of the Royal College of Physicians of London*, 2 vols. (London, 1964–6); R. S. Roberts, "The Personnel and Practice of Medicine in Tudor and Stuart England," *Medical History* 6 (1962):363–82, and 8 (1964):217–34. Two valuable treatments of attempts to reform the medical profession during the English Revolution are Charles Webster, *The Great Instauration: Science, Medicine, and Reform, 1626–1660* (New York, 1976), Chap. 4; Christopher Hill, *Change and Continuity in Seventeenth-Century England* (Cambridge, Mass., 1975), Chap. 7. Three contemporary sources deserve special mention because of the light they throw on the therapeutic pluralism of the early seventeenth century: John Cotta, *A Short Discouerie of the vnobserued dangers of seuerall sorts of ignorant and vnconsiderate Practisers of Physicke in England* (London, 1612), Charles Goodall, *The Royal*

College of Physicians of London (London, 1684), and E. Poeton, "The Vrinall cract in the carriage" and "The winnowing of white Witchcraft" in Sloane MS 1954.

9   Thomas, *Religion and Magic*, esp. Chaps. 2, 3, 9, 12, 15.

10 Writers who emphasize the anxieties of the godly are Max Weber, *The Protestant Ethic and the Spirit of Capitalism*, trans. Talcott Parsons (New York, 1958), pp. 95–139; Erich Fromm, *The Fear of Freedom* (London, 1960), Chap. 3; S. E. Sprott, *The English Debate on Suicide* (La Salle, Ill., 1961), Chap. 2. Scholars who stress the solace Puritanism provided are Michael Walzer, "Puritanism as a Revolutionary Ideology," *History and Theory* 3 (1963):59–90; idem, *The Revolution of the Saints* (New York, 1969), pp. 200–10, 309, 313; William Haller, *The Rise of Puritanism* (New York, 1957), Chap. 1, esp. p. 27.

11 For a selection of autobiographical accounts of Puritans' anxieties before and after their conversions, see n. 215.

12 The best discussions of medieval and Renaissance cosmology remain C. S. Lewis, *The Discarded Image* (Cambridge, 1964); E. M. W. Tillyard, *The Elizabethan World Picture* (New York, n.d.); and especially Hardin Craig, *The Enchanted Glass* (Oxford, 1952).

13 Information about patients' habits of consultation is very scattered. Napier sometimes noted that his clients had been treated by another physician or folk healer; he recorded such information for 79 of his mentally disturbed patients. Pelling and Webster mention many practitioners who offered or could have offered more than one service: "Medical Practitioners," pp. 184–7, 198–200, 208–10, 216, 222–6, 227–34. Contemporary complaints about the common people's preference for consulting the physicians' rivals include Cotta, *Short Discouerie*; Francis Bacon, *The Advancement of Learning and New Atlantis*, ed. Thomas Case (London, 1969), pp. 129–30; Burton, *Anatomy of Melancholy*, 2:7; Jonathan Goddard, *A Discourse setting forth the unhappy condition of the practice of physick in London* (London, 1670), pp. 19–20; *The Present Ill State of Physick in this Nation* (n.p., ca. 1704–6), pp. 32–3; *The Fundamental Laws of physick* (London, 1711), pp. 2–6. See also Bernard Capp, *Astrology and the Popular Press: English Almanacs 1500–1800* (London, 1979), p. 110.

14 For general treatments of Elizabethan psychology see Lawrence Babb, *The Elizabethan Malady* (East Lansing, Mich., 1951), esp. Chap. 1; Kocher, *Science and Religion*, Chaps. 11, 14; John Bamborough, *The Little World of Man* (London, 1951); Herschel Baker, *The Image of Man* (New York, 1961), Chap. 17; Tillyard, *Elizabethan World Picture*; Craig, *Enchanted Glass*, Chaps. 1, 2, 5. Its medieval background is well described by Judith S. Neaman, "The Distracted Knight: A Study of Insanity in the Arthurian Romance" (Ph.D. diss., Columbia University, 1968); Lewis, *Discarded Image*; Walter Clyde Curry, *Chaucer and the Medieval Sciences*, 2nd ed. (New York, 1960), Chaps. 1, 11.

15 Burton, *Anatomy of Melancholy*, 1:155. Cf. John Davies, *Nosce Teipsum* in his *Complete Poems*, ed. Alexander B. Grosart, 2 vols. (London, 1876), 1:1–123.

16 Timothy Bright, *A Treatise of Melancholie*, ed. Hardin Craig (New York, 1940), p. 40. Cf. Joseph Hall, *Works*, 12 vols. (Oxford, 1837), 8:174.

17 Burton, *Anatomy of Melancholy*, 1:130. For the importance of the idea of man as a microcosm see Kocher, *Science and Religion*, Chap. 11; Tillyard, *Elizabethan World Picture*, Chap. 7.

18 Burton, *Anatomy of Melancholy*, 1:130–3. Cf. Babb, *Elizabethan Malady*, p. 18.

19 Andreas Laurentius [André Du Laurens], *A Discourse of the Preservation of the Sight*, ed. Sanford V. Larkey, Shakespeare Association Facsimiles, No. 15 (London, 1938), p. 81; Anthony Michael Platt and Bernard L. Diamond, "The Origins and Development of the 'Wild Beast' Concept of Mental Illness and Its Relationship to Theories of Criminal Responsibility," *Journal of the History of the Behavioral Sciences* 1 (1965):355–67; Doob, *Nebuchadnezzar's Children*, Chap. 2.

20 Burton, *Anatomy of Melancholy*, 1:157–62.

21 Phrases indicating that patients were disturbed in their senses appear in 27.9% of Napier's consultations with mopish patients; equivalents appear in just 13.3% of

all his consultations with mentally disturbed clients. See Chapter 4, under "Mopishness: a discarded image."

22 Burton, *Anatomy of Melancholy*, 1:159–62. See also Bamborough, *Little World of Man*, pp. 36–8; Babb, *Elizabethan Malady*, pp. 3–4.

23 Burton, *Anatomy of Melancholy*, 1:165.

24 Burton, *Anatomy of Melancholy*, 1:162–9. See also Babb, *Elizabethan Malady*, pp. 4–5.

25 Ashml. 227, f. 117 (Maddison).

26 Burton, *Anatomy of Melancholy*, 1:255. See also Babb, *Elizabethan Malady*, pp. 42–7.

27 Levinus Lemnius, quoted by Babb, *Elizabethan Malady*, p. 29. See also Burton, *Anatomy of Melancholy*, 1:374–8; Babb, *Elizabethan Malady*, pp. 27–9; Bamborough, *Little World of Man*, pp. 88–9.

28 Burton, *Anatomy of Melancholy*, 1:257–8.

29 Baker, *Image of Man*, p. 276.

30 Baker, *Image of Man*, Chap. 17; Bamborough, *Little World of Man*, Chaps. 4, 5; Bright, *Treatise of Melancholie*, pp. 39–67; Kocher, *Science and Religion*, Chap. 14; Babb, *Elizabethan Malady*, pp. 1–38.

31 Thomas Wright, *The Passions of the Minde in generall* (London, 1604), pp. 61, 63. See also Burton, *Anatomy of Melancholy*, 1:259–61; Lily B. Campbell, *Shakespeare's Tragic Heroes: Slaves of Passion* (New York, 1930); Babb, *Elizabethan Malady*, pp. 12–17.

32 Babb, *Elizabethan Malady*, p. 15; Burton, *Anatomy of Melancholy*, 1:261–2, 335–9 (the quoted passage is on p. 337).

33 See, e.g., Ashml. 228, f. 34 (Haddell); Ashml. 238, f. 14 (Sherly); Ashml. 194, f. 5 (Belamye); Ashml. 214, f. 238 (Silby); Ashml. 202, f. 110 (Hartlye); Ashml. 211, f. 202 (Barber); Ashml. 228, f. 69 (Burman); Ashml. 214, f. 324 (Wright); Ashml. 194, f. 367 (Banks); Ashml. 404, f. 165ᵛ (Wright); Ashml. 232, f. 151 (Cheynie); Ashml. 200, f. 17ᵛ (Britton); Ashml. 217, f. 22 (Kay).

34 Ashml. 197, f. 130 (Goodyere); Ashml. 200, f. 106 (Weston).

35 Ashml. 228, f. 34 (Haddell).

36 John Graunt, *Natural and Political Observations . . . Upon the Bills of Mortality* (London, 1662), p. 32 and the table following p. 70.

37 Cotta, *Short Discouerie*, pp. 51–3; Burton, *Anatomy of Melancholy*, 1:255–6.

38 Richard Hunter and Ida Macalpine, comps., *Three Hundred Years of Psychiatry, 1535–1860* (London, 1963), p. 111.

39 Ashml. 230, f. 162 (Neighbor); Ashml. 416, f. 235 (Wooden).

40 Wright, *Passsions of the Minde*, p. 61; Burton, *Anatomy of Melancholy*, 1:252–3, 259–62; Babb, *Elizabethan Malady*, Chap. 2; Kocher, *Science and Religion*, pp. 292–3.

41 Burton, *Anatomy of Melancholy*, 1:161.

42 Davies, *Complete Poems*, 1:73.

43 Wright, *Passions of the Minde*, p. 4.

44 Tillyard, *Elizabethan World Picture*, pp. 75, 94–9; Theodore Spencer, *Shakespeare and the Nature of Man* (New York, 1942), pp. 136–49; Hill, *Change and Continuity*, p. 189; Earl of Clarendon [Edward Hyde], *Selections from Clarendon* (London, 1968), pp. 249–50 and passim.

45 Quoted in Bamborough, *Little World of Man*, p. 39. For two descriptions of madness preceding death in Simon Forman's practice see Ashml. 234, f. 43ᵛ; Ashml. 226, f. 102ᵛ.

46 Henry Foley, ed., *Records of the English Province of the Society of Jesus*, 7 vols. (London, 1877–83), 1:345.

47 Andrew B. Appleby, "Nutrition and Disease: The Case of London, 1550–1750," *Journal of Interdisciplinary History* 6 (1975):1–22; Paul A. Slack, "Some Aspects of Epidemics in England, 1485–1640" (D. Phil., diss., Oxford University, 1972), p. 252; Thomas, *Religion and Magic*, pp. 3–14.

48 Thomas Nashe, *The Terrors of the Night* in his *The Unfortunate Traveller and Other*

Works, ed. J. B. Steane (Harmondsworth, 1972), p. 217. See also Burton, *Anatomy of Melancholy*, 1:250, 374–82, 398–404.

49 Thomas Adams, *Mystical Bedlam*, in Herschel Baker, ed., *The Later Renaissance in England* (Boston, 1975), p. 541.

50 Characteristic lists of the symptoms of frenzy and madness may be found in Andrew Boorde, *Brevuary of Helthe* (London, 1557), pp. lxxv, lxxxxii^v (*sic*); Philip Barrough, *The Methode of Phisick* (London, 1596), pp. 21–4, 44–5; John Archer, *Every Man his own Doctor* (London, 1673), pp. 125–7. Napier diagnosed 10 patients as frenzied and 2 as suffering from mania.

51 William Lilly, *Christian Astrology* (London, 1647), pp, 264–6; Ashml. 403, ff. 168^v–9^v (a copy of Simon Forman's astrological textbook, owned and annotated by Napier).

52 Ashml. 240, f. 104^v.

53 Ashml. 363, ff. 138^v–45^v.

54 For exemplary cases in which the distinction between delirium and madness was ignored see Ashml. 408, f. 176^v (anonymous, Sir Thomas Snagg's gamekeeper); Ashml. 220, f. 159^v (Thomson); Ashml. 220, f. 4 (Caynee); Ashml. 239, f. 146^v (Whyting). Many of the medicaments Napier used were believed to be effective against mental and physical diseases.

55 Babb, *Elizabethan Malady*, pp. 24–6, 48, 96–100, 122–3, 134, 182, 184.

56 Burton, *Anatomy of Melancholy*, 1:300–30, esp. 300–5.

57 Ashml. 233, f. 144^v (Gadstone). See also Ashml. 213, f. 170 (George); Ashml. 235, f. 103 and Ashml. 218, f. 131 (Baker); Ashml. 408, f. 117^v (Birthmore); Ashml. 413, f. 189 (Carrington); Ashml. 211, f. 344 (Fouke); Ashml. 214, f. 259 (Grave); Ashml. 232, f. 450 (Hill); Ashml. 402, f. 27 (Hustwate); Ashml. 227, ff. 39–39^v (Hutchinson); Ashml. 224, ff. 157^v–8 (Richardson); Ashml. 406, f. 80^v (Smith); Ashml. 229, f. 253 (Soule); Ashml. 402, f. 137^v (Strait).

58 For laymen and women perplexed by reading scripture see Ashml. 201, f. 102^v (Symons); Ashml. 223, f. 115^v (Collyn); Ashml. 414, f. 153^v (Marchall); Ashml. 223, f. 161^v (Sambrook); Ashml. 194, f. 8 (Whitter); Ashml. 406, f. 33^v (Kays). For clients disordered by the suspect arts of astrology, arithmetic, and geomancy see Ashml. 217, f. 11 (Hardinge); Ashml. 407, f. 4^v (Franklin); Ashml. 410, f. 183 (Spring). Napier's own opinions of the mental powers of women is epitomized in his denial that the word of God can be edifying "when it cometh out of a conjurer's mouth, a woman's, a witch's, an idiot's, or a madman's mouth" (Ashml. 194, f. 8). Addiction to reading is mentioned in the cases of 11 disturbed women.

59 Frequent complaints common to men and women included insomnia (411 cases), stomach problems (166), general discomfort (107), short-windedness (32), other chest complaints (65), "rising" sensations (50), "rising" stomach (37), trembling (114), ringing ears (29), headaches (53), vertigo (66), swooning (35), and weakness (76).

60 Levinus Lemnius, *The Touchstone of Complexions* (London, 1576), pp. 84–5; Hunter and Macalpine, *Psychiatry*, pp. 22–3; Babb, *Elizabethan Malady*, pp. 9–17, 100–1, 125.

61 Wright, *Passions of the Minde*, pp. 37 and 38. See also Bamborough, *Little World of Man*, pp. 89–90; Blagrave, *Blagrave's Physick*, pp. 184–5; Du Laurens, *Preservation of Sight*, p. 97; Babb, *Elizabethan Malady*, pp. 16–17.

62 Simon Forman used complexions more enthusiastically; see his medical practice, 1596–1601: Ashml. 234, 226, 195, 219, 236, 411.

63 Babb, *Elizabethan Malady*, pp. 7, 38–9, 139. Hunter and Macalpine, *Psychiatry*, pp. 3, 28, 36, 122, 148, 192, 214, 223, 225, 234, 254. For the practice of other contemporary physicians see, e.g. [Daniel Oxenbridge], *General Observations and prescriptions in the practice of physick* (London, 1715), pp. 6–22; William Salmon, *Iatrica: seu Praxis Medendi. The Practice of Curing Diseases* (London, 1694), pp. 771–7; F. N. L. Poynter and W. J. Bishop, eds., *A Seventeenth Century Doctor and His Patients: John Symcotts, 1592?–1662*, Beds. Historical Record Society, 31 (1950):52, 65–7; John Hall, *Select Observations on English Bodies* (1657), facsimile

in Harriet Joseph, *Shakespeare's Son-in-law: John Hall, Man and Physician* (Hamden, Conn., 1964), pp. 23–4, 26–7, 29–30, 37–8, 41–3, 74–5, 174–8. Numerous unprinted medical casebooks in the Sloane Manuscripts in the British Library also provide evidence that Napier's medical treatments for mental disorder were typical. See, e.g., Henry Power's notes on his medical practice: Sloane MSS 1339 (esp. ff. 77ᵛ–81, 97–8ᵛ), 1340–51, 1353–8.

64 Examples of Napier's use of *hiera logadii* are in Ashml. 193, f. 307; Ashml. 199, f. 132ᵛ; Ashml. 203, f. 7ᵛ; Ashml. 238, f. 82; Ashml. 221, ff. 46ᵛ, 206ᵛ, 276ᵛ; see also Ashml. 1386, f. 231; Ashml. 228, f. 85ᵛ. For the antiquity of the preparation and Ptolemy's enthusiasm see Du Laurens, *Preservation of Sight*, p. 110; Burton, *Anatomy of Melancholy*, 2:233. A list of the drugs Napier frequently used and their functions is in Ashml. 1488, ff. 141–4. I have relied chiefly upon contemporary and near-contemporary sources to identify the ingredients and effects of these preparations. References to *hiera logadii* in three useful and convenient works are Royal College of Physicians of London, *Pharmacopoeia Londinensis of 1618*, ed. George Urdange (Madison, Wisc., 1944), p. 87; William Salmon, *Pharmacopoeia Londinensis* (London, 1716), p. 586; Joseph Hill, *A History of the Materia Medica* (London, 1751), pp. 449–51, 559–62, 772–76.

65 Ashml. 193, f. 307; Ashml. 409, f. 126ᵛ; Royal College, *Pharmacopoeia*, p. 180; Salmon, *Pharmacopoeia*, p. 7; Hill, *Materia Medica*, pp. 415–17, 500–3, 546–9; Du Laurens, *Preservation of Sight*, p. 110; Burton, *Anatomy of Melancholy*, 1:233.

66 R. S. Roberts, "The Early History of the Import of Drugs into Britain," in F. N. L. Poynter, ed., *The Evolution of Pharmacy in Britain* (London, 1965).

67 Burton, *Anatomy of Melancholy*, 2:228.

68 Leslie G. Matthews, *History of Pharmacy in Britain* (Edinburgh, 1962), pp. 41–55. See Ashml. 177, f. 128ᵛ, for the drugs Napier purchased. In later years Napier employed a London apothecary named Harryson, Ashml. 223, f. 123.

69 Clark, *Royal College of Physicians*, 1:218–27, 265–72; Roberts, "Personnel and Practice," II, pp. 226–9.

70 Alan G. Debus, *The Chemical Philosophy: Paracelsian Science and Medicine in the Sixteenth and Seventeenth Centuries*, 2 vols. (New York, 1977), 1:58–9; Walter Pagel, *Paracelsus* (Basel, 1958), pp. 126–58.

71 Full discussions of Paracelsus' work and reputation are Debus, *Chemical Philosophy*, Vol. 1, and Pagel, *Paracelsus*.

72 This is a crude synthesis of a controversial topic. For the reception of Paracelsianism before 1640 see Charles Webster, "Alchemical and Paracelsian Medicine," in Webster, *Health, Medicine and Mortality*; Alan G. Debus, *The English Paracelsians* (London, 1965), pp. 145–67; George Urdange, Introduction, Royal College, *Pharmacopoeia*, pp. 43–6, 59–64. For the significance of Paracelsianism during the Interregnum and afterward see Webster, *Great Instauration*, Chap. 4, esp. pp. 273–88, 311–17, 322–3; P. M. Rattansi, "Paracelsus and the Puritan Revolution," *Ambix* 11 (1963):24–32; Theodore M. Brown, "The College of Physicians and the Acceptance of Iatromechanism in England, 1665–1695," *Bulletin of the History of Medicine*, 64 (1970):12–30; P. M. Rattansi, "The Helmontian-Galenist Controversy in Restoration England," *Ambix* 12 (1964):1–23; Hill, *Change and Continuity*, Chap. 7.

73 Quoted in Debus, *Chemical Philosophy*, 1:178.

74 Napier used antimonial compounds more than the other mineral medicines; see, e.g., Ashml. 222, f. 2; Ashml. 231, f. 63ᵛ; Ashml. 221, f. 206ᵛ; Ashml. 404, f. 252. He occasionally prescribed mercury preparations as well; see, e.g., Ashml. 416, f. 354. The chemical preparations he employed were often in the official pharmacopoeia. Compare the drugs in the cases just cited with Royal College, *Pharmacopoeia*, pp. 87, 165; Debus, *English Paracelsians*, pp. 152–3. For a folk remedy see Ashml. 202, f. 84.

75 Napier's extensive alchemical papers are described in William H. Black, comp., *A Descriptive, Analytical and Critical Catalogue of the Manuscripts Bequeathed Unto the University of Oxford by Elias Ashmole* (Oxford, 1845), and are listed in its index, W. D. Macray, *Index to the Catalogue of the Manuscripts of Elias Ashmole*

(Oxford, 1866), p. 115. For Robeson and Gravius see Black, *Ashmole Manuscripts*, and Webster, "Alchemical and Paracelsian Medicine," p. 311. A list of the many alchemical works Napier possessed can be reconstructed from Black, *Ashmole Manuscripts*, and from the lists of books lent that Napier often included in his medical notebooks. His interest in Bacon and Lull is evident from annotations of manuscripts of their works and from his record of a conversation with John Dee, Ashml. 1488, art. II, f. 21ᵛ.

76 Many of Forman's alchemical manuscripts and books are listed by Black, *Ashmole Manuscripts*. The importance of his library is emphasized by Webster, "Alchemical and Paracelsian Medicine," pp. 310–11. For Napier's purchase of the collection see Ashml. 227, ff. 85ᵛ, 103; Ashml. 275, ff. 103, 108, 119, 171ᵛ, and esp. 275.

77 Ashml. 1458, f. 11. For a collection of Napier's own notes about making chemical medicines see Ashml. 1730, ff. 1ᵛ–52ᵛ, 83ᵛ–84.

78 "Mr. Tomson of Watton wrote unto [me] a pitiful letter, lamenting his vain experiments in the philosopher's stone, desiring me to help him to some of the elixer vitae which Thomas Robson told him he had almost finished . . . To whom I returned a long letter to dissuade him from meddling with things so chargeable and so uncertain" (Ashml. 198, f. 49).

79 Ashml. 1408, ff. 205–27.

80 See, e.g., Ashml. 228, f. 228; Ashml. 194, ff. 65 and esp. 393. Napier used formal medical language often in the early years of his practice, banished it from his vocabulary during the middle years, and resumed it during the mid-1620s.

81 Ashml. 1386, f. 231, cf. Royal College, *Pharmacopoeia*, pp. 154, 161.

82 Characteristic of the remedies for melancholy that Napier collected are Ashml. 1386, ff. 227, 229, 231; Ashml. 1453, f. 105; Ashml. 1473, ff. 21, 91, 114, 115, 124, 145, 146, 331, 375, 489, 500, 565, 575, 593, 691, 729, 731, 738; Ashml. 1488, art. II, f. 53; Ashml. 416, ff. 117, 439.

83 Burton, *Anatomy of Melancholy*, 2:240–1, 225–34.

84 Du Laurens, *Preservation of Sight*, pp. 111, 113–5; Burton, *Anatomy of Melancholy*, 2:251; Charles Goodall, *The Colledge of Physicians vindicated* (London, 1676), pp. 117–18.

85 Hill remarks that opium was reintroduced into general practice by Felix Platter in the sixteenth century; the increasing trade in exotic drugs from the Levant made it widely available in the next century: Hill, *Materia Medica*, p. 782; Roberts, "Early History of the Import of Drugs." Laudanum was included in the offical dispensary, Royal College, *Pharmacopoeia*, p. 61.

86 See, e.g., Oxenbridge, *General Observations*, pp. 6–8; Salmon, *Iatrica*, pp. 774, 776, 777; Hall, *Select Observations*, pp. 24, 143.

87 For Napier's use of *confectio hamech* and antimony see, e.g., Ashml. 409, f. 126ᵛ; Ashml. 193, f. 307; Ashml. 222, f. 2; Ashml. 231, f. 63ᵛ. See also Royal College, *Pharmacopoeia*, pp. 43–6, 59–64, 160, 163, 165, 180; Sloane MS 1340, f. 11ᵛ.

88 Representative prescriptions for wealthy patients are in Ashml. 239, f. 77 (Curson); Ashml. 237, f. 191ᵛ; Ashml. 1457, f. 20 (Throgmorton). Alternative prescriptions for malignant fever, one "for rich people" and one "for very poor people" are in Ashml. 237, f. 191ᵛ The controversy surrounding the *aurum potabile* is summarized by Debus, *Chemical Philosophy*, pp. 184–5.

89 For orders to bleed mentally disturbed patients see, e.g., Ashml. 193, f. 119; Ashml. 199, f. 139; Ashml. 214, ff. 156, 420; Ashml. 229, ff. 27, 166ᵛ; Ashml. 409, f. 59 (cephalic); Ashml. 199, f. 132ᵛ; Ashml. 231, f. 63ᵛ (saphenous); Ashml. 194, f. 65 (hemorrhoidal).

90 Thomas Brian, *The Pisse-Prophet, or, Certain Pissepot Lectures* (London, 1637), pp. 11–12. Cf. Burton, *Anatomy of Melancholy*, 2:237.

91 Ashml. 413, f. 26 (Purbeck).

92 Ashml. 224, f. 190ᵛ (Purbeck).

93 Ashml. 413, ff. 104, 198 (Purbeck).

94 Du Laurens, *Preservation of Sight*, p. 111.

95 Ashml. 220, f. 14 (Glassenbery).

96 John Hayward, *Sanctuarie of a Troubled Soule*, 2nd ed. (London, 1650), sig. A6^v. A more complex and influential criticism of contemporary medical therapy was Bacon, *Advancement of Learning*, pp. 133–5.

97 Webster, *Great Instauration*, Chap. 4, esp. pp. 250–73; Hill, *Change and Continuity*, Chap. 7.

98 Ashml. 402, f. 53 (Purbeck).

99 Ashml. 229, f. 39^v (Martyns in Houghton). Cf. Ashml. 193, f. 273^v (Hatch).

100 A medical historian cautions me that purging and bloodletting are effective therapies in rare instances and that a few chemical and herbal medicines did relieve certain illnesses. Contemporaries, however, seldom identified correctly the circumstances in which these treatments were potent, and they made very broad claims for their efficacy.

101 Burton, *Anatomy of Melancholy*, 1:256–7.

102 Burton, *Anatomy of Melancholy*, 2:18–19.

103 Jerome Frank, *Persuasion and Healing*, rev. ed. (New York, 1974), Chap. 6; Thomas, *Religion and Magic*, pp. 209–11.

104 For Napier's use of amulets see the notes Ashmole made on the subject, Ashml. 421, ff. 171–171^v, 144–5. For other physicians' views and practices see Thomas, *Religion and Magic*, pp. 634–5.

105 For Napier see, e.g., Ashml. 211, f. 143 (Rombold); Ashml. 410, f. 100 (Sallock); Ashml. 198, f. 186 (Simpson). The principles of timing treatments astrologically are expounded in Forman's textbook of astrological physic, Ashml. 363, ff. 159–75. Thomas notes that the timing of purging and phlebotomy was commonly included in popular astrological almanacs, *Religion and Magic*, pp. 295, 297.

106 Burton, *Anatomy of Melancholy*, 1:217; Kocher, *Science and Religion*, pp. 292–3.

107 Burton, *Anatomy of Melancholy*, 2; Kocher, *Science and Religion*, pp. 292–3.

108 Burton, *Anatomy of Melancholy*, 2:119–26. Madmen, conversely, were to be isolated, to avoid excitement, and to remain in dark and quiet places.

109 Burton, *Anatomy of Melancholy*, 3:204–26.

110 See later in this chapter, pp. 221–2.

111 John Spencer, *A Discourse of Divers Petitions* (London, 1641), pp. 64–5.

112 Hunter and Macalpine, *Psychiatry*, p. 191.

113 Michael Dalton, *The Countrey Iustice*, 3rd ed. (London, 1626), p. 162; Edmund Wingate, *Justice Revived: Being the Whole Office of a Country Justice of the Peace* (London, 1661), p. 28.

114 Hunter and Macalpine, *Psychiatry*, pp. 6, 239.

115 Burton, *Anatomy of Melancholy*, Vol. 2.

116 Andrew T. Scull, "Museums of Madness: The Social Organization of Insanity in Nineteenth-Century England" (Ph.D. diss., Princeton University, 1974), Chaps. 3 and 4; William L. Parry-Jones, *The Trade in Lunacy* (London, 1972), Chap. 8; Peter McCandless, "Insanity and Society: A Study of the English Lunacy Reform Movement, 1815–1870" (Ph.D. diss., University of Wisconsin–Madison, 1974), Chap. 1.

117 Webster, *Great Instauration*, Chap. 4; Brown, "College of Physicians"; Owsei Temkin, *Galenism: Rise and Decline of a Medical Philosophy* (Ithaca, 1973), Chap. 4; Michael V. DePorte, *Nightmares and Hobbyhorses: Swift, Sterne, and Augustan Ideas of Madness* (San Marino, Calif., 1974), pp. 12–25.

118 Brown, "College of Physicians," esp. p. 29.

119 Cotta, *Short Discouerie*, p. 59.

120 Burton, *Anatomy of Melancholy*, 2:7; Thomas, *Religion and Magic*, Chaps. 7, 8. Cf. Bacon, *Advancement of Learning*, pp. 128–29.

121 Edward Jorden, *A briefe discourse of a disease Called the Suffocation of the Mother* (London, 1603), sig. A2; Ilza Veith, *Hysteria: The History of a Disease* (Chicago, 1965), Chap. 7.

122 Cotta, *Short Discouerie*, pp. 55–8. Cf. Jorden, *Briefe discourse*, esp. pp. 15–16; Richard Bernard, *A Guide to Grand-Iury Men* (London, 1624), pp. 11–18.

123 Cotta, *Short Discouerie*, pp. 66–7; John Cotta, *The Infallible True and Assured*

Witch (London, 1624), pp. 69–77; Bernard, *Guide to Grand-Iury Men*, pp. 49–52; William Drage, *Daimonomageia: A Small Treatise of Sicknesses and Diseases from Witchcraft and Supernatural Causes* (London, 1665), pp. 3–10; James I, *Daemonologie* (London, 1597), pp. 70–1; Richard Baxter, *The Cure of Melancholy and Over-much Sorrow, By Faith and Physic* (1682) in his *Practical Works*, ed. William Orme, 23 vols. (London, 1830), 17:274; Kocher, *Science and Religion*, pp. 141–2; Thomas, *Religion and Magic*, pp. 477–8, 480, 574.

124 Thomas, *Religion and Magic*, pp. 497, 537–8, 548, 573, 574; Kocher, *Science and Religion*, pp. 137–8.

125 Ashml. 224, f. 335 (Sussex); C. L. Ewen, *Witchcraft in the Star Chamber* (n.p., 1938), pp. 60–1.

126 Ashml. 227, f. 259ᵛ (Scrope). For other references to Sunderland's illness and Napier's treatments see Ashml. 421, ff. 162ᵛ–4; Ashml. 227, f. 254; Ashml. 232, f. 423; Ashml. 405, ff. 57ᵛ, 62, 63ᵛ, 69ᵛ, 72ᵛ, 79ᵛ, 113ᵛ, 212ᵛ–13, 255ᵛ, 284ᵛ, 285ᵛ, 294, 310; Ashml. 407, ff. 8ᵛ, 77, 93, 166ᵛ; Ashml. 410, ff. 2–5, 17ᵛ, 20, 22ᵛ–3, 25ᵛ, 27ᵛ, 28, 32ᵛ, 33ᵃ, 36ᵛ, 37ᵛ, 127ᵛ, 130ᵛ, 186; Ashml. 194, ff. 2, 11.

127 Hugh Ross Williamson, *George Villiers* (London, 1940), pp. 268–9; *Calendar of State Papers Domestic, 1623–5*, pp. 485, 476; *Calendar of State Papers Domestic, 1625–6*, p. 363; *Historical Manuscripts Commission*, Report 60, *Earl of Mar and Kellie*, 2:220; William Laud, *Works*, 7 vols. (Oxford, 1847–60), 3:156–7; 7:623.

128 Thomas, *Religion and Magic*, pp 480–1.

129 Nathaniel Bacon, *A Relation of the Fearfvll Estate of Francis Spira* (London, 1638). There were eleven editions of this book in the seventeenth century. For other references to the story see Robert Bolton, *Instructions For a Right comforting Afflicted Consciences*, 2nd ed. (London, 1635), pp. 18–20, 83, 126; Samuel Ward, *Sermons and Treatises*, ed. J. C. Ryle (Edinburgh, 1862), p. 59; Brink, Introduction, in Trosse, *Life of Trosse*, pp. 17–19. For other famous cases and their influence see Thomas, *Religion and Magic*, pp. 481–2, 490.

130 Ashml. 217, f. 93 (March). See also Ashml. 413, f. 198 (Collins); Ashml. 235, f. 28 (Cox); Ashml. 212, f. 26 (Garret); Ashml. 410, ff. 146, 154 (Harrys); Ashml. 215, f. 141ᵛ (Worlye). In two cases, spirits ordered clients to pray, a command that contrasted so strongly with the malevolence of most apparitions that it convinced Napier that one of his patients, the Earl of Sunderland, was suffering from strange fancies rather than genuine intimations of the supernatural: Ashml. 425, f. 11ᵛ (Austen); Ashml. 410, f. 66ᵛ (Scrope).

131 See Chapter 4, pp. 133–4.

132 Ashml. 227, f. 213 (Ringe).

133 Ashml. 410, ff. 41ᵛ, 42ᵛ, 44 (Ringe).

134 Ashml. 410, f. 195 (Ringe).

135 Thomas, *Religion and Magic*, pp. 474–6.

136 Ashml. 216, f. 119 (Brawbrook).

137 Ashml. 222, f. 146ᵛ (Perkins). See also Ashml. 413, f. 104ᵛ (Spenloe).

138 Ashml. 412, ff. 152–152ᵛ (Dudley).

139 Ashml. 409, ff. 59, 65 (Edwards); Ashml. 220, f. 21ᵛ (Byrge); Ashml. 218, ff. 23ᵛ, 24ᵛ (Freeman); Ashml. 203, f. 105 (Martyn); Ashml. 203, f. 7ᵛ (Smith); Ashml. 214, f. 202 (anonymous).

140 Ashml. 227, ff. 237ᵛ–8ᵛ (Langly).

141 Ashml. 218, ff. 188ᵛ–9 (Cleaver).

142 Ashml. 409, f. 65 (Edwards).

143 Ashml. 239, f. 31 (Pattiforde).

144 Ashml. 405, f. 253 (Seabrooke).

145 Ashml. 416, f. 329 (James).

146 Ashml. 215, f. 64 (Dwyn).

147 Ashml. 198, f. 55 (Bodington).

148 Ashml. 404, f. 114ᵛ (Rawlings).

149 Ashml. 413, f. 168 (Howe). For similar descriptions of symptoms see also Ashml. 196, f. 58ᵛ (Hoddle); Ashml. 223, f. 32ᵛ (Edwards); Ashml. 235, f. 146ᵛ (Bullocke); Ashml. 223, f. 180ᵛ (Markes); Ashml. 239, f. 41 (Turny); Ashml. 196, f. 151 (Pitkin).

150 For spirits who were small animals see Ashml. 409, f. 83ᵛ (Payne); Ashml. 215, f. 36 (Haynes); Ashml. 181, f. 120 (Holland); Ashml. 413, f. 168 (Howe); Ashml. 405, f. 207ᵛ (Pearce); Ashml. 193, f. 222 (Devenall); Ashml. 201, f. 229ᵛ (Kent); Ashml. 233, f. 139 (Deary); Ashml. 404, ff. 114ᵛ, 145ᵛ (Rawlings); Ashml. 230, f. 161 (Hascar); Ashml. 218, f. 208ᵛ (Shronte); Ashml. 212, f. 381 (Smyth).

151 For discussions of "familiars" and visions precisely like those of Napier's patients see Rossell Hope Robbins, *The Encyclopedia of Witchcraft and Demonology* (New York, 1959), pp. 190–3; G. L. Kittredge, *Witchcraft in Old and New England* (New York, 1972), Chap. 10; Alan Macfarlane, *Witchcraft in Tudor and Stuart England* (New York, 1970), index s.v. "familiar"; C. L'Estrange Ewen, *Witchcraft and Demonianism* (London, 1933), index s.v. "familiars"; Thomas, *Religion and Magic*, pp. 445–6; *The Wonderful Discoverie of the Witchcrafts of Margaret and Phillipa Flower* (London, 1619), p. 10; *A True and Perfect Relation of the Witches that Were Arraigned, Tryed and Convicted Last Sessions Holden at St. Edmunds-bury in Suffolk* (London, 1645).

152 Contemporary beliefs about the Devil's powers are summarized effectively by Thomas, *Religion and Magic*, pp. 469–77.

153 Ashml. 227, f. 94ᵛ (Chalice); Ashml. 218, f. 42ᵛ (Southan).

154 Characteristic descriptions of the Devil are Ashml. 203, f. 105 (Martyn); Ashml. 203, f. 134ᵛ (Rhead); Ashml. 198, f. 19ᵛ (Course); Ashml. 198, f. 186 (Simpson); Ashml. 230, f. 177 (Smith); Ashml. 193, f. 97ᵛ (Dee); Ashml. 213, f. 124ᵛ (Spark); Ashml. 228, f. 151ᵛ (Ringe).

155 Ashml. 220, ff. 29ᵛ–30 (Holder). See also Ashml. 414, f. 16 (Underhill); Ashml. 198, f. 73 (Clarke); Ashml. 220, f. 64ᵛ (W. Smith); Ashml. 203, f. 256 (Scot).

156 Nashe, *Traveller and Other Works*, p. 213.

157 Robbins, *Encyclopedia of Witchcraft*, pp. 94–6; Thomas, *Religion and Magic*, pp. 477–83.

158 Robbins, *Encyclopedia of Witchcraft*, pp. 168–9; Wallace Notestein, *A History of Witchcraft in England* (New York, 1968), Chaps. 6 and 7. *Witchcraft in Northamptonshire* (1612; reprint ed., Wilbarston, Northants., 1867).

159 Ashml. 416, f. 99 (Howett); cf. Ashml. 224, f. 132ᵛ (Lowys). See also Ashml. 408, f. 165; Ashml. 201, ff. 160, 167ᵛ, 186, 230 (Sanders).

160 Ashml. 1730, f. 251.

161 Burton, *Anatomy of Melancholy*, 1:183. Cf. Hall, *Works*, 8:88.

162 Macfarlane, *Witchcraft in England*, Chaps. 7 and 8; Thomas, *Religion and Magic*, pp. 184, 185–7, 208, 249, 265, 544, 545, 548–50, 553.

163 This treatment of the controversy involving Darrell is based largely on Thomas, *Religion and Magic*, pp. 483–92, and Kocher, *Science and Religion*, pp. 127–45.

164 Kocher, *Science and Religion*, p. 132; John Deacon and John Walker, *Dialogicall Discourses of Spirits and Devils* (London, 1601), p. 325.

165 Deacon and Walker, *Dialogicall Discourses*, p. 160.

166 Deacon and Walker, *Dialogicall Discourses*, pp. 206–7.

167 Reginald Scot, *The Discoverie of Witchcraft* (1584; reprint ed., Carbondale, Ill., 1964), Books 1–3, esp. pp. 64–9.

168 Bernard, *Guide to Grand-Iury Men*, pp. 11–18, 29–52, 74, 204.

169 Thomas, *Religion and Magic*, pp. 486–92; Garfield Tourney, "The Physician and Witchcraft in Restoration England," *Medical History* 16 (1972):143–55.

170 Thomas, *Religion and Magic*, pp. 476–7, 577–8, 580–1. See also Joseph Glanvill, *Saducismus Triumphatus*, ed. Coleman O. Parsons (Gainesville, Fla., 1966), pp. 65–129; Hall, *Works*, 8:89; Ashml. 194, f. 119 (Cathorne).

171 Thomas, *Religion and Magic*, Chaps. 17 and 18 (note esp. p. 583); Macfarlane, *Witchcraft in England*, Chaps. 12, 15, and 16.

172 See Appendix E, Table E.3.

173 Ashml. 218, f. 233ᵛ (Paul).

174 Ashml. 228, f. 232 (Woodrosse). See also Ashml. 237, ff. 166, 171ᵛ (Butler); Ashml. 211, f. 240 (Pluntre).

175 Ashml. 406, f. 202 (Turvey).

176 Macfarlane, *Witchcraft in England*, pp. 180–2, Table 19.

177 Ashml. 220, f. 24 (King).

178 Macfarlane, *Witchcraft in England*, p. 182.
179 Ashml. 207, f. 232 (Morgan); Ashml. 414, ff. 25ᵛ–6 (Enfild).
180 Ashml. 414, f. 5 (James).
181 Ashml. 220, f. 135ᵛ (Maunfield).
182 Macfarlane, *Witchcraft in England*, pp. 192–5; Thomas, *Religion and Magic*, pp. 543–6.
183 Ashml. 235, ff. 186ᵛ–92ᵛ.
184 Ashml. 214, f. 75.
185 Ashml. 235, f. 192ᵛ.
186 Ashml. 222, f. 195, 196 (Jennings); British Library, Add. MS 36674, ff. 134–7; Ewen, *Witchcraft and Demonianism*, p. 134.
187 Ashml. 213, f. 61 (Child).
188 Ashml. 220, f. 129ᵛ (anonymous).
189 The woman told Napier that a minister had found her to be possessed by three spirits, whom he had named, Ashml. 213, f. 61 (Child).
190 Ashml. 405, ff. 90ᵛ, 95 (Robinson).
191 Ashml. 200, f. 232ᵛ (Belcher). The trial is described in Ewen, *Witchcraft and Demonianism*, pp. 206–7, 209–12.
192 For some of the folklore about detecting witchcraft that Napier collected see Ashml. 1473, ff. 390, 410, 658; Ashml. 1488, art. 2, f. 15ᵛ; British Library, Add. MS 36674, ff. 145–145ᵛ.
193 Ashml. 199, f. 140.
194 Ashml. 421, f. 171. See also Ashml. 410, f. 100 (Sallock); Ashml. 211, f. 143 (Rumball); Ashml. 198, f. 186 (Simpson); Ashml. 235, f. 186ᵛ (Hueson).
195 Ashml. 421, ff. 144–5, 166, 171–171ᵛ; Ashml. 200, f. 175; Ashml. 431, f. 152; Ashml. 363, f. 71ᵛ; Sloane MS 3822, ff. 6–9, 22–3, 80–80ᵛ, 89ᵛ. For notes about timing the use of sigils see the cases cited in n. 194. Sloane MS 3822, f. 89ᵛ contains Forman's revealing instructions about how to make and use an amulet "for madness" written out in Napier's hand.
196 Ashml. 421, f. 171.
197 Ashml. 431, f. 152; Sloane MS 3822, ff. 35–35ᵛ.
198 Although Napier's inconsistency in recording all the remedies he prescribed makes reliable statistics unobtainable, a count of the cases in which he dispensed amulets illustrates his habits clearly enough. Contrast the proportion of consultations containing notes about amulets in which supernatural causes were likely with the proportion of consultations in which they were less likely: tempted to suicide, 20.3%; religious symptoms, 13.3%; demonism suspected, 15.2%; witchcraft feared, 16.3%; mad or lunatic, 8.8%; melancholy, 8.7%; mopish, 8.8%.
199 Ashml. 1473, ff. 619, 659; Thomas, *Religion and Magic*, pp. 186–7.
200 William Lilly, *History of His Life and Times* (London, 1715), pp. 53–4; Ashml. 235, f. 116ᵛ (Olive).
201 Ashml. 421, f. 158. For some other prayers and exorcisms Napier used see Ashml. 1790, f. 113ᵛ; Ashml. 182, ff. 167ᵛ–70; Ashml. 198, f. 187; Ashml. 237, unfoliated (between ff. 167–8); Ashml. 1432, art. 7, f. 15ᵛ (a traditional charm); Ashml. 1473, f. 658.
202 Ashml. 431, f. 171; Ashml. 1490, f. 119.
203 Ashml. 412, f. 256ᵛ (Franklin).
204 Ashml. 213, f. 96 (Musgrave).
205 Ashml. 199, f. 57 (Norman).
206 Thomas, *Religion and Magic*, p. 207.
207 Thomas, *Religion and Magic*, pp. 486–9.
208 Ashml. 232, f. 79 (Wheelowes).
209 Blagrave, *Blagrave's Physick*, pp. 168–73 (the quote is on p. 172).
210 The most influential Puritan advocates of "practical divinity" were Richard Greenham, Richard Sibbes, William Perkins, Robert Bolton, and Richard Baxter; see Richard Greenham, *The Workes* (London, 1612); Richard Sibbes, *The Complete Works*, ed. Alexander Balloch Grosart, 7 vols. (Edinburgh, 1862–4),

esp. Vol. 1; William Perkins, *A Golden chaine* [and other treatises] (Cambridge, 1600); Bolton, *Right comforting*; and Richard Baxter, *Gildas Salvianus; The First Part; i.e. The Reformed Pastor* (London, 1656) for their views. The best discussion of their rhetorical and psychological techniques is Haller, *Rise of Puritanism*, Chaps. 1 and 4. My debt to Haller's work is very great. Brian Opie, "Foundations of Style in the Elizabethan Sermon" (Ph.D. diss., Edinburgh University, 1972), and Brink, Introduction, in Trosse, *Life of Trosse*, pp. 15–29, are also useful.

211 Robert Yarrow, *Soveraigne Comforts for a Trovbled Conscience* (London, 1634), pp. 29–30; Bolton, *Right comforting*, pp. 198–9; Sibbes, *Complete Works*, 1:48.

212 Bolton, *Right comforting*, pp. 202–3; Samuel Hoard, *The Soules miserie and recoverie* (London, 1636), pp. 205–6; John Sym, *Lifes Preservative against self-killing* (London, 1637), p. 248; Richard Baxter, *The Signs and Causes of Melancholy*, ed. Samuel Clifford (London, 1716), pp. 98–9, 106–8; Sibbes, *Complete Works*, 1:136.

213 Haller, *Rise of Puritanism*, p. 33; Thomas Wilson, *Saints by Calling* (London, 1620), pp. 195–205, and *A Sermon of the Spiritual Combat* in his *Jacob's Ladder* (London, 1611).

214 John Bunyan, *Grace Abounding to the Chief of Sinners and Pilgrim's Progress*, ed. Roger Sharrock (London, 1966), pp. 1–105, 231–5; Owen C. Watkins, *The Puritan Experience* (London, 1972), pp. 8–11, 13.

215 George Fox, *The Journal of George Fox*, ed. John L. Nickalls (Cambridge, 1952), pp. 1–6; [Henry Walker], comp., *Spirituall Experiences of Sundry Beleevers* (London, 1652), pp. 6, 18–19, 26, 34–35, 43, 47, 82, 135, 138, 143, 258, 290, 358–9; Vavasour Powell, *The Bird in the Cage, Chirping* (London, 1653), p. 138; B. S. Capp, *The Fifth-Monarchy Men* (London, 1972), pp. 94–6; Dean Ebner, *Autobiography in Seventeenth-Century England* (The Hague, 1971), pp. 28, 29.

216 Haller, *Rise of Puritanism*, pp. 27, 33.

217 Wilson, *Saints by Calling*, p. 17. Samuel Clarke, *The Lives of sundry eminent persons* (London, 1683), p. 74; Sibbes, *Complete Works*, 1:148–53, 4:59–74, 83, 88–96, 7:48–64; M. M. Knappen, ed., *Two Elizabethan Puritan Diaries* (Gloucester, Mass., 1966), p. 65; Haller, *Rise of Puritanism*, Chap. 3; Watkins, *Puritan Experience*, p. 13; J. Sears McGee, "Conversion and the Imitation of Christ in Anglican and Puritan Writing," *Journal of British Studies* 15 (1976):24–5; Norman Pettit, *The Heart Prepared: Grace and Conversion in Puritan Spiritual Life* (New Haven, 1966), Chaps. 1 and 3.

218 Watkins, *Puritan Experience*, p. 13.

219 Richard Capel, *Tentations*, 4th ed. (London, 1650), pp. 23, 25; Sibbes, *Complete Works*, 1:160–1; Opie, "Foundations of Elizabethan Sermon," p. 427.

220 Wilson, *Saints by Calling*, pp. 30, 42–3, 111–12, 142, 145–6, 166–7; Clarke, *Lives of sundry persons*, pp. 70–1; Capel, *Tentations*, pp. 192–4; Perkins, *Golden chaine*, p. 667; Arthur Hildersham quoted in David Stannard, "Death and Dying in Puritan New England," *American Historical Review*, 78 (1973):1311.

221 Sibbes, *Complete Works*, 1:148 and 148–54 generally.

222 George Herbert, *Remains, 1652* (Menston, 1970), pp. 66, 67–8.

223 For a range of such cases see Ashml. 233, f. 21^v (Bregrave); Ashml. 405, f. 102 (Derrick); Ashml. 223, f. 19^v (Goodspeed); Ashml. 414, f. 55^v (Gregory); Ashml. 222, f. 135 (Harvey); Ashml. 218, f. 219^v (Nueman); Ashml. 232, f. 339 (Odor); Ashml. 214, f. 409 (Sallys); Ashml. 194, f. 174 (Smith); Ashml. 413, f. 188^v (Pathoe); Ashml. 224, f. 56 (Peacock); Ashml. 201, f. 53^v (Tins); Ashml. 223, f. 143^v (Zayer); Ashml. 218, ff. 157^v–8 (Allyn); Ashml. 233, f. 144^v (anonymous); Ashml. 410, f. 107 (Pawlyn).

224 Ashml. 194, f. 8 (Whitter).

225 Ashml. 217, f. 133^b (Abbot). See also Ashml. 340, f. 169 (Hills); Ashml. 223, f. 161^v (Sambrook); Ashml. 233, f. 144^v (Gadstone); Ashml. 227, f. 9^v (Faldoe).

226 Ashml. 406, f. 33^v (Kays).

227 Ashml. 410, f. 126^v, and Ashml. 406, f. 22^v (Astill).

228 Ashml. 214, f. 324 (Bonner).

229 Ashml. 235, f. 125^v (Laurenc).
230 Burton, *Anatomy of Melancholy*, 3:426.
231 Wilson, *Saints by Calling*, p. 17.
232 Ashml. 221, f. 74 (Hill).
233 Ashml. 228, f. 151^v (Ringe). Cf. Ashml. 212, f. 324 (Hectour).
234 Ashml. 402, f. 9 (Wasley); Ashml. 199, f. 2^v (Lockley). According to Aubrey, Napier prayed for each of his patients: John Aubrey, *Three Prose Works*, ed. John Buchanan-Brown (Carbondale, Ill., 1972), p. 101. He seems to have recommended recitation rather than extemporaneous prayer; he advised Purbeck, for example, to recite a psalm morning and evening and he wrote out a book of set prayers for Sunderland's use: Ashml. 413, f. 5^v (Purbeck); Ashml. 421, f. 163 (Scrope). For other cases involving prayers see Ashml. 244, f. 5 (Abbot); Ashml. 229, f. 251 (Greene); Ashml. 222, f. 7 (Hobbs); Ashml. 406, f. 369 (Grant); Ashml. 233, f. 143^v (Lancford); Ashml. 216, f. 198 (Hearne); Ashml. 217, f. 115 (Jus); Ashml. 222, f. 47 (Sanders); Ashml. 404, fragment pinned to f. 306 (Earell).
235 J. Sears McGee, *The Godly Man in Stuart England* (New Haven, 1976), pp. 54–67; idem, "Conversation in Anglican and Puritan Writing," pp. 27–33. For similar treatments of Anglican attitudes toward spiritual counseling see Thomas Wood, *English Casuistical Divinity in the Seventeenth Century* (London, 1952), Chap. 3; H. R. McAdoo, *The Structure of Caroline Moral Theology* (London, 1949), pp. 120–31. Napier's preference for comforting speeches that dwelt on God's mercy rather than troubling matters such as predestination was shared by other conservatives, such as Robert Burton and Jeremy Taylor, who composed set speeches for ministers to use when they counseled spiritually distressed people, Burton, *Anatomy of Melancholy*, 3:409, 427; Jeremy Taylor, *The Whole Works*, ed. R. Heber, 2nd ed., rev. by Charles Page Eden and Alexander Taylor, 10 vols. (London, 1850–54), 3:152–5. These two influential divines also emphasized the importance of formal religious exercises as a means to ease religious distress, Burton, *Anatomy of Melancholy*, 3:427; Taylor, *Whole Works*, 3:152. Taylor, in contrast to some Puritan writers, claimed that the regenerate man is no longer much troubled by "a contention within him concerning good or bad," *Whole Works*, 7:371–2.
236 Ashml. 212, ff. 313, 334.
237 Burton, *Anatomy of Melancholy*, 1:199–200; Sibbes, *Complete Works*, 1:136.
238 Richard Baxter, *The Practical Works*, ed. William Orme, 23 vols. (London, 1830), 17:278.
239 Burton, *Anatomy of Melancholy*, 3:370.
240 Burton, *Anatomy of Melancholy*, 3:372. Henry Howard, Earl of Northampton, John Harvey, Francis Bacon, John Donne, and Jeremy Taylor all made similar attacks on religious enthusiasts before 1650: Babb, *Elizabethan Malady*, pp. 51–2; Truman Guy Steffan, "The Social Argument against Enthusiasm (1650–1660)," *Studies in English*, No. 21 (1941):45–8. Identical reasoning was apparently used by French Catholics to discredit Protestant enthusiasts during the same period, but I can find no evidence of direct influence on English writers: John F. Sena, "Melancholic Madness and the Puritans," *Harvard Theological Review* 66 (1973):297. See also George Rosen, "Enthusiasm: 'a dark lanthorn of the spirit,'" *Bulletin of the History of Medicine* 42 (1968):393–421.
241 Burton, *Anatomy of Melancholy*, 3:399–400. See also Taylor, *Whole Works*, 9:272; McGee, "Conversion in Anglican and Puritan Writing," pp. 26–7; Wood, *English Casuistical Divinity*, pp. 132–4. For religious melancholy see Brink, Introduction, in Trosse, *Life of Trosse*, pp. 20–31; Babb, *Elizabethan Malady*, pp. 47–54.
242 Sibbes, *Complete Works*, 2:456; 7:212.
243 Bolton, *Right comforting*, pp. 204–12.
244 Yarrow, *Soveraigne Comforts*, pp. 15–16.
245 George Williamson, "The Restoration Revolt against Enthusiasm," *Studies in*

Philology 30 (1933):571–603; Steffan, "Social Argument," pp. 39–63; Sena, "Melancholic Madness"; Rosen, "Enthusiasm"; DePorte, *Nightmares and Hobby-horses*, pp. 33, 37–43, 58, 65; Jackson I. Cope, *Joseph Glanvill, Anglican Apologist* (St. Louis, 1956), pp. 30–2, 40–1, 53–8, 65, 73–9, 83, 146–7, 157, 159–65; Phillip Harth, *Swift and Anglican Rationalism* (Chicago, 1961); Hillel Schwartz, *Knaves, Fools, Madmen, and that Subtile Effluvium: A Study of the Opposition to the French Prophets in England, 1706–1710* (Gainesville, Fla., 1978), Chap. 2; John Walsh, "Methodism and the Mob in the Eighteenth Century," in *Popular Belief and Practice*, Studies in Church History, 8, ed. G. J. Cuming and Derek Baker (Cambridge, 1972), pp. 213–28; Margaret C. Jacob, *The Newtonians and the English Revolution, 1689–1720* (Ithaca, 1976), esp. pp. 18, 22–71.

Among the most notable attacks on enthusiastic madness were Henry More, *Enthusiasmus Triumphatus* (London, 1656); Meric Casaubon, *A Treatise concerning Enthusiasme*, ed. Paul J. Korshin (Gainesville, Fla., 1970), esp. pp. 106–17, 145–6, 159–64, 171–6; Thomas Sprat, *History of the Royal Society*, ed. Jackson I. Cope (St. Louis, 1959), pp. 152–3, 356–78, 403–12, esp. 359; George Hickes, *The Spirit of Enthusiasm exorcised* (London, 1680); John Locke, *An Essay Concerning Human Understanding*, ed. A. C. Fraser, 2nd ed., 2 vols. (New York, 1959), 1:209–10; The Earl of Shaftsbury, *Characters of Men, Manners, Opinions, Times, etc.*, ed. John M. Robertson, 2 vols. (London, 1900), 1:5–39; Jonathan Swift, *A Tale of a Tub and other Satires*, ed. Kathleen Williams (London, 1975), pp. 102–14, 167–90; Edmund Gibson, *A Caution against enthusiasm*, 7th ed. (London, 1751); Theophilus Evans, *The History of Modern Enthusiasm*, 2nd ed. (London, 1757); George Lavington, *The Enthusiasm of Methodists and Papists Compared*, 3 parts in 2 vols. (London, 1754), Pt. 1:6, 7, 15, 37, 61, 63; Pt. 2:title page, xxiii, xxv, 1–2, 9, 39–40, 53, 56–9, 84–5; Pt. 3:C2, C3ᵛ–C4ᵛ, 2–3, 5, 10–16, 23, 36, 38, 54–5, 59, 65–9, 81–2, 93–104, 158; Joseph Trapp, *The Nature, Folly, Sin, and Danger of being righteous Over-much*, 2nd ed. (London, 1739), esp. pp. 13–17; Thomas Church, *Remarks on the Reverend Mr. John Wesley's last journal* (London, 1745), esp. pp. 67–76.

246 For attacks on the healing activities of Dissenters see Hickes, *Spirit of Enthusiasm*, pp. 13, 21–7, 40, 44–5; Evans, *History of Modern Enthusiasm*, pp. 130–33; Church, *Remarks on Wesley's last journal*, pp. 68–9; Lavington, *Enthusiasm of Methodists*, Pt. 2:139–57; Pt. 3:C2, 23–30, 33–69, 93–104, 117–135, 158–198. Revealing incidents in the same vein are reported by Oliver Heywood, *His Autobiography, Diaries, Anecdote and Event Books*, ed. J. Horsfall Turner, 4 vols. (Bingley and Brighouse, 1881–85), 4:280–1; Thomas Woodcock, *Extracts from the Papers of Thomas Woodcock*, ed. G. C. Moore, Camden Society, 3rd ser. 8 (1907):55–56; McAdoo, *Structure of Caroline Moral Theology*, pp. 66, 96–7, notes the decline of Anglican casuistry after 1660.

247 Bacon, *Advancement of Learning*, p. 130.

248 Webster, *Great Instauration*, Chap. 4; Hill, *Change and Continuity*, Chap. 7. For criticisms of orthodox medicine after the Restoration see Marchmont Needham, *Medela Medicinae. A plea For the Free Profession and a Renovation of the Art of Physick* (London, 1665); Adrian Huyberts, *A Corner-Stone Laid towards the Building of a New colledge (that is to say, a new Body of Physicians) in London* (London, 1675); Gideon Harvey, *The Conclave of physicians* (London, 1683).

249 Brown, "College of Physicians." See also George Castle, *The Chemical Galenist* (London, 1667), esp. p. 196; Robert Sprackling, *Medela ignorantiae: Or A Just and plain Vindication of Hippocrates and Galen from The groundless Imputations of M.N.* (London, 1665), pp. 45–6; Goodall, *Colledge of Physicians*, pp. 49–55 (note also the contradictory remarks on pp. 69–76, 85–156). All of these authors condemned their opponents as enthusiasts, Castle, *Chemical Galenist*, pp. A6; Sprackling, *Medela ignorantiae*, pp. 81, 157–8; Goodall, *Colledge of Physicians*, p. 157.

250 James Howell, *Epistolae Ho-Elianae*, ed. Joseph Jacobs (London, 1890), p. 527; Morris Palmer Tilley, *A Dictionary of Proverbs in England in the Sixteenth and Seventeenth Centuries* (Ann Arbor, Mich., 1950), p. 537; R. Flecknoe, *Sixtynine*

Enigmatical Characters (London, 1665), p. 101. Cf. Peter Shaw [M.D.], *The Reflector: representing Human Affairs, As they are; and may be improved* (London, 1750), pp. 225–31.

251 Capp, *Astrology and the Popular Press*, p. 110.

252 Needham, *Medela Medicinae*, p. 405.

253 Baxter, *Gildas Salvianus*, pp. 77, 94. Baxter became the most famous Restoration physician of the soul. Samuel Clifford, who collected Baxter's scattered comments about the nature and cure of melancholy, remarked that "multitudes of melancholy persons of all sorts, learned and unlearned, rich and poor, for many years together, made their continual application to him for advice" (*Signs and Causes of Melancholy*, pp. x–xi). Two notable divines who followed his example were Heywood, *Autobiography, Diaries*, 4:index s.v. "melancholy"; Henry Newcome, *The Diary*, ed. Thomas Heywood, Chetham society, 28 (1849):55–8, 74–7, 92, 132, 133, 140, 186, 193, 216.

254 *The Records of a Church of Christ in Bristol, 1640, 1687*, ed. Roger Hayden, Bristol Record Society Publications, 27 (1974):139–41; Thomas, *Religion and Magic*, pp. 482–87; Michael R. Watts, *The Dissenters: From the Reformation to the French Revolution* (Oxford, 1978), pp. 314–15; John Wesley, *The Works*, 14 vols. (Grand Rapids, Mich., 1958–59), 3:140–4.

255 Fox, *Book of Miracles*, pp. 3, 9, 37, 40, 43, 60, 69–70, 90, 92, 109, 114, 115, 118, 121, 122, 123, 124, 127, 128, 132, 135, 140, 143; Fox, *Journal*, pp. 42–4, 139, 171, 230, 652, 742. The Quakers preserved Fox's concern for the insane and his healing methods in the eighteenth century, Fox, *Book of Miracles*, p. 98, n.; Isabel McKenzie, *Social Activities of the English Friends* (New York, 1935), Pt 2.

256 For the attitudes toward medicine of some of the leading Dissenting thaumaturgists see Baxter, *Cure of Melancholy by Faith and Physic*; Fox, *Book of Miracles*, pp. 48–58; Wesley, *Works*, 2:39, 58, 78, 456 (esp. p. 456); 3:237, 243; 12:83; George Whitefield, *George Whitefield's Journals* (n.p., 1960), pp. 266–71. Many Nonconformist divines who were ejected from their livings at the Restoration turned to medical practice, Huyberts, *Corner-Stone*, p. 19; Watts, *Dissenters*, p. 344. The Quakers commended medicine as an art compatible with their religious mission (Fox, *Book of Miracles*, pp. 54–5; Watts, *Dissenters*, p. 344).

257 Woodcock, *Woodcock Papers*, pp. 55–6.

258 Heywood, *Autobiography, Diaries*, 2:280–1. For another propaganda triumph scored by a sectarian thaumaturgist see Fox, *Book of Miracles*, pp. 121–2.

259 Wesley, *Works*, 1:155–6, 214, 218, 218–19, 270; 2:70–1, 354, 354–5, 456; 3:237, 383–4; 5:450–4; 6:356–8; 7:315; Whitefield, *Journals*, pp. 255, 266–71.

260 Thomas, *Religion and Magic*, pp. 349–56, 640–7, 656–63; Webster, *Great Instauration*, Chap. 4; Hill, *Change and Continuity*, Chap. 7; Christopher Hill, *World Turned Upside Down* (Harmondsworth, 1976), pp. 87–93, 287–300; Rattansi, "Paracelsus and the Puritan Revolution," pp. 24–32; Capp, *Astrology and the Popular Press*, pp. 67–101, 247–55, 261–2, and esp. 281; Clark, *Royal College*, 1:303–75; 2:427–613, esp. 540–2; Bernice Hamilton, "The Medical Professions in the Eighteenth Century," *Economic History Review*, 2nd ser., 4 (1951):141–69.

261 Edward Hughes, "The Professions in the Eighteenth Century," in *Aristocratic Government and Society in Eighteenth-Century England*, ed. Daniel A. Baugh (New York, 1975), pp. 184–8, 195–7; Norman Sykes, *Church and State in England in the XVIIIth Century* (Cambridge, 1934), Chap. 5.

262 Thomas, *Religion and Magic*, Chap. 18; Tourney, "The Physician and Witchcraft," pp. 143–55; Wesley, *Works*, 3:308–18, 383–4; 4:72; Levington, *Enthusiasm of Methodists*, Pt. 3:117–18. Cf. Richard Mead, *The Works* (Edinburgh, 1775), pp. 465–6, 470–77.

263 Parry-Jones, *Trade in Lunacy*.

264 The contribution of the Dissenting therapeutic tradition has been neglected by historians. Quakers were conspicuous among the early champions of lunacy reform in England: Samuel Tuke, *Description of the Retreat*, eds. Richard Hunter and Ida Macalpine (London, 1964); William F. Bynum, "Rationales for Therapy in British Psychiatry: 1780–1835," *Medical History*, 18 (1974):318–28, esp. 326;

Andrew T. Scull, *Museums of Madness: The Social Organization of Insanity in Nineteenth-Century England* (London, 1979), pp. 67–70, 107–113, 134; Parry-Jones, *Trade in Lunacy*, pp. 192–8; Hunter and Macalpine, *Psychiatry*, pp. 191, 475; Vieda Skultans, *Madness and Morals: Ideas on Insanity in the Nineteenth Century* (London, 1975), pp. 10–20, 135–56; idem, *English Madness: Ideas on Insanity, 1580–1890* (London, 1979), pp. 52–68. McCandless, "Insanity and Society," is a lucid survey of English lunacy reform.

Manuscript sources

1. Bodleian Library (Oxford)

Ashmole Manuscripts

The Ashmole Manuscripts are fully described in William H. Black, comp., *A Descriptive, Analytical and Critical Catalogue of the Manuscripts Bequeathed . . . by Elias Ashmole* (Oxford, 1845). The descriptions of categories of manuscripts containing large numbers of volumes, such as Richard Napier's medical practice, adhere to the format in W. D. Macray's *Index to the Catalogue of the Manuscripts of Elias Ashmole* (Oxford, 1866).

a. Manuscripts of Richard Napier (alias Sandy)
   Medical and Astrological Practice

1597	175
1597–1598	182
July 1598–Feb. 1600	228
1598–1629 (loose notes)	181
1599–1619 (loose notes)	204
1599–1624 (loose notes)	240
1599–1631 (loose notes)	174
Feb. 1600–Dec. 1600	202
Jan. 1601–Mar. 1602	404
Mar. 1602–Feb. 1603	221
Feb. 1603–Feb. 1604	197
Feb. 1603–Apr. 1605	207
Mar. 1604–Mar. 1605	415
Mar. 1605–Dec. 1605	216
Dec. 1605–Apr. 1606 (some later)	215
Oct. 1606–Jan. 1608	193
Jan. 1608–Apr. 1609	229

Sept. 1608–Feb. 1609	338
Feb. 1609–Sept. 1610 (some later)	335
Apr. 1609–Mar. 1610	203
Nov. 1609–Nov. 1610	329
Mar. 1610–Jan. 1611	239
Mar. 1610–May 1611	334
Jan. 1611–Feb. 1612	200
Feb. 1612–Dec. 1612	409
Dec. 1612–Aug. 1613	199
May 1614–Apr. 1615	237
Apr. 1615–Feb. 1616	196
Feb. 1616–Sept. 1616	408
Sept. 1616–June 1617	198
June 1617–Feb. 1618	220
Feb. 1618–Aug. 1618	201
Aug. 1618–May 1619	230
May 1619–Sept. 1619	235
Sept. 1619–Apr. 1620	213
Apr. 1620–Nov. 1620	414
Nov. 1620–May 1621	233
June 1621–Feb. 1622	231
Feb. 1622–July 1622	223
July 1622–Feb. 1623	222
Mar. 1623–Oct. 1623	218
Oct. 1623–June 1624	413
June 1624–Mar. 1625	402
Mar. 1625–Aug. 1625	217
Sept. 1625–Feb. 1627	224
Feb. 1627–Nov. 1627	227
Nov. 1627–Jan. 1628	410
Apr. 1628–Dec. 1628	405
Dec. 1628–May 1629	407
May 1629–Dec. 1629	406
Dec. 1629–June 1630	194
June 1630–Nov. 1630	238
Nov. 1630–July 1631	232
July 1631–Mar. 1632	212
Mar. 1632–Sept. 1632	416
Sept. 1632–Apr. 1633	214
Apr. 1633–Oct. 1633	211

Medical Papers *(cont.)*

2. British Library (London)

Sloane Manuscripts

The Sloane manuscripts are briefly described in Samuel Ayscough, *A Catalogue of the Manuscripts Preserved in the British Museum* (London, 1782). They contain many medical and astrological practice books, a selection of which is listed below. The descriptions of categories of manuscripts containing many items are meant to match the relevant headings in Edward E. J. Scott, *Index to the Sloane Manuscripts in the British Museum* (London, 1904), in which individual citations may be found.

a. Manuscripts Pertaining to Richard Napier and his Circle

Notes about Magic, Astrology and Religion by Richard Napier and Simon Forman	3822, 3854
Magical Treatises Copied by Richard Napier and Sir Richard Napier	3884
Magical Treatise Copied by Sir Richard Napier *(Picatrix)*	3679
Magical Treatises Copied by Gerence James	3826
Magical and Alchemical Tracts Copied by Thomas Robson	1744
Closely Related Magical Tracts Collected by Elias Ashmole	3821, 3824–5, 3846, 3849–51, 3853, 3857, 3885
Medical Recipes by Richard Napier	519, 1087
References to Sir Richard Napier	519, 856, 1087, 1708, 2251, 3679
Simon Forman's Treatise of Astrological Medicine (cf. Ashmole 363, 389, 403)	99
Simon Forman's Groundes of Physicke	2250
Astrological Schemes by Simon Forman	3822
Letter from Thomas Napier to Ashmole	3822
Medical and Astrological Notes by Arthur Dee	1902

b. Medical and Astrological Manuscripts

Medical Treatises by E. Poeton	1954

Medical Notes of Henry Powers, M.D.	1351, 1353–8
Anonymous Medical and Astrological Collections (Sixteenth and Seventeenth Centuries)	14, 69, 171, 426, 461, 462, 1055, 1087, 1295, 1476, 1492, 2529, 2595, 2817, 3169, 3288, 3722, 3857

Additional Manuscripts

Notes on Magic, Alchemy and Witchcraft by Richard Napier and Simon Forman	36674
William Coles's *Collections of Various Kinds,* Vol. 33 (Notes on the Purbeck Affair)	5834
Whether it be Dampnation for a man to kill himself (Anonymous, ?1578)	27632
Case Book of a Hampshire Physician (1565–1573)	23023

Lansdowne Manuscripts

Burghley Papers: Letters Written by Mad People	42, 99

3. Public Records Office (London)

Court of Wards and Liveries

Entry Books of Petitions and Compositions for Wardship	Wards 9/214–220 Wards 10/27
Feodaries' Surveys	Wards 5/1, 3, 30, 52

Chancery

Inquisitions Post Mortem, Series II (Inquisitions on Idiots and Lunatics)	C 142
Commissions and Inquisitions of Lunacy, 1627–1932 (Petty Bag Office)	C 211

Court of King's Bench (Crown Side)

Ancient Indictments, 1597–1643 (Coroners' Inquisitions)	KB 9/692–826

Court of Star Chamber, James I
 Proceedings to Recover the Goods of
  Alleged Suicides STAC 8/1-3
Miscellaneous
 Index of Lunacy Inquisitions in C 211 Index 17612

4. Buckinghamshire County Record Office (Aylesbury)

Uthwatt of Great Linford Papers
 Financial Records of Richard Napier and
  Sir Richard Napier D/U/1
Ecclesiastical Records, Archdeaconry of Buckingham
  Act Books, 1630–1635 D/A/C 1-6
 Parish Register of Great Linford
  (Transcript) D/A/T 123

5. Bedfordshire County Record Office (Luton)

Francklin Papers
 Papers on the Lunacy of Edmund
  Francklin FN 1060-1084

6. Lancashire County Record Office (Preston)

 Quarter Sessions Order Book QSO 2/31

7. Essex County Record Office (Chelmsford)

 Transcript of Coroners' Inquests QBIA 693/II
 Terling Parish Register

8. Guildhall Library (London)

 Nehemiah Wallington, *A record of* Guildhall
  the Mercies of God; or a thankful Library MS
  Remembrance* 204

Index of printed sources

The following list gives the page and note where the first full citation to printed sources referred to in the notes may be found. Works are listed by their author's name, except in the cases of anonymous works, for which short titles are given, and some collections of records, for which appropriate headings are given. Where more than one work by an author has been cited, separate sources are indicated by keywords from the short titles.

General index

Purbeck, John Villiers, Viscount, 21–2,
49, 92, 152, 192, 199
purges, *see* medicines
Puritanism: and anxiety, 177
Puritans: on conduct, 3, 80, 85, 93–4, 98,
103, 104; in Napier's vicinity, 22–3,
30–1, 68–9; reject magic, 23–4, 25; and
religious melancholy, 223–5; and religious psychology, 217–19; and spiritual
healing, 9, 176–7, 206, 217–20; on suicide, 171

Quakers, 9, 170, 174, 208, 225, 228, 230

rage, sign of madness, 140, 141–2; *see also*
violence
Raleigh, Sir Walter, 187; widow of, 50
Raphael, Archangel: Napier conjures, 16,
17–19, 157, 210; prophecy by, 18
Rawlins, Stephan, wife of, 100
Red Lion Inn, mistress of, 82
religion: and rates of mental disorder, 68–
9
religious controversy, 9, 17, 156, 170,
171, 206–9, 223–6, 227–31; *see also* enthusiasm, religious; religious melancholy
religious melancholy, 223–5
religious psychology, popular: functions,
167–70, 202–4, 216–17; and medical
psychology, 167–70; Puritans' use of, 3,
218–19; survival, 171–2; symbolism of,
xiii, 144–5, 167, 175, 202–4, 216–17;
see also demonology; demons; Devil;
spirits, good
restraint: of lunatics, 141–2
Rhodes, Mistress Elizabeth, 146
Rhodes, Lady Margaret, 146
Rice, Sara, 154
Richardson, Thomas, wife of, 144
Ringe, Jane, 221–2
Ringe, William, 155–6, 201–2
Robinson, Mistress Mary, 101, 212
Robson, Thomas, 189
Rothwell, Northants., 69
Rowly, Matthew, 83
Rutland, George Manners, Earl of, and
family, 49

Sanderson, Bishop Robert, 25
Sandie, *see* Napier
Sandys, Archbishop Edwin, 91
Satan, *see* Devil
Savage, Joan, 130
Savil, Alice, 84, 134
Sceavington, John, 67
science, rise of, 9, 32, 197–8, 226–7, 229;
see also medical psychology; medicine;

secularization
Scot, Reginald, 155, 207
sects: thaumaturgy, 9–10
secularization, 2, 9–11, 170–2, 229–31
Selbee, Ellen, 158
senses: functions and disorders, 162–3,
179–80; *see also* mind
servants, 50, 51, 75, 96; treatment of, 85–
8; vs. laborers, 262, n. 59
service: extent of custom, 85–6, 88, 268,
n. 57
sex, premarital, 91–2
sex ratios, 36–8, 73–4, 232–5
sexual abuse: of servants, 87–8; fear of,
106
Shakespeare, William, 89; *As You Like It*,
89–90; *Hamlet*, 162–3; *King John*, 183;
King Lear, 44; *The Tempest*, 162
Shepherd, Michael, 35–6, 43
Sherington, Bucks., 68
Shorter, Edward, 80–1
Sibbes, Richard, 224–5
sigils, *see* amulets
Simpson, Joan, 144
skepticism, 155, 198–9, 206–7, 208, 212–
13, 230
Skynner, Christopher, 106
Smith, Ann, 131
Smith, Elizabeth, 109
Smith, John, 44, 140
Smith, Sir Thomas, 85
Smyth, John, 88
social status: and mental disorder, 33–4,
34–5, 48–54, 161–2; repudiated by in-
sane, 126, 128–31
sorrow, 157, 158–60, 181–2; *see also* fear;
grief; passion
Southan, Guiles, 134, 204
Southcott, Joanna, 172
Southern, R. W., 164
speech: of the insane, *see* language
Spencer, Frances, 103
Spencer, Master George, 152
Spencer, John, 95–6, 131
Spencer, Sir Robert, 49
Spira, Francis, 200
spirits, animal, 182–3
spirits, evil, *see* demons
spirits, good, 167
spiritual afflictions, 168–9, 174, 220–1,
223; *see also* judgments
spiritual healing: by Anglicans, 195–6; by
Dissenters, 9–11, 177, 225, 227–9; duty
of clergy, 218, 220; popular approval,
227, 229; *see also* exorcism; Jesuits;
Nonconformists; Puritans; Quakers;
sects
Stafford, Young Mistress, 97